Nutrition for Musculoskeletal Health

Nutrition for Musculoskeletal Health

Editors

Matteo Cesari
Emanuele Marzetti

MDPI • Basel • Beijing • Wuhan • Barcelona • Belgrade • Manchester • Tokyo • Cluj • Tianjin

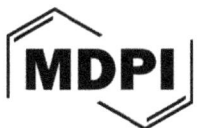

Editors
Matteo Cesari
University of Milan
Italy
IRCCS Istituti Clinici
Scientifici Maugeri
Italy

Emanuele Marzetti
Università Cattolica del Sacro Cuore
Italy
Fondazione Policlinico Universitario
Agostino Gemelli IRCCS
Italy

Editorial Office
MDPI
St. Alban-Anlage 66
4052 Basel, Switzerland

This is a reprint of articles from the Special Issue published online in the open access journal *Nutrients* (ISSN 2072-6643) (available at: https://www.mdpi.com/journal/nutrients/special_issues/Nutrition_Musculoskeletal_Health).

For citation purposes, cite each article independently as indicated on the article page online and as indicated below:

LastName, A.A.; LastName, B.B.; LastName, C.C. Article Title. *Journal Name* **Year**, *Article Number*, Page Range.

ISBN 978-3-03943-234-9 (Hbk)
ISBN 978-3-03943-235-6 (PDF)

© 2020 by the authors. Articles in this book are Open Access and distributed under the Creative Commons Attribution (CC BY) license, which allows users to download, copy and build upon published articles, as long as the author and publisher are properly credited, which ensures maximum dissemination and a wider impact of our publications.

The book as a whole is distributed by MDPI under the terms and conditions of the Creative Commons license CC BY-NC-ND.

Contents

About the Editors vii

Preface to "Nutrition for Musculoskeletal Health" ix

Stephanie A. Lee, Caroline Sypniewski, Benjamin A. Bensadon, Christian McLaren,
William T. Donahoo, Kimberly T. Sibille and Stephen Anton
Determinants of Adherence in Time-Restricted Feeding in Older Adults: Lessons from a Pilot Study
Reprinted from: *Nutrients* **2020**, *12*, 874, doi:10.3390/nu12030874 1

Riccardo Calvani, Leocadio Rodriguez-Mañas, Anna Picca, Federico Marini, Alessandra Biancolillo, Olga Laosa, Laura Pedraza, Jacopo Gervasoni, Aniello Primiano, Giorgia Conta, Isabelle Bourdel-Marchasson, Sophie C. Regueme, Roberto Bernabei, Emanuele Marzetti, Alan J. Sinclair, Giovanni Gambassi and on behalf of the European MID-Frail Consortium
Identification of a Circulating Amino Acid Signature in Frail Older Persons with Type 2 Diabetes Mellitus: Results from the Metabofrail Study
Reprinted from: *Nutrients* **2020**, *12*, 199, doi:10.3390/nu12010199 11

Anna Picca, Francesca Romana Ponziani, Riccardo Calvani, Federico Marini, Alessandra Biancolillo, Hélio José Coelho-Junior, Jacopo Gervasoni, Aniello Primiano, Lorenza Putignani, Federica Del Chierico, Sofia Reddel, Antonio Gasbarrini, Francesco Landi, Roberto Bernabei and Emanuele Marzetti
Gut Microbial, Inflammatory and Metabolic Signatures in Older People with Physical Frailty and Sarcopenia: Results from the BIOSPHERE Study
Reprinted from: *Nutrients* **2020**, *12*, 65, doi:10.3390/nu12010065 23

Floris K. Hendriks, Joey S.J. Smeets, Frank M. van der Sande, Jeroen P. Kooman and Luc J.C. van Loon
Dietary Protein and Physical Activity Interventions to Support Muscle Maintenance in End-Stage Renal Disease Patients on Hemodialysis
Reprinted from: *Nutrients* **2019**, *11*, 2972, doi:10.3390/nu11122972 39

Charlotte Beaudart, Dolores Sanchez-Rodriguez, Médéa Locquet, Jean-Yves Reginster, Laetitia Lengelé and Olivier Bruyère
Malnutrition as a Strong Predictor of the Onset of Sarcopenia
Reprinted from: *Nutrients* **2019**, *11*, 2883, doi:10.3390/nu11122883 53

Mudan Cai and Eun Jin Yang
Hochu-Ekki-To Improves Motor Function in an Amyotrophic Lateral Sclerosis Animal Model
Reprinted from: *Nutrients* **2019**, *11*, 2644, doi:10.3390/nu11112644 67

Claudia Romano, Giovanni Corsetti, Vincenzo Flati, Evasio Pasini, Anna Picca, Riccardo Calvani, Emanuele Marzetti and Francesco Saverio Dioguardi
Influence of Diets with Varying Essential/Nonessential Amino Acid Ratios on Mouse Lifespan
Reprinted from: *Nutrients* **2019**, *11*, 1367, doi:10.3390/nu11061367 79

Yoshitaka Ohno, Koki Ando, Takafumi Ito, Yohei Suda, Yuki Matsui, Akiko Oyama, Hikari Kaneko, Shingo Yokoyama, Tatsuro Egawa and Katsumasa Goto
Lactate Stimulates a Potential for Hypertrophy and Regeneration of Mouse Skeletal Muscle
Reprinted from: *Nutrients* **2019**, *11*, 869, doi:10.3390/nu11040869 99

Domenico Azzolino, Pier Carmine Passarelli, Paolo De Angelis, Giovan Battista Piccirillo, Antonio D'Addona and Matteo Cesari
Poor Oral Health as a Determinant of Malnutrition and Sarcopenia
Reprinted from: *Nutrients* **2019**, *11*, 2898, doi:10.3390/nu11122898 . . . . **109**

Donatella Granchi, Nicola Baldini, Fabio Massimo Ulivieri and Renata Caudarella
Role of Citrate in Pathophysiology and Medical Management of Bone Diseases
Reprinted from: *Nutrients* **2019**, *11*, 2576, doi:10.3390/nu11112576 . . . . **127**

About the Editors

Matteo Cesari, MD, Ph.D., is Associate Professor of Geriatrics at the University of Milan, and Head of the Geriatric Unit at the IRCCS Istituti Clinici Scientifici Maugeri (Milan, Italy). His research activities are focused on the frailty condition and strategies aimed at preventing the disabling cascade. Dr. Cesari has currently published more than 460 articles in peer-reviewed scientific journals, 21 book chapters, and numerous other publications; more than 200 abstracts of his have been accepted at National and International meetings. Overall, Dr. Cesari's current h-index is 71. He is listed by Clarivate Analytics among the worldwide Highly Cited Researchers (http://highlycited.com). Dr. Cesari is Editor-in-Chief of *The Journal of Frailty & Aging*, and Senior Associate Editor of the *Journal of the American Medical Directors Association* [JAMDA]. Dr. Cesari also serves as a consultant for the World Health Organization on the themes of aging and integrated care in older people.

Emanuele Marzetti, MD, Ph.D., is a board certified Geriatrician, Clinical Assistant Professor in Geriatrics, and the leader of the Orthogeriatric Unit at the Department of Geriatrics, Neurosciences and Orthopedics (Fondazione Policlinico Universitario "Agostino Gemelli" IRCCS, Università Cattolica del Sacro Cuore, Rome, Italy). He received his MD and PhD degrees at the Università Cattolica del Sacro Cuore, and postdoctoral training in biochemistry of aging at the University of Florida (Gainesville, FL, USA). Dr. Marzetti serves as an Associate Editor for *Experimental Gerontology*, *The Journal of Frailty & Aging*, *JCSM Clinical Reports*, and *Frontiers in Medicine*. His research focuses on the mechanisms responsible for skeletal muscle and cardiovascular aging, with a special interest in mitochondrial pathophysiology, biomarker discovery, and the factors involved in the pathogenesis of frailty and disability in old age.

Preface to "Nutrition for Musculoskeletal Health"

Malnutrition, mostly in the form of undernutrition, is highly prevalent among older adults, especially in those who are institutionalized. The development of malnutrition during aging is often the consequence of multiple concurring factors, including reduced appetite, sensory impairment (in particular, taste and smell abnormalities), poor oral health, dysphagia, changes in gastrointestinal function and motility, comorbidities, medications, social isolation, inactivity, depression, poverty, etc. Regardless of the underlying cause(s), malnutrition increases the risk of adverse health-related events, among which, musculoskeletal conditions (sarcopenia and osteoporosis) are especially worrisome.

The purpose of this book was to convene experts and opinion leaders in nutrition and the musculoskeletal system to provide a multifaceted and comprehensive view of the impact of malnutrition on musculoskeletal health during and in the setting of specific disease conditions. The book showcases original articles and reviews addressing this subject through pre-clinical, clinical, and translational approaches. Nutritional interventions aimed at improving overall and musculoskeletal health in both humans and experimental models are also presented. Selected contributions illustrate the prospect of using circulating amino acids, either alone or in combination with inflammatory biomolecules and gut microbiota composition, as biomarkers for sarcopenia. The variety of topics and the interdisciplinary content make the book appealing to a large readership, from clinicians interested in implementing nutritional interventions in their daily practice to researchers who may take cues for future studies on the subject.

Lastly, we would like to take the opportunity to thank the contributors, the reviewers, and the MDPI editorial staff, whose scientific excellence, time, and dedication made this book a reality.

Matteo Cesari, Emanuele Marzetti
Editors

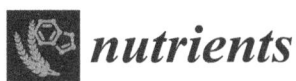

Article

Determinants of Adherence in Time-Restricted Feeding in Older Adults: Lessons from a Pilot Study

Stephanie A. Lee [1],*, Caroline Sypniewski [1], Benjamin A. Bensadon [1], Christian McLaren [1], William T. Donahoo [2], Kimberly T. Sibille [1] and Stephen Anton [1,3],*

1. Department of Aging and Geriatric Research, Institute on Aging, University of Florida, Gainesville, FL 32610, USA; csypniewski@ufl.edu (C.S.); bensadon@ufl.edu (B.A.B.); mclaren@ufl.edu (C.M.); ksibille@ufl.edu (K.T.S.)
2. Department of Medicine, University of Florida, Gainesville, FL 32610, USA; troy.donahoo@medicine.ufl.edu
3. Department of Clinical and Health Psychology, University of Florida, Gainesville, FL 32610, USA
* Correspondence: Stephanie.lee2@valpo.edu (S.A.L.); santon@ufl.edu (S.A.); Tel.: +352-273-7514 (S.A.)

Received: 12 February 2020; Accepted: 17 March 2020; Published: 24 March 2020

Abstract: Time-restricted feeding (TRF) is a type of intermittent fasting in which no calories are commonly consumed for approximately 12–18 hours on a daily basis. The health benefits of this eating pattern have been shown in overweight adults, with improvements in cardiometabolic risk factors as well as the preservation of lean mass during weight loss. Although TRF has been well studied in younger and middle-aged adults, few studies have evaluated the effects of TRF in older adults. Thus, the goal of this study was to evaluate older-adult perspectives regarding the real-world advantages, disadvantages, and challenges to adopting a TRF eating pattern among participants aged 65 and over. A four-week single-arm pre- and post-test design was used for this clinical pilot trial TRF intervention study. Participants were instructed to fast for approximately 16 h per day with the daily target range between 14 and 18 h. Participants were provided with the TRF protocol at a baseline visit, along with a pictorial guide that depicted food items and beverages that were allowed and not allowed during fasting windows to reinforce that calorie-containing items were to be avoided. The trial interventionist called each participant weekly to promote adherence, review the protocol, monitor for adverse events, and provide support and guidance for any challenges faced during the intervention. Participants were instructed to complete daily eating time logs by recording the times at which they first consumed calories and when they stopped consuming calories. At the end of the intervention, participants completed an exit interview and a study-specific Diet Satisfaction Survey (Table 1) to assess their satisfaction, feasibility, and overall experience with the study intervention. Of the 10 participants who commenced the study (mean age = 77.1 y; 6 women, 4 men), nine completed the entire protocol. Seven of the ten participants reported easy adjustment to a 16-hour fast and rated the difference from normal eating patterns as minimal. Eight participants reported no decrease in energy during fasting periods, with greater self-reported activity levels in yardwork and light exercise. Adverse events were rare, and included transient headaches, which dissipated with increased water intake, and dizziness in one participant, which subsided with a small snack. The findings of the current trial suggest that TRF is an eating approach that is well tolerated by most older adults. Six participants, however, did not fully understand the requirements of the fasting regimen, despite being provided with specific instructions and a pictorial guide at a baseline visit. This suggests that more instruction and/or participant contact is needed in the early stages of a TRF intervention to promote adherence.

Keywords: weight loss; intermittent fasting; fat loss; sarcopenia; body composition

1. Introduction

Aging is often associated with a host of biological changes that contribute to a progressive decline in cognitive and physical function, frequently leading to a loss of independence and increased risk of mortality. The life expectancy of adults in many industrialized countries continues to increase [1], with persons aged ≥65 years representing the fastest growing segment of the US population [2]. While prolongation of life remains an important public health goal, of even greater significance is the extension of healthspan, often defined as continued intact functional capacity, and delay of the physiological changes that result in disease and disability [3,4]. For these reasons, there is a longstanding interest in understanding the biopsychosocial and functional determinants of successful aging [5]. Although many factors can contribute to functional decline, loss of muscle mass (sarcopenia) in particular, has been consistently linked to functional decline during aging [6].

Globally, sarcopenia has become a major health challenge, and is now recognized as a medical condition across the world [7,8]. In a recent multi-ethnic study (MEMOSA—Multi-Ethnic Molecular determinants of Sarcopenia) involving participants from Singapore, the UK, and Jamaica [9], the genome-wide transcriptomic profiles of skeletal muscle biopsies in 119 older men diagnosed with sarcopenia compared with age-matched controls were examined using high-coverage RNA sequencing. The novel and important finding of this study was that mitochondrial bioenergetic dysfunction was the strongest molecular signature of sarcopenia in men irrespective of ethnicity. Specifically, sarcopenia was associated with major impairments of oxidative phosphorylation, mitochondrial dynamics, and mitochondrial quality. Such findings strongly suggest links between mitochondrial health, muscle quality, and physical function in older adults.

Exercise is widely known to improve mitochondrial health, potentially by providing a hormetic challenge that induces mitochondrial biogenesis [10]. Another potential intervention strategy for enhancing the metabolic flexibility of the mitochondria is intermittent fasting (IF), or more specifically, time-restricted feeding (TRF) [11]. This type of eating pattern involves a cessation in caloric intake commonly for 12–18 hours daily and has been shown to be sufficient to induce the metabolic switch from glucose to ketones as a source of energy for the mitochondria [12–14]. Specifically, this shift in metabolism takes place when nutrient availability is low and occurs at the point of negative energy balance when liver glycogen stores are depleted and fatty acids are mobilized (typically beyond 12 h after cessation of caloric intake) [15,16].

In contrast to traditional caloric restriction paradigms, food is not consumed during designated fasting time periods but is typically not restricted during designated eating time periods. The length of the fasting time period can also vary but is frequently 12 or more continuous hours. There are many types of intermittent fasting approaches, but the two most popular and well-studied approaches are alternate day fasting (ADF) or alternate day modified fasting (ADMF) and TRF. Alternate day or alternate day modified fasting involves consuming no or very little food on fasting days and then alternating with a day of unrestricted food intake or a "feast" day. Time-restricted feeding interventions differ from ADF interventions in that individuals engage in daily fasts between 14 and 18 hours. Findings from a recent review indicate participants generally have high levels of adherence (range = 77% to 98%) with no serious adverse events to fasting regimens ranging in duration from two weeks to one year [17].

Several clinical trials now indicate that a TRF eating pattern can reduce fat mass with retention of lean mass in younger and middle-aged adults [18–21]; however, the effects of TRF are not well understood in adults aged 65 and older. We recently reported that a four-week TRF eating pattern was sufficient to induce weight loss and produce small but clinically meaningful improvements in physical function in overweight older adults [22]. Although these findings are promising, they are limited by the short duration of the intervention. Therefore, the present study aimed to better understand factors affecting adherence and feasibility of TRF in an older adult population.

2. Methods

As described previously [22], ten overweight, sedentary, older adults aged 65 and older with mild to moderate functional limitations were recruited to participate in the *Time to Eat* pilot study. All participants were living independently in the community. Primary outcomes were feasibility, tolerability, and safety in overweight, sedentary older adults over four weeks using a single-arm pre–post design. Secondary outcomes included changes in body weight, waist circumference, cognitive and physical function, health-related quality of life, and adverse events [22]. The overarching goal of the present study was to evaluate participant perspectives who were enrolled in the *Time to Eat* pilot study regarding the real-world advantages, disadvantages, and challenges to adopting a TRF eating pattern via weekly phone interviews, a diet satisfaction survey, and an exit interview during the study.

2.1. Intervention

A four-week TRF single-arm clinical pilot trial was employed to test the study objectives. All participants were asked to abstain from any caloric intake during the targeted fasting window of 16 continuous hours and consume ad libitum during the eating window. Fasting times were chosen by the participant and were allowed to vary each day. The first week involved a gradual increase to a full 16-hour fasting period (Days 1–3 fast for 12–14 hours per day, Days 4–6 fast for 14–16 hours per day, Days 7–28 fast for 16 hours per day). Participants were encouraged to hydrate during fasting times. There were no dietary restrictions on the amount or types of food consumed during the 8-h feeding window, and participants were allowed to choose a time frame that best fit their lifestyle.

To promote adherence to the intervention, participants were provided with directions on how to follow the TRF protocol at the baseline visit. During this visit, participants received a pictorial flyer for future reference which depicted food items that were allowed and not allowed during fasting windows. On the flyer, "Go Foods" were written in green (water, diet soda, unsweetened teas, sugar free gum, black coffee) and "No Foods" were written in red (anything with calories, including coffee creamer, sweet teas, alcohol, snacks, drinks with calories). Participants also received an eating time log, which they were instructed to complete by recording the times when they first consumed calories and when they stopped consuming calories each day.

The trial interventionist called each participant weekly to promote adherence, review the protocol, monitor for adverse events, and provide support and guidance for any challenges faced during the intervention. A semi-structured, open-ended interview guide was used for the calls to inquire about daily activities, changes to normal routine, and any changes in health. During the call, the eating time log was reviewed, and support and guidance were provided for any challenges faced due to the intervention. An intervention-specific interview guide was used to routinely monitor adherence and adverse events, and to obtain direct participant feedback at multiple time points throughout the trial. The same questions were asked during each call, and calls concluded with open discussion. Participant answers and comments were documented during the phone calls. The questions asked during each phone call are displayed in Figure S1.

2.2. Adherence

Self-reported adherence to the study intervention was measured using the eating time log. Participants were considered adherent if they fasted between 14–18 hours per day during weeks two through four of the intervention. For this intervention, participants were allowed to pick the times of day in which they fasted as well as their eating window.

2.3. Outcome Measures

Diet Satisfaction Survey. At the end of the intervention, participants completed a study-specific Diet Satisfaction Survey (Table 1) to assess their satisfaction, feasibility, and overall experience with the study intervention. The Diet Satisfaction Survey contained 22 items and categorically measured respondents' attitudes by asking the extent to which they agreed or disagreed with a particular statement on a 5-point Likert scale (strongly disagree, disagree, neutral, agree, and strongly agree). The scores were summed and questions were grouped into one of three domains: biological, psychological, and socio-environmental.

Table 1. Participant responses to the Diet Satisfaction Survey.

Questions	Strongly Disagree (%)	Disagree (%)	Neutral (%)	Agree (%)	Strongly Agree (%)
Biological					
It was difficult to eat enough calories within the 8 hour window.	3(33)	4(44)	1(11)	1(11)	0(0)
I would eat more than normal amount of food during feeding period.	1(11)	5(56)	2(22)	1(11)	0(0)
I was uncomfortably hungry while fasting	0(0)	7(78)	1(11)	0(0)	1(11)
I had less energy than usual while fasting.	3(33)	5(56)	0(0)	0(0)	1(11)
I had difficulty falling asleep, staying asleep, or waking during fasting.	2(22)	3(33)	3(33)	1(11)	0(0)
Psychological					
Fasting became more difficult as the study went on.	4(44)	2(22)	1(11)	1(11)	1(11)
Fasting became easier as the study went on.	0(0)	2(22)	1(11)	3(33)	3(33)
My mood improved while intermittent fasting.	0(0)	2(22)	6(67)	0(0)	1(11)
My mood worsened while intermittent fasting.	2(22)	1(11)	5(56)	1(11)	0(0)
Fasting was more difficult than others previously tried.	2(22)	3(33)	3(33)	0(0)	1(11)
My overall quality of life improved during the IF diet.	0(0)	2(22)	6(67)	1(11)	0(0)
I could continue to IF for 6 months.	1(11)	2(22)	0(0)	6(67)	0(0)
I could continue to IF for 12 months.	2(22)	2(22)	1(11)	4(44)	0(0)
I could continue to IF for 24 months.	3(33)	1(11)	3(33)	2(22)	0(0)
I plan to continue IF after this study.	0(0)	2(22)	2(22)	5(56)	0(0)
I would participate in this study again.	1(11)	1(11)	1(11)	5(56)	1(11)
Socio-environmental					
I consumed all of my calories in one sitting.	3(33)	4(44)	1(11)	1(11)	0(0)
Fasting periods made tasks and work and home more difficult.	2(22)	3(33)	2(22)	1(11)	1(11)
Fasting periods negatively impacted my Social life.	2(22)	3(33)	2(22)	2(22)	0(0)
It was inconvenient to restrict my food intake to an 8-hour time frame.	0(0)	4(44)	1(11)	3(33)	1(11)
If recommended by their doctor, I think people would follow the IF diet.	0(0)	0(0)	4(44)	5(56)	0(0)
I would recommend this study to a friend.	1(11)	0(0)	2(22)	4(44)	2(22)

Exit Interview. Exit interviews were also conducted in person by the study interventionist during the follow-up assessment visits. Interview format mirrored that of the weekly phone calls and included additional questions measuring interest and the likelihood of continuing the TRF eating pattern. The interview concluded by allowing the participant to offer future suggestions and modifications if desired. The Specific Exit Interview Questions asked are displayed in Figure S2.

2.4. Analyses

Using the information obtained during the weekly phone calls and exit interviews, participant views on the perceived advantages, disadvantages, and challenges to adopting the TRF regimen were explored through qualitative analyses to better understand how older adults can successfully adopt TRF. A constant-comparison coding process was used to categorize and compare interview data for analysis purposes [23]. A trained researcher (SL) open-coded each interview and mapped data within the three primary constructs of the biopsychosocial model (biological, psychological, socio-environmental) to systematically categorize these three primary factors in their interactions in the TRF intervention. Open coding was completed by hand instead of using data mining software in order to take on the full context of the interviews. Positive and negative categories within each of the three primary themes were documented.

3. Results

Nine of the ten participants who commenced the study (mean age = 77.1 y; 6 women, 3 men) completed the entire protocol. One participant was considered non-adherent as the participant did not complete phone calls during the intervention or post-intervention assessments. However, this participant did complete an exit interview but not the Diet Satisfaction Survey post intervention. Thus, exit interviews were completed with all 10 participants who were enrolled in this study. Four participants completed all three weekly phone calls with the interventionist, three participants completed two calls, one participant completed one call near study end due to the wrong phone number being provided, and one participant did not complete any phone calls due to being on vacation.

Self-reported mean adherence to the TRF regimen was 84%, measured by daily eating time logs [22]. Few adverse events were reported during this intervention. Specifically, two participants experienced headaches during fasting periods, which resolved following an increase in water intake. One participant experienced dizziness, which resolved after having a small snack.

Over the four-week TRF intervention, the average reported start time for the participant eating period was 10:21 AM (range = 6:56 AM–1:25 PM) and the average reported stop time was 6:38 PM (range = 5:08 PM–9:00 PM), respectively. During week 1, the average reported start time of the first meal was 9:23 AM. During weeks 2 to 4, the start time of the eating period shifted later in the morning by a little over an hour, with participants reporting an average start time of 10:33 AM during week 4. The average eating stop time occurred 27 minutes earlier over the four-week study, concluding at 6:49 PM during week 1 and at 6:22 PM during week 4. The self-selected start and stop times for each participant's eating window are displayed in Figure 1.

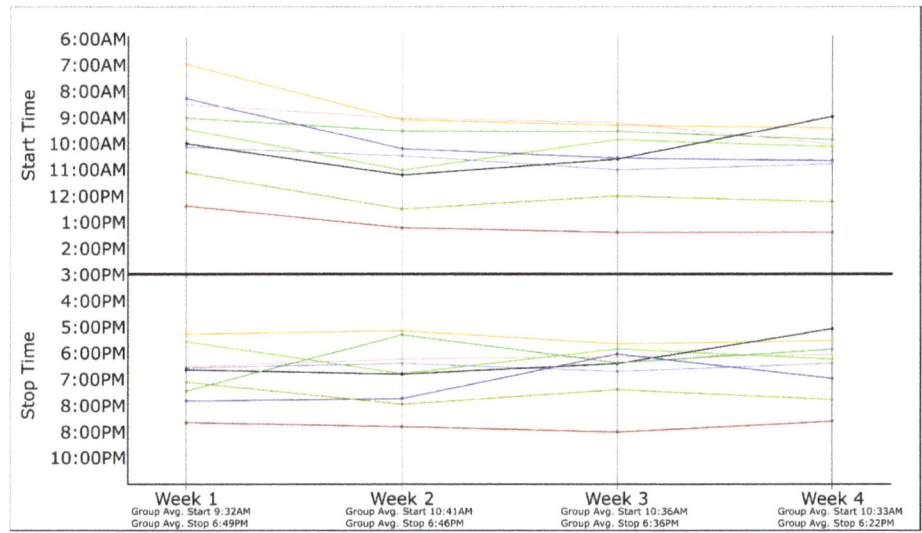

Figure 1. Self-selected start and stop times for each participant's eating window. N = 9 for each of the four weeks. Each participant's average weekly self-reported start/stop times are indicated by differing colors, with each line representing a single participant. The time between "Start Time" and "Stop Time" is indicative of each participant's eating window.

Participant answers to the questions on the Diet Satisfaction Survey revealed specific adherence-related barriers and facilitators within each of the three primary domains (biological, psychological, social) of the biopsychosocial model. Summed scores and percentages are shown in Table 1.

3.1. Biological Factors

Five participants reported easy adjustment to a 16-h fast, agreeing that fasting got easier as the study went on. Seven participants reported that it was not difficult to eat enough calories within the 8-h window. After the first few days of fasting, only one participant reported uncomfortable hunger during the study, but this participant misunderstood the protocol and was only eating one meal a day. Six of the nine participants stated that overeating was not problematic during the eating window and two participants neither agreed nor disagreed. Normal energy levels were retained throughout the intervention, with eight of the nine participants reporting "disagree" when asked if energy levels decreased while fasting. Only one participant indicated that fasting interfered with normal sleep patterns. Participant responses to the five questions within the biological domain of the Diet Satisfaction Survey are displayed in Figure S3.

3.2. Psychological Factors

Subjective mood and quality of life were unaffected in six of the nine participants, and seven participants expressed eagerness to participate in a similar study again. Despite this, participant comprehension of the TRF protocol was lower than expected, with many participants not fully understanding instructions regarding calorie consumption during fasting times. For example, during weekly phone calls, some participants stated they ate snacks in the evening before bed but did not record this in their eating window. Additionally, low-calorie foods were often confused with no-calorie foods, and not recorded even after the interventionist reiterated that any food item with calories must be documented. One participant misunderstood the regimen and only consumed one meal per day throughout the study, which was not revealed until the exit interview. Additionally, five participants thought that TRF was being examined solely for weight loss despite the interventionist explaining that other health outcomes were being evaluated. Due to this misunderstanding, two participants focused on consuming small or low-calorie foods during the eating window rather than eating as normal.

Six of nine participants agreed that they could adhere to the TRF eating pattern for six months, however, this number gradually decreased when asked about the feasibility of maintaining a TRF eating pattern for 12 or 24 months. Six of the participants agreed that fasting became easier over the study period, while two disagreed and one neither agreed nor disagreed. Five of the nine participants stated that they would continue fasting after concluding the study, while two had no preference and two indicated they would not continue. Participant responses to the ten questions within the psychological domain of the Diet Satisfaction Survey are displayed in Figure S4.

3.3. Socio-Environmental Factors

Family support was central to participant adherence. Although not formally enrolled in the trial, the spouses of participants often altered their eating patterns to accompany their partner. Seven participants were able to space out their meals during their chosen eight-hour eating window rather than consuming all daily calories in one sitting, with four participants reporting inconvenience in eating all of their meals during the eating window. Environmental challenges to TRF adherence included social events during which food was served outside the participant's eating window, as well as changes in work schedules that interfered with the timing of meals. Regular doctor appointments for the participant or their spouse requiring long commutes also extended fasting times beyond the 14-18 hour goal for a few individuals. Additionally, several participants reported that they would not want to follow this eating pattern during holidays or vacations. Notwithstanding these challenges, only one participant stated they would not recommend TRF to a friend, and five believed people would follow this eating pattern if recommended by their healthcare provider. Participant responses to the seven questions within the socio-environmental domain of the Diet Satisfaction Survey are displayed in Figure S5.

4. Discussion

The findings of the current trial suggest that TRF is an eating approach that is well tolerated by most older adults. However, six participants did not fully understand the requirements of the fasting regimen, despite being provided with specific instructions and a pictorial guide at a baseline visit. Among these six participants, three reported consuming snacks during fasting periods, two participants confused low-calorie with no-calorie items, and one participant thought they were only allowed to eat one meal a day. Thus, these findings suggest that more instruction and/or participant contact is needed in the early stages of a TRF intervention to promote adherence.

Most participants reported limited physical discomfort caused by this eating pattern. After the first few days of fasting, only one participant reported discomfort related to hunger, and this was likely due to misunderstanding the eating pattern directions. The few reported side effects included transient headaches which dissipated with increased water intake, and dizziness in one participant which subsided with a small snack.

While it is challenging to separately measure biological, psychological, and socio-environmental factors related to eating, energy, and satiety, our findings suggest each domain is relevant to TRF adherence. From a biological perspective, all but one participant perceived they were consuming the same or higher amount of calories as they did prior to beginning the intervention. It is also noteworthy that eight out of nine participants disagreed that fasting decreased energy levels, with greater self-reported activity levels in both yardwork and light exercise. Eight participants indicated on the Diet Satisfaction Survey that the TRF intervention did not negatively affect their sleep, with only one participant reporting that fasting interfered with their normal sleep patterns.

From a psychological perspective, most participants also expressed positive attitudes on the phone calls throughout the study and seven of the nine participants reported feeling eager, motivated and excited to continue with the intervention. Many had heard of IF regimens and wanted to experience this eating pattern. Despite this, participant comprehension of the TRF protocol was lower than anticipated, with six participants not fully understanding instructions regarding avoiding calorie consumption during fasting times. Two participants also had difficulty differentiating foods and beverages with low versus no calories. Additionally, participants were initially inaccurate and inconsistent when reporting their food intake times. To maximize protocol comprehension, it is recommended that future interventions provide even more frequent contact (e.g., bi-weekly) during the initial intervention period to ensure the participant understands the protocol. Similar to calorie restriction interventions, ongoing contact is advisable and can equip participants with adherence promoting behavioral modification techniques and strategies, and continued monitoring for adverse events.

Socio-environmental factors also served as both barriers and facilitators to adherence. Consistent with prior literature [24], participants were often positively influenced by their partners. Many participants reported receiving significant support from spouses, some of whom even changed their eating patterns to be in synchrony with them during the intervention. These reports were highly encouraging, as successful behavior modification requires disrupting the socio-environmental factors that cue habitual behavior [25], and spousal eating times represent an important factor that could cue eating in the participants [26]. On the other hand, a few socio-environmental factors emerged as barriers to adherence. Also consistent with previous studies [27–29], pressures from work, long commutes, vacations, and social engagements represented barriers to adherence to intervention for some participants.

Despite strong evidence indicating that lifestyle intervention programs involving diet, exercise, and behavior modification can reduce risk factors for many chronic diseases and improve physical function, long-term adherence to lifestyle interventions to date is notoriously low [30]. Consequently, the "adherence problem" represents an important challenge to weight loss interventions [30]. Findings from a recent review of 27 studies indicate that participants generally have high levels of adherence (range = 77% to 98%) to different types of fasting regimens, including ADF and TRF [17]. Thus, future trials are needed to evaluate the potential that this eating pattern may have for enhancing long-term weight loss.

There were a few notable strengths of this study. First, participants received personalized attention throughout the intervention, which allowed for discussion of individual challenges and tailored solutions to help participants adopt this new eating pattern. This contact was provided through weekly phone calls to check on their adherence and assist them in problem-solving any challenges they were experiencing following the intervention. Second, adherence was carefully tracked throughout the study, as participants reported the time of their first and last meal in an eating time log each day. The participants then reported their daily start and stop times during weekly phone calls and adjustments were discussed if needed. Third, adverse events were assessed, and potential solutions were offered during the calls. We also conducted exit interviews to obtain each participant's perspective on what challenges and what changes, if any, they would recommend the intervention in future trials.

There were also several limitations to this study, including difficulty in contacting some participants via telephone during the intervention. Additionally, only one coder was used for analysis, and triangulation was not used to cross-check data collection. In future studies, a second coder will be used to verify the coding scheme. As this was a pre–post pilot study of short duration, a small sample size was used, which limits the generalizability of the results as well as our ability to make conclusive statements. Response bias is also a possible limitation of this study, as participants may have only reported what they thought the interventionist wanted to hear in the interviews, or second-guessed what the interventionist was asking and altered their answers. Individual interpretation of the questions asked on the Diet Satisfaction Survey may have also varied. Future studies should utilize larger sample sizes to ensure sufficient power to detect both pre–post differences and between-group differences.

5. Conclusions

Most (6 of 10) participants appreciated the simplicity of the time-restricted eating pattern and reported willingness to continue this eating pattern with slight modification such as decreased daily fasting times or a weekly "unrestricted feeding" day. Comprehension of the fasting regimen and guidelines varied, indicating more participant contact and/or education is needed during the initial stages of the intervention. Additionally, baseline group instruction about the protocol with weekly in-person group sessions may enhance understanding and social support. Motivation to follow the protocol was strongly guided by weight loss, as many participants thought this was the goal of the study. Interventions with older adults should consider these factors to optimally support lifestyle modification and protocol adherence.

Clinical Implications

This study provides exciting preliminary data on the potential beneficial effects and feasibility of TRF in older adults with very few risks associated with the intervention. In addition to the previously reported weight loss outcome and high adherence to the intervention [22], most participants adjusted relatively easily to the fasting window of 14–18 hours. Adverse effects were rare and were quickly remedied. No decrease in energy during the fasting time was reported by eight participants. There was also a carry-over effect, with some family members participating and a high likelihood the participants would recommend this intervention to a friend. While these findings are promising, more work needs to be done before a TRF intervention can be effectively implemented into clinical practice. The primary challenge relates to the participants' initial misunderstanding of what they were and were not allowed to consume during the 14–18 hour fasting period. The addition of dietary monitoring in which participants record their food intake, as well as the start and stop times, may be one approach to enhance adherence levels. This approach has proven essential for most behavioral weight loss programs, so it may be beneficial to helping older adults understand the key distinction between the fasting and non-fasting time periods. Other common adherence barriers expressed by participants included program adherence during social events, changes in work schedule, or vacations.

Nevertheless, there is more opportunity to overcome these barriers due to the flexibility of TRF and the ultimate ability to focus on a yes or no behavior (eating vs. fasting) rather than consciously eating less or counting calories with traditional diets.

Supplementary Materials: The following are available online at http://www.mdpi.com/2072-6643/12/3/874/s1, Figure S1: Time to eat pilot study—Weekly follow-up progress notes. Figure S2: Exit Interview Questions. Figure S3: Participant responses to the five questions within the biological domain of the Diet Satisfaction Survey, Figure S4: Participant responses to the ten questions within the psychological domain of the Diet Satisfaction Survey., Figure S5: Participant responses to the seven questions within the socio-environmental domain of the Diet Satisfaction Survey.

Author Contributions: Conceptualization, S.A.L. and S.A.; methodology, S.A.; formal analysis, S.A.L.; original draft preparation, S.A.L.; writing—Review and editing, C.S., C.M., S.A., B.A.B., K.T.S., W.T.D.; visualization, C.S., C.M.; supervision, S.A.; funding acquisition, S.A. All authors have read and agreed to the published version of the manuscript.

Funding: This research received no external funding.

Acknowledgments: The authors would like to express their appreciation to the participants and research associates who made it possible to complete this research project. This research was supported by the NIH-funded Claude D. Pepper Older Americans Independence Center (P30AG028740).

Conflicts of Interest: The authors declare no conflicts of interest.

References

1. Kontis, V.; Bennett, J.E.; Mathers, C.D.; Li, G.; Foreman, K.; FMedSci, M.Z. Future life expectancy in 35 industrialised countries: Projections with a Bayesian model ensemble. *Lancet* **2017**, *389*, 1323–1335. [CrossRef]
2. Reider, L. *Life Expectancy and Assessment of Functional Status in Older Patients, in Acetabular Fractures in Older Patients*; Springer: Cham, Switzerland, 2020; pp. 5–19.
3. Katz, S.; Branch, L.G.; Branson, M.H.; Papsidero, J.A.; Beck, J.C.; Greer, D.S. Active life expectancy. *N. Engl. J. Med.* **1983**, *309*, 1218–1224. [CrossRef]
4. Crimmins, E.M. Lifespan and healthspan: Past, present, and promise. *Gerontologist* **2015**, *55*, 901–911. [CrossRef] [PubMed]
5. Anton, S.D.; Woods, A.J.; Ashizawa, T.; Barb, D.; Buford, T.W.; Carter, C.S.; Clark, D.J.; Cohen, R.A.; Corbett, D.B.; Cruz-Almeida, Y.; et al. Successful aging: Advancing the science of physical independence in older adults. *Ageing Res. Rev.* **2015**, *24*, 304–327. [CrossRef] [PubMed]
6. Buford, T.W.; Anton, S.D.; Judge, A.R.; Marzetti, E.; Wohlgemuth, S.E.; Carter, C.S.; Leeuwenburgh, C.; Pahor, M.; Manini, T.M. Models of accelerated sarcopenia: Critical pieces for solving the puzzle of age-related muscle atrophy. *Ageing Res. Rev.* **2010**, *9*, 369–383. [CrossRef] [PubMed]
7. Cruz-Jentoft, A.J.; Bahat, G.; Bauer, J.; Boirie, Y.; Bruyère, O.; Cederholm, T.; Cooper, C.; Landi, F.; Rolland, Y.; Sayer, A.A. Sarcopenia: Revised European consensus on definition and diagnosis. *Age Ageing* **2019**, *48*, 601. [CrossRef]
8. Vellas, B.; Fielding, R.A.; Bens, C.; Bernabei, R.; Cawthon, P.M.; Cederholm, T.; Cruz-Jentoft, A.J.; Del Signore, S.; Donahue, S.; Morley, J.; et al. Implications of icd-10 for sarcopenia clinical practice and clinical trials: Report by the international conference on frailty and sarcopenia research task force. *J. Frailty Aging* **2018**, *7*, 2–9.
9. Migliavacca, E.; Tay, S.K.H.; Feige, J.N. Mitochondrial oxidative capacity and NAD(+) biosynthesis are reduced in human sarcopenia across ethnicities. *Nat. Commun.* **2019**, *10*, 5808. [CrossRef]
10. Musci, R.V.; Hamilton, K.L.; Linden, M.A. Exercise-induced mitohormesis for the maintenance of skeletal muscle and healthspan extension. *Sports* **2019**, *7*, 170. [CrossRef]
11. Lettieri Barbato, D.; Tatulli, G.; Aquilano, K.; Ciriolo, M.R. Mitochondrial Hormesis links nutrient restriction to improved metabolism in fat cell. *Aging* **2015**, *7*, 869–881. [CrossRef]
12. Di Francesco, A. A time to fast. *Science* **2018**, *362*, 770–775. [CrossRef] [PubMed]
13. Mattson, M.P.; Allison, D.B.; Fontana, L.; Harvie, M.; Longo, V.D.; Willy, J.; Mosley, M.M.; Notterpek, L.; Ravussin, E.; Scheer, F.A.J.K.; et al. Meal frequency and timing in health and disease. *Proc. Natl. Acad. Sci. USA* **2014**, *111*, 16647–16653. [CrossRef]

14. Anton, S.D.; Moehl, K.; Donahoo, W.T.; Marosi, K.; Lee, S.A.; Mainous, A.G., III; Leeuwenburgh, C.; Mattson, M.P. Flipping the metabolic Switch: Understanding and applying the health benefits of fasting. *Obesity* **2018**, *26*, 254–268. [CrossRef] [PubMed]
15. Longo, V.D.; Mattson, M.P. Fasting: Molecular mechanisms and clinical applications. *Cell Metab.* **2014**, *19*, 181–192. [CrossRef] [PubMed]
16. Klein, S.; Wolfe, R.R. Carbohydrate restriction regulates the adaptive response to fasting. *Am. J. Physiol.* **1992**, *262*, E631–E636. [CrossRef] [PubMed]
17. Welton, S.; Minty, R.; O'Driscoll, T.; Willms, H.; Poirier, D.; Madden, S.; Len, K. Intermittent fasting and weight loss: Systematic review. *Can. Fam. Phys.* **2020**, *66*, 117–125.
18. Moro, T.; Tinsley, G.; Bianco, A.; Marcolin, G.; Pacelli, Q.F.; Battaglia, G.; Palma, A.; Gentil, P.; Neri, M.; Paoli, A. Effects of eight weeks of time-restricted feeding (16/8) on basal metabolism, maximal strength, body composition, inflammation, and cardiovascular risk factors in resistance-trained males. *J. Transl. Med.* **2016**, *14*, 290. [CrossRef]
19. Carlson, O.; Martin, B.; Stote, K.S.; Golden, E.; Maudsley, S.; Najjar, S.N.; Ferrucci, L.; Ingram, D.K.; Longo, D.L.; Rumpler, W.V.; et al. Impact of reduced meal frequency without caloric restriction on glucose regulation in healthy, normal-weight middle-aged men and women. *Metabolism* **2007**, *56*, 1729–1734. [CrossRef]
20. Stote, K.S.; Baer, D.J.; Spears, K.; Paul, D.R.; Harris, G.K.; Rumpler, W.V.; Strycula, P.; Najjar, S.S.; Ferrucci, L.; Ingram, D.K. A controlled trial of reduced meal frequency without caloric restriction in healthy, normal-weight, middle-aged adults. *Am. J. Clin. Nutr.* **2007**, *85*, 981–988. [CrossRef]
21. Tinsley, G.M.; Forsse, J.S.; Butler, N.K.; Paoli, A.; Bane, A.A.; Bounty, P.M.L.; Morgan, G.B.; Grandjean, P.W. Time-restricted feeding in young men performing resistance training: A randomized controlled trial. *Eur. J. Sport Sci.* **2017**, *17*, 200–207. [CrossRef]
22. Anton, S.D.; LEE, S.A.; Donahoo, W.T.; McLaren, C.; Manini, T.; Leeuwenburgh, C.; Pahor, M. The effects of time restricted feeding on overweight, older adults: A pilot study. *Nutrients* **2019**, *11*, 1500. [CrossRef]
23. Anderson, A.R.; Jack, S.L. An introduction to the constant comparative technique. In *Hallbook of Qualitative Research Techniques and Analyses in Entrepreneurships*; Edward Elgar Publishing: Troutham, UK, 2015.
24. Jackson, S.E.; Steptoe, A.; Wardle, J. The influence of partner's behavior on health behavior change: The english longitudinal study of ageing. *JAMA Intern. Med.* **2015**, *175*, 385–392. [CrossRef] [PubMed]
25. Verplanken, B.; Wood, W. Intervention to break and create consumer habits. *J. Public Policy Market.* **2006**, *25*, 90–103. [CrossRef]
26. Marshall, D.W.; Anderson, A.S. Proper meals in transition: Young married couples on the nature of eating together. *Appetite* **2002**, *39*, 193–206. [CrossRef] [PubMed]
27. Burgess, E.; Hassmen, P.; Pumpa, K.L. Determinants of adherence to lifestyle intervention in adults with obesity: A systematic review. *Clin. Obes.* **2017**, *7*, 123–135. [CrossRef] [PubMed]
28. Venditti, E.M.; Wylie-Rosett, J.; Delahanty, L.M.; Mele, L.; Hoskin, M.A.; Edelstein, S.L. Short and long-term lifestyle coaching approaches used to address diverse participant barriers to weight loss and physical activity adherence. *Int. J. Behav. Nutr. Phys. Act.* **2014**, *11*, 16. [CrossRef]
29. Leone, L.A.; Ward, D.S. A mixed methods comparison of perceived benefits and barriers to exercise between obese and nonobese women. *J. Phys. Act. Health* **2013**, *10*, 461–469. [CrossRef]
30. Middleton, K.R.; Anton, S.D.; Perri, M.G. Long-term adherence to health behavior change. *Am. J. Lifestyle Med.* **2013**, *7*, 395–404. [CrossRef]

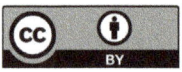

© 2020 by the authors. Licensee MDPI, Basel, Switzerland. This article is an open access article distributed under the terms and conditions of the Creative Commons Attribution (CC BY) license (http://creativecommons.org/licenses/by/4.0/).

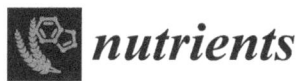

Article

Identification of a Circulating Amino Acid Signature in Frail Older Persons with Type 2 Diabetes Mellitus: Results from the Metabofrail Study

Riccardo Calvani [1,2], Leocadio Rodriguez-Mañas [3], Anna Picca [1,2], Federico Marini [4], Alessandra Biancolillo [5], Olga Laosa [6], Laura Pedraza [6], Jacopo Gervasoni [1,2], Aniello Primiano [1,2], Giorgia Conta [4], Isabelle Bourdel-Marchasson [7], Sophie C. Regueme [7], Roberto Bernabei [1,2], Emanuele Marzetti [1,2,*], Alan J. Sinclair [8], Giovanni Gambassi [1,2] and on behalf of the European MID-Frail Consortium

[1] Università Cattolica del Sacro Cuore, 00168 Rome, Italy; riccardo.calvani@gmail.com (R.C.); anna.picca1@gmail.com (A.P.); jacopo.gervasoni@policlinicogemelli.it (J.G.); anielloprim@gmail.com (A.P.); Roberto.Bernabei@unicatt.it (R.B.); giovanni.gambassi@unicatt.it (G.G.)
[2] Fondazione Policlinico Universitario "Agostino Gemelli" IRCCS, 00168 Rome, Italy
[3] Servicio de Geriatría, Hospital Universitario de Getafe, 28905 Madrid, Spain; leocadio.rodriguez@salud.madrid.org
[4] Department of Chemistry, Sapienza Università di Roma, 00185 Rome, Italy; federico.marini@uniroma1.it (F.M.); giorgia.conta@uniroma1.it (G.C.)
[5] Department of Physical and Chemical Sciences, Università degli Studi dell'Aquila, 67100 L'Aquila, Italy; alessandra.biancolillo@univaq.it
[6] Foundation for Biomedical Research, Hospital Universitario de Getafe, 28905 Madrid, Spain; olga.laosa@salud.madrid.org (O.L.); laura.pedraza@salud.madrid.org (L.P.)
[7] Centre Hospitalier Universitaire de Bordeaux, 33000 Bordeaux, France; isabelle.bourdel-marchasson@chu-bordeaux.fr (I.B.-M.); sophie.regueme@chu-bordeaux.fr (S.C.R.)
[8] Foundation for Diabetes Research in Older People, Diabetes Frail Ltd., Luton LU1 3UA, UK; sinclair.5@btinternet.com
* Correspondence: emanuele.marzetti@policlinicogemelli.it; Tel.: +39-0630155559; Fax: +39-063051911

Received: 20 December 2019; Accepted: 9 January 2020; Published: 12 January 2020

Abstract: Diabetes and frailty are highly prevalent conditions that impact the health status of older adults. Perturbations in protein/amino acid metabolism are associated with both functional impairment and type 2 diabetes mellitus (T2DM). In the present study, we compared the concentrations of a panel of circulating 37 amino acids and derivatives between frail/pre-frail older adults with T2DM and robust non-diabetic controls. Sixty-six functionally impaired older persons aged 70+ with T2DM and 30 age and sex-matched controls were included in the analysis. We applied a partial least squares-discriminant analysis (PLS-DA)-based analytical strategy to characterize the metabotype of study participants. The optimal complexity of the PLS-DA model was found to be two latent variables. The proportion of correct classification was 94.1 ± 1.9% for frail/pre-frail persons with T2DM and 100% for control participants. Functionally impaired older persons with T2DM showed higher levels of 3-methyl histidine, alanine, arginine, glutamic acid, ethanolamine sarcosine, and tryptophan. Control participants had higher levels of ornithine and taurine. These findings indicate that a specific profile of amino acids and derivatives characterizes pre-frail/frail older persons with T2DM. The dissection of these pathways may provide novel insights into the metabolic perturbations involved in the disabling cascade in older persons with T2DM.

Keywords: aging; metabolomics; systems biology; personalized medicine; metabolism; frailty; sarcopenia; muscle wasting; precision medicine; metabolic profiling

1. Introduction

Type 2 diabetes mellitus (T2DM) is a chronic condition frequently occurring in old age [1,2]. T2DM is associated with higher risk of negative outcomes, including disability and mortality [3]. T2DM-related complications are especially prevalent in older adults and account for the increasing costs of T2DM [4]. Frailty defines a geriatric syndrome characterized by reduced ability to cope with life stressors and increased risk of adverse events (e.g., falls, delirium, loss of independence, mortality) [5,6]. T2DM and frailty are intimately related and share common features, including complex pathophysiology and heterogeneous phenotypes [7], that challenge their management [5,8].

Muscle failure, both in its metabolic and functional manifestations, is a hallmark of T2DM and frailty [7,9]. The progressive and generalized loss of muscle mass, strength, and function with age, termed sarcopenia, fuels a self-reinforcing cycle in which structural, metabolic, and endocrine perturbations in muscle exacerbate T2DM-related signs and symptoms [10]. T2DM further promotes the decline in muscle mass and function [11,12] which, in turn, aggravates functional impairment [13].

The central role of muscle wasting in frailty and T2DM may guide the identification of novel biomarkers and possibly new treatment targets for the two conditions [14–16]. In this context, circulating amino acids are promising candidates given their sensor-transducer-effector role in systemic metabolism, muscle homeostasis, and physical function [17–20]. Moreover, amino acids are involved in processes critical to the development and progression of frailty and T2DM, such as inflammation, glucose homeostasis, and redox regulation [21–23].

Targeted metabolomics allowed identifying specific amino acid profiles that were associated with insulin resistance and risk of developing T2DM in independent cohorts across US, Europe, and China [24–27]. A plasma amino acid signature, together with specific circulating lipid species, was linked to glucose dyshomeostasis and impaired insulin sensitivity in older adults from the Baltimore Longitudinal Study of Aging (BLSA) [28]. In addition, distinct patterns of circulating amino acids were associated with frailty and/or muscle-related parameters (mass, turnover, performance) in older individuals at risk for frailty [29–32]. Finally, within the "BIOmarkers associated with Sarcopenia and PHysical frailty in EldeRly pErsons" (BIOSPHERE) study, a combination of serum amino acids and derivatives was identified that characterized the metabotype of older adults with physical frailty and sarcopenia (PF&S) [17].

Here, we sought to define the circulating amino acid profile of frail/pre-frail older adults with T2DM (F-T2DM). Our approach, described in the context of the "Metabolic biomarkers of frailty in older people with type 2 diabetes mellitus" (MetaboFrail) study, coupled targeted metabolomics with a chemometric modeling strategy [16]. Through this innovative biomarker discovery strategy, we identified a specific profile of serum amino acids in F-T2DM older people. These findings may offer new insights into the metabolic perturbations associated with the disabling cascade in older persons with T2DM.

2. Materials and Methods

2.1. Study Population

MetaboFrail was developed as an ancillary study of the "Multi-modal Intervention in Diabetes in Frailty" (MID-Frail) project [16,33,34]. The latter was a cluster-randomized multicenter clinical trial that evaluated the effectiveness of a multicomponent intervention (mainly based on resistance exercise and lifestyle counseling) on improving physical performance compared with usual care in F-T2DM older adults from seven European countries (ClinicalTrials.gov identifier: NCT01654341) [16,33]. For the present study, a subgroup of MID-Frail participants recruited in Spanish and French study centers were enrolled. The main eligibility criteria were: (a) age at screening 70 years or older; (b) T2DM diagnosis from at least two years; and (c) being pre-frail or frail according to Fried's criteria [35]. The main exclusion criteria were: (a) poor cognition operationalized as a Mini Mental State Examination score <20 [36]; (b) severe disability defined as a Barthel index score <60 [37]; critical conditions and/or major illnesses with a life expectancy <6 months; (c) inability or unwillingness to provide informed consent. Control participants were enrolled at the Università Cattolica del Sacro Cuore (Rome, Italy) and had the following characteristics: 70+ years of age, no T2DM, and no functional impairment. The study protocol was approved by local ethics committees according to both national and international laws. Prior to enrolment, all participants provided written informed consent. The study was conducted in agreement with legal requirements and international norms (Declaration of Helsinki, 1964).

2.2. Blood Collection and Determination of Serum Concentrations of Amino Acids and Derivatives

Blood samples were collected after overnight fasting. For serum separation, blood samples were kept on ice for about 30 min until clotting and were subsequently centrifuged at 1000× g for 10 min at 4 °C. Serum samples were eventually aliquoted and stored at −80 °C until analysis.

Concentrations of 37 amino acids and derivatives were determined in serum by ultraperformance liquid chromatography/mass spectrometry (UPLC/MS), as described previously [17]. Briefly, 50 µL of sample was added to 100 µL 10% (w/v) sulfosalicylic acid containing an internal standard mix (50 µM; Cambridge Isotope Laboratories, Inc., Tewksbury, MA, USA) and centrifuged at 1000× g for 15 min. Ten µL of the resulting supernatant were mixed with 70 µL of borate buffer and 20 µL of AccQ Tag reagents (Waters Corporation, Milford, MA, USA) and heated at 55 °C for 10 min. Samples were eventually loaded onto a CORTECS UPLC C18 column 1.6 µm 2.1 × 150 mm (Waters Corporation) for chromatographic separation (ACQUITY H-Class, Waters Corporation, Milford, MA, USA). Elution was performed at 500 µL/min flow rate with a linear gradient (9 min) from 99:1 to 1:99 water 0.1% formic acid/acetonitrile 0.1% formic acid. Analytes were detected on an ACQUITY QDa single quadrupole mass spectrometer equipped with electrospray source operating in positive mode (Waters Corporation, Milford, MA, USA). Amino acid controls (MCA laboratory of the Queen Beatrix Hospital, Winterswijk, The Netherlands) were used to monitor the analytic process.

2.3. Statistical Analysis

The normal distribution of data was ascertained through the Kolmogorov-Smirnov test. Comparisons between F-T2DM and control participants for normally distributed continuous variables were performed by t-test statistics. The non-parametric test Mann-Whitney U was applied to assess differences for non-normally distributed continuous data. Differences in categorical variables between groups were determined via χ^2 statistics. Descriptive analyses were performed using the GraphPrism 5.03 software (GraphPad Software, Inc., San Diego, CA), with statistical significance set at $p < 0.05$.

2.4. Partial Least Squares-Discriminant Analysis and Double Cross-Validation Procedures

In order to unveil possible differences in circulating amino acid patterns between F-T2DM and control participants, a multivariate classification strategy based on partial least squares-discriminant analysis (PLS-DA) modeling was adopted [38]. PLS-DA is a classification method particularly suited for dealing with highly correlated predictors, as it is based on projecting the predictors (measured variables) onto a reduced subspace of latent variables (LVs; directions in space) of highest covariance with the responses, i.e., providing the maximum separation between classes. In order to validate the results of PLS-DA modeling and rule out the possibility that good results were obtained because of chance correlation, a procedure based on repeated double cross-validation (DCV) and permutation tests was used [39,40]. DCV consists of spitting the samples to obtain two cross-validation loops, an internal loop for model building/model selection and an outer loop that mimics external (test set) validation. The DCV procedure is repeated a sufficient number of times such that estimates do to depend on one specific sample splitting. This allows evaluating the consistency of model parameters and the confidence intervals for model predictions. To assess the statistical significance of the obtained predictions, the figures of merit which summarize the classification accuracy in repeated DCV [i.e., number of misclassifications (NMC), area under the receiver operating characteristic curve (AUROC), and discriminant (DQ2)] are compared with their distribution under the null hypothesis, which is estimated non-parametrically through permutation tests with 1000 randomizations. A more detailed description of the procedure can be found elsewhere [41]. PLS-DA and DCV were run under Matlab R2015b environment by means of in-house written functions (freely downloadable at: https://www.chem.uniroma1.it/romechemometrics/research/algorithms/plsda/).

3. Results

3.1. Study Population

The present investigation included 66 F-T2DM older adults and 30 age and sex-matched robust, non-diabetic controls. The main characteristics of the two groups are reported in Table 1. F-T2DM and control participants were comparable for age, sex distribution, and number of diseases. F-T2DM older adults showed higher body mass index relative to controls. As expected, a significant difference was found in physical functional between groups, as indicated by the scores on the short physical performance battery (SPPB).

Table 1. Main characteristics of study participants.

	F-T2DM ($n = 66$)	Controls ($n = 30$)	p
Age, years (mean ± SD)	76.5 ± 14.5	74.6 ± 4.3	0.46
Sex (female), n (%)	32 (48)	16 (53)	0.82
BMI, kg/m^2 (mean ± SD)	29.2 ± 4.9	26.7 ± 2.4	0.01
SPPB score (mean ± SD)	8.6 ± 2.9	11.3 ± 0.9	<0.0001
Number of diseases (mean ± SD) §	2.8 ± 1.0	2.9 ± 2.0	0.86

§ Includes hypertension, coronary artery disease, prior stroke, peripheral vascular disease, diabetes, chronic obstructive pulmonary disease, and osteoarthritis; Abbreviations: BMI, body mass index; F-T2DM, frail/pre-frail older adults with type 2 diabetes mellitus; SD, standard deviation; SPPB, short physical performance battery.

3.2. Identification of Circulating Amino Acid Profiles

In the present study, we aimed at identifying profiles of circulating amino acids that discriminate older persons with F-T2DM from functionally intact non-diabetic peers. Among the available statistical options, we selected a PLS-DA-based strategy for its ability to handle multiple interdependent variables. The best PLS-DA model was built using two LVs. As indicated by the stringent DCV applied, the classification performance of the model was almost perfect. Indeed, the proportion of correct classification of participants was 96.6 ± 1.5% over the calibration sets (95.0 ± 2.2% for cases and 100.0 ± 0.0% for controls), 96.6 ± 1.5% (95.0 ± 2.2% for cases and 100.0 ± 0.0% for controls) in the internal DCV loop (i.e., the one used for model selection), and 95.9 ± 1.3% (94.1 ± 1.9% for cases and 100.0 ± 0.0% for controls) in the outer DCV loop, which accounts for the results of repeated external validation.

The remarkable classification performance of the PLS-DA model can be appreciated by inspecting the projection of study participants over the space spanned by the two LVs (Figure 1).

A sharp separation between F-T2DM participants and controls is evident. To ensure the reliability of our findings against the possibility of chance correlations, DCV results of the PLS-DA model were compared with the distributions of specific figures of merit under the null hypothesis. As depicted in Figure 2, for all of the figures considered (i.e., NMC, AUROC, and DQ2), values obtained from the unpermuted dataset fell outside the corresponding null hypothesis distribution, indicating a p value <0.05.

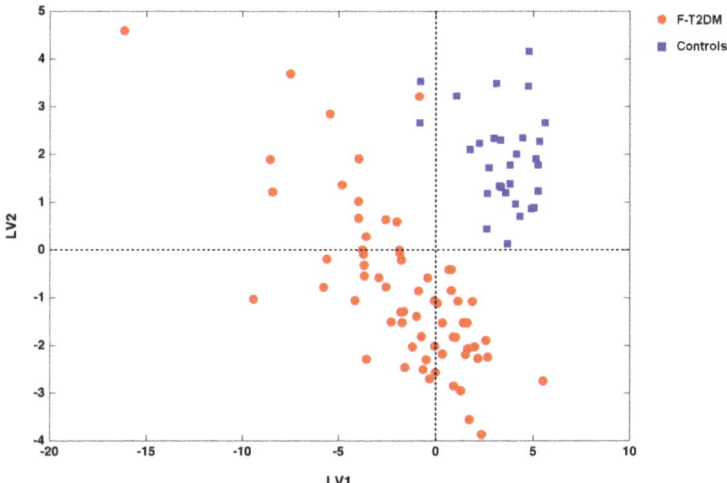

Figure 1. Scores plot showing the separation of frail/pre-frail older adults with type 2 diabetes mellitus (F-T2DM) from control participants according to the serum concentrations of amino acids and derivatives in the space spanned by the two latent variables (LV1 and LV2), as determined by partial least squares-discriminant analysis.

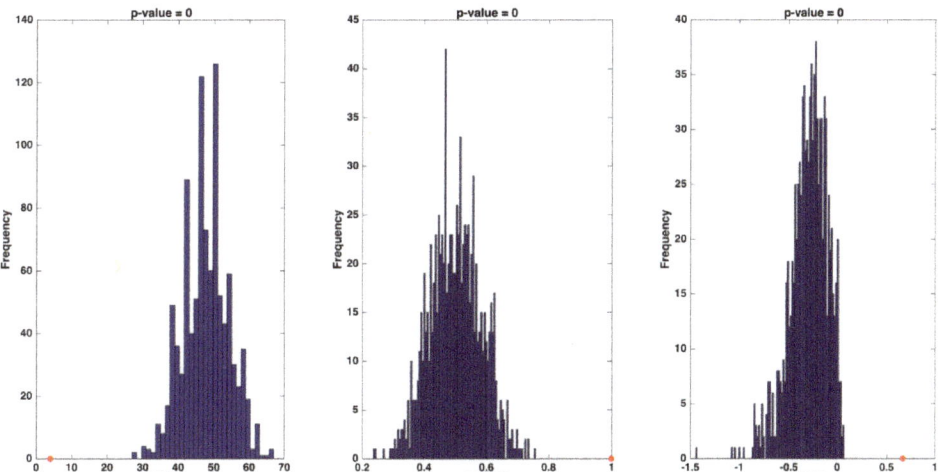

Figure 2. Distribution of values of number of misclassifications (NMC), area under the receiver operating characteristic curve (AUROC), and discriminant Q2 (DQ2) under their respective null hypothesis as estimated by permutation tests (blue histograms) and the corresponding values obtained by the partial least squares-discriminant analysis model on unpermuted data (red circles). Values obtained on the real dataset (red circles) fall outside of the corresponding null hypothesis distribution (blue histograms), corresponding to a $p < 0.05$.

The identification of the metabolites with the greatest discriminating power was accomplished by inspecting variable importance in projection (VIP) indices. Table 2 reports variables with a VIP value higher than 1.

Table 2. Serum concentrations of discriminant biomolecules as resulted from partial least squares-discriminant analysis.

Analytes	F-T2DM (n = 66)	Controls (n = 30)
3-methylhistidine	7.8 ± 4.2	5.2 ± 2.5
Alanine	542.3 ± 165.8	384.3 ± 98.3
Arginine	168.3 ± 91.2	103.7 ± 31.2
Ethanolamine	11.5 ± 3.4	9.0 ± 2.2
Glutamic acid	130.0 ± 66.8	54.3 ± 21.3
Ornithine	103.2 ± 37.6	109.4 ± 25.0
Sarcosine	2.5 ± 0.9	1.6 ± 0.6
Taurine	100.4 ± 49.0	189.5 ± 47.2
Tryptophan	66.2 ± 23.4	62.0 ± 13.1

Data are shown as mean ± standard deviation. Concentrations are expressed in μmol/L.

F-T2DM participants showed higher serum levels of 3-methyl histidine, alanine, arginine, ethanolamine, glutamic acid, sarcosine, and tryptophan. Instead, controls were characterized by higher circulating levels of ornithine and taurine. Serum concentrations of non-discriminant analytes in the two participant groups are listed in Table S1.

4. Discussion

Over the last few years, analytical platforms have been developed together with sophisticated computational algorithms to allow the study of complex diseases in unprecedented detail [42]. This new healthcare paradigm, called personalized or precision medicine, incorporates "omics" technologies to unveil the inner biological properties of morbid conditions [42] and devise innovative diagnostics and interventions tailored to the needs of single individuals [42,43]. Metabolomics, by virtue of its privileged position at the interface between biological pathways and clinical manifestations of healthy/disease conditions [44], are improving our understanding of "normal" physiology and the pathophysiology of many disorders, including frailty and T2DM [15,45,46]. These premises led to the design of the MetaboFrail study [16].

In the present investigation, we applied targeted metabolomics to characterize the circulating amino acid profile of functionally impaired older persons with T2DM. Our major finding was that a specific pattern of amino acids discriminated F-T2DM older people from age- and sex-matched controls. The amino acid signature of F-T2DM participants included higher circulating levels of 3-methyl histidine, alanine, arginine, ethanolamine, glutamic acid, sarcosine, and tryptophan.

The presence of 3-methyl histidine among the most relevant predictors supports the involvement of muscle wasting in frailty [30]. Indeed, 3-methyl histidine derives from the post-translational methylation of histidine moieties of actin and myosin [47,48]. Hence, 3-methyl histidine has been proposed as a biomarker of myofibrillar proteolysis and skeletal muscle loss [49]. Interestingly, 3-methyl histidine is also a marker of increased protein catabolism in T2DM [50].

Alanine and glutamic acid are crucial intermediates of muscle energy metabolism and liver-muscle metabolic interchange under both physiologic and pathologic conditions [51–53]. Perturbations in alanine and glutamate circulating pool may be indicative of skeletal muscle dysfunction, and are commonly encountered in age-related chronic conditions and models of muscle atrophy [54,55]. Notably, both alanine and glutamic acid levels were positively associated with insulin resistance and risk of T2DM in several independent study cohorts [56–58].

Arginine metabolism involves the cooperation of various organs, including kidneys, muscles, gut, and liver [59]. Major pathways in arginine metabolism include muscle protein breakdown and its de novo synthesis from citrulline [59]. Arginine is involved in nitric oxide as well as urea and polyamine synthesis, and research focus has recently been directed towards the determination of the pathophysiological role of arginine and its metabolites in aging and age-related chronic diseases [60]. Noticeably, our findings mirror the higher levels of arginine and lower concentrations of its urea-cycle companion ornithine found in Chinese adults with T2DM [61]. Higher concentrations of another intermediate of urea-cycle, i.e., citrulline, defined the serum amino acid profile of older people with PF&S [17]. Further investigations on arginine/nitrogen interorgan networks are needed to explain the results found in F-T2DM older adults.

Sarcosine, the N-methylated derivative of glycine, is an important intermediate of one-carbon metabolism [62]. Recent studies have investigated the association between sarcosine levels and age-related conditions in humans with conflicting results [63–66]. In a comparative metabolomics analysis, circulating sarcosine was found to be reduced with aging and increased by dietary restriction in both rodents and humans [67]. Conversely, elevated urine sarcosine levels were associated with incident T2DM [68], and higher serum concentrations of sarcosine characterized the metabotype of older adults with PF&S [17]. Collectively, these findings suggest that perturbations in folate/one-carbon metabolism may play a role in frailty and T2DM as well as in other age-related conditions.

Ethanolamine is a crucial intermediate of the CDP-ethanolamine pathway, the main route of phosphatidylethanolamine synthesis, and modulates lipid metabolism and the turnover of biological membranes [69]. Recently, a critical role for skeletal muscle phospholipid metabolism has been described in the regulation of both insulin sensitivity and contractile function [70]. Moreover, the ethanolamine/phosphatidylethanolamine synthesis dyad is directly involved in autophagy regulation, thereby modulating anti-aging properties of this cellular process [71]. Interestingly, perturbations in the CDP-ethanolamine pathway were associated with altered mitochondrial biogenesis in mouse models of muscle atrophy [71], while higher circulating levels of ethanolamine were found in older adults with PF&S [17].

Tryptophan is an essential amino acid that exerts multiple roles in growth, mood, behavior, and immune responses [72]. Tryptophan is metabolized via two major pathways, the tryptophan-kynurenine and the tryptophan-methoxyndole pathways, that lead to the production of NAD, serotonin, and melatonin [72]. Alterations in tryptophan metabolism have been described in the context of frailty and T2DM [73,74]. In particular, tryptophan and its associated metabolites have been associated with insulin resistance and incident T2DM in independent cohorts [74,75]. Moreover, higher circulating levels of tryptophan were associated with low muscle quality in a large cohort of men and women enrolled in the BLSA [32].

Non-frail non-T2DM controls were characterized by higher serum levels of taurine. Taurine is the most abundant free amino acid in several organs, including the skeletal muscle that contains approximately 70% of total body taurine [76]. Taurine has multiple regulatory effects and its role in osmoregulation, modulation of inflammatory response, protection against oxidative stress, and stimulation of cellular quality control processes is widely acknowledged [76,77]. Taurine deficiency is commonly encountered in people with T2DM [78,79], and its supplementation has been proposed as a strategy against T2DM complications, including retinopathy, nephropathy, neuropathy, atherosclerosis, and cardiomyopathy [80]. Recently, taurine supplementation has also been proposed as a possible remedy against sarcopenia [81]. The causes of taurine depletion in F-T2DM older adults are multifaceted and may include decreased dietary intake, reduced intestinal absorption, renal wasting, and inflammation [77].

Unexpectedly, branched-chain amino acids (BCAAs) were not found to be discriminant by the PLS-DA classification model. BCAAs are metabolic rheostats that modulate whole-body and tissular metabolism [20]. Recent evidence suggests that BCAAs may have a Janus-like behavior in F-T2DM older adults. Indeed, while BCAA-induced activation of the mammalian target of rapamycin (mTOR) in skeletal myocytes may contrast sarcopenia and functional decline in advanced age [20,31], other studies found an association between higher circulating levels of BCAAs and insulin resistance or T2DM in older adults [24–27]. The low discriminant power of BCAAs in MetaboFrail might therefore reflect the dual effect of BCAAs in F-T2DM older people.

Although innovative, the present investigation has some limitations that should be mentioned. The study sample was quite small while the dataset comprised numerous variables. To cope with this issue, we adopted a PLS-DA-based strategy which is particularly suited for handling matrices populated by highly correlated variables. The MetaboFrail study enrolled older adults from three European countries; thus, a validation study in other ethnic groups is warranted. Eating habits may affect circulating amino acid levels, but diet was not objectively assessed in our study sample. However, it has recently been reported that differences in blood amino acid concentrations do not necessarily mirror those of amino acid intakes [82]. As commonly occurs in biomarker discovery studies, although a large number of candidates were investigated, we could not evaluate all possible mediators involved in frailty and T2DM.

In conclusion, in the present investigation, we showed the existence of a specific amino acid signature in F-T2DM older persons. Our novel approach enabled us to obtain new insights into the pathophysiology of the two conditions. In particular, a relevant role for perturbations in muscle metabolism and muscle-liver interorgan communication was highlighted. The longitudinal implementation of our analytical strategy could allow validating novel sets of biomarkers and identifying new targets for interventions.

Supplementary Materials: The following are available online at http://www.mdpi.com/2072-6643/12/1/199/s1; Table S1: Serum concentrations of non-discriminant amino acids and derivatives in frail/pre-frail participants with type 2 diabetes mellitus (F-T2DM) and controls.

Author Contributions: Conceptualization, A.P. (Anna Picca), E.M., and R.C.; methodology, A.P. (Aniello Primiano), G.C., and J.G.; software, A.B. and F.M.; validation, A.P. (Anna Picca), E.M., and R.C.; formal analysis, A.B. and F.M.; investigation, A.P. (Anna Picca), E.M., and R.C.; resources, A.J.S., G.G., L.R.-M., and R.B.; data curation, A.P. (Anna Picca) and R.C.; writing—original draft preparation, E.M. and R.C.; writing—review and editing, A.P. (Anna Picca), F.M., I.B.-M., L.P., O.L., R.C., and S.C.R.; supervision, A.J.S., G.G., L.R.-M., and R.B.; funding acquisition, A.J.S., G.G., L.R.-M., and R.B. All authors have read and agreed to the published version of the manuscript.

Funding: This work was supported by grants from the European Commission - EU 7th Framework Programme (Contract N° 278803), and Innovative Medicine Initiative-Joint Undertaking (IMI-JU #115621). The work was also partly supported by the nonprofit research foundation "Centro Studi Achille e Linda Lorenzon". The funders had no role in study design, data collection and analysis, preparation of the manuscript, or decision to publish.

Acknowledgments: The authors thank Luca Mariotti for his precious technical and administrative support.

Conflicts of Interest: A.J.S., E.M., L.R.-M., R.B., and R.C are partners of the SPRINTT Consortium, which is partly funded by the European Federation of Pharmaceutical Industries and Associations (EFPIA). R.C. served as a consultant for Abbott, Novartis, and Nutricia. E.M. served as a consultant for Abbott, Biophytis, Nestlè, Novartis, and Nutricia.

References

1. Sinclair, A.; Dunning, T.; Rodriguez-Mañas, L. Diabetes in older people: New insights and remaining challenges. *Lancet Diabetes Endocrinol.* **2015**, *3*, 275–285. [CrossRef]
2. Cho, N.H.; Shaw, J.E.; Karuranga, S.; Huang, Y.; da Rocha Fernandes, J.D.; Ohlrogge, A.W.; Malanda, B. IDF Diabetes Atlas: Global estimates of diabetes prevalence for 2017 and projections for 2045. *Diabetes Res. Clin. Pract.* **2018**, *138*, 271–281. [CrossRef] [PubMed]
3. GBD 2017 Disease and Injury Incidence and Prevalence Collaborators; James, S.L.; Abate, D.; Abate, K.H.; Abay, S.M.; Abbafati, C.; Abbasi, N.; Abbastabar, H.; Abd-Allah, F.; Abdela, J.; et al. Global, regional, and national incidence, prevalence, and years lived with disability for 354 diseases and injuries for 195 countries and territories, 1990–2017: A systematic analysis for the Global Burden of Disease Study 2017. *Lancet* **2018**, *392*, 1789–1858. [CrossRef]
4. Kalyani, R.R.; Golden, S.H.; Cefalu, W.T. Diabetes and Aging: Unique Considerations and Goals of Care. *Diabetes Care* **2017**, *40*, 440–443. [CrossRef] [PubMed]
5. Cesari, M.; Calvani, R.; Marzetti, E. Frailty in Older Persons. *Clin. Geriatr. Med.* **2017**, *33*, 293–303. [CrossRef] [PubMed]
6. Clegg, A.; Young, J.; Iliffe, S.; Rikkert, M.O.; Rockwood, K. Frailty in elderly people. *Lancet* **2013**, *381*, 752–762. [CrossRef]

7. El Assar, M.; Laosa, O.; Rodríguez Mañas, L. Diabetes and frailty. *Curr. Opin. Clin. Nutr. Metab. Care* **2019**, *22*, 52–57. [CrossRef]
8. LeRoith, D.; Biessels, G.J.; Braithwaite, S.S.; Casanueva, F.F.; Draznin, B.; Halter, J.B.; Hirsch, I.B.; McDonnell, M.E.; Molitch, M.E.; Murad, M.H.; et al. Treatment of Diabetes in Older Adults: An Endocrine Society* Clinical Practice Guideline. *J. Clin. Endocrinol. Metab.* **2019**, *104*, 1520–1574. [CrossRef]
9. Sinclair, A.J.; Rodriguez-Mañas, L. Diabetes and Frailty: Two Converging Conditions? *Can. J. Diabetes* **2016**, *40*, 77–83. [CrossRef]
10. Larsson, L.; Degens, H.; Li, M.; Salviati, L.; Lee, Y., II; Thompson, W.; Kirkland, J.L.; Sandri, M. Sarcopenia: Aging-Related Loss of Muscle Mass and Function. *Physiol. Rev.* **2019**, *99*, 427–511. [CrossRef]
11. Guerrero, N.; Bunout, D.; Hirsch, S.; Barrera, G.; Leiva, L.; Henríquez, S.; De la Maza, M.P. Premature loss of muscle mass and function in type 2 diabetes. *Diabetes Res. Clin. Pract.* **2016**, *117*, 32–38. [CrossRef] [PubMed]
12. Park, S.W.; Goodpaster, B.H.; Strotmeyer, E.S.; Kuller, L.H.; Broudeau, R.; Kammerer, C.; de Rekeneire, N.; Harris, T.B.; Schwartz, A.V.; Tylavsky, F.A.; et al. Accelerated Loss of Skeletal Muscle Strength in Older Adults With Type 2 Diabetes: The Health, Aging, and Body Composition Study. *Diabetes Care* **2007**, *30*, 1507–1512. [CrossRef] [PubMed]
13. Landi, F.; Calvani, R.; Cesari, M.; Tosato, M.; Martone, A.M.; Bernabei, R.; Onder, G.; Marzetti, E. Sarcopenia as the Biological Substrate of Physical Frailty. *Clin. Geriatr. Med.* **2015**, *31*, 367–374. [CrossRef] [PubMed]
14. Calvani, R.; Marini, F.; Cesari, M.; Tosato, M.; Anker, S.D.; von Haehling, S.; Miller, R.R.; Bernabei, R.; Landi, F.; Marzetti, E.; et al. Biomarkers for physical frailty and sarcopenia: State of the science and future developments. *J. Cachexia. Sarcopenia Muscle* **2015**, *6*, 278–286. [CrossRef] [PubMed]
15. Picca, A.; Coelho-Junior, H.J.; Cesari, M.; Marini, F.; Miccheli, A.; Gervasoni, J.; Bossola, M.; Landi, F.; Bernabei, R.; Marzetti, E.; et al. The metabolomics side of frailty: Toward personalized medicine for the aged. *Exp. Gerontol.* **2019**, *126*, 110692. [CrossRef] [PubMed]
16. Calvani, R.; Rodriguez-Mañas, L.; Picca, A.; Marini, F.; Biancolillo, A.; Laosa, O.; Pedraza, L.; Gervasoni, J.; Primiano, A.; Miccheli, A.; et al. The "Metabolic biomarkers of frailty in older people with type 2 diabetes mellitus" (MetaboFrail) study: Rationale, design and methods. *Exp. Gerontol.* **2020**, *129*, 110782. [CrossRef] [PubMed]
17. Calvani, R.; Picca, A.; Marini, F.; Biancolillo, A.; Gervasoni, J.; Persichilli, S.; Primiano, A.; Coelho-Junior, H.; Bossola, M.; Urbani, A.; et al. A Distinct Pattern of Circulating Amino Acids Characterizes Older Persons with Physical Frailty and Sarcopenia: Results from the BIOSPHERE Study. *Nutrients* **2018**, *10*, 1691. [CrossRef]
18. Pasini, E.; Corsetti, G.; Aquilani, R.; Romano, C.; Picca, A.; Calvani, R.; Dioguardi, F.S. Protein-Amino Acid Metabolism Disarrangements: The Hidden Enemy of Chronic Age-Related Conditions. *Nutrients* **2018**, *10*, 391. [CrossRef]
19. Lu, Y.; Karagounis, L.G.; Ng, T.P.; Carre, C.; Narang, V.; Wong, G.; Tan, C.T.Y.; Zin Nyunt, M.S.; Gao, Q.; Abel, B.; et al. Systemic and Metabolic Signature of Sarcopenia in Community-Dwelling Older Adults. *J. Gerontol. Ser. A* **2019**. [CrossRef]
20. Neinast, M.; Murashige, D.; Arany, Z. Branched Chain Amino Acids. *Annu. Rev. Physiol.* **2019**, *81*, 139–164. [CrossRef]
21. Zhenyukh, O.; Civantos, E.; Ruiz-Ortega, M.; Sánchez, M.S.; Vázquez, C.; Peiró, C.; Egido, J.; Mas, S. High concentration of branched-chain amino acids promotes oxidative stress, inflammation and migration of human peripheral blood mononuclear cells via mTORC1 activation. *Free Radic. Biol. Med.* **2017**, *104*, 165–177. [CrossRef] [PubMed]
22. Yoon, M.-S. The Emerging Role of Branched-Chain Amino Acids in Insulin Resistance and Metabolism. *Nutrients* **2016**, *8*, 405. [CrossRef] [PubMed]
23. Yang, Q.; Vijayakumar, A.; Kahn, B.B. Metabolites as regulators of insulin sensitivity and metabolism. *Nat. Rev. Mol. Cell Biol.* **2018**, *19*, 654–672. [CrossRef] [PubMed]
24. Wang, T.J.; Larson, M.G.; Vasan, R.S.; Cheng, S.; Rhee, E.P.; McCabe, E.; Lewis, G.D.; Fox, C.S.; Jacques, P.F.; Fernandez, C.; et al. Metabolite profiles and the risk of developing diabetes. *Nat. Med.* **2011**, *17*, 448–453. [CrossRef] [PubMed]
25. Wang-Sattler, R.; Yu, Z.; Herder, C.; Messias, A.C.; Floegel, A.; He, Y.; Heim, K.; Campillos, M.; Holzapfel, C.; Thorand, B.; et al. Novel biomarkers for pre-diabetes identified by metabolomics. *Mol. Syst. Biol.* **2012**, *8*, 615. [CrossRef] [PubMed]

26. Floegel, A.; Stefan, N.; Yu, Z.; Mühlenbruch, K.; Drogan, D.; Joost, H.-G.; Fritsche, A.; Häring, H.-U.; Hrabě de Angelis, M.; Peters, A.; et al. Identification of serum metabolites associated with risk of type 2 diabetes using a targeted metabolomic approach. *Diabetes* **2013**, *62*, 639–648. [CrossRef]
27. Chen, T.; Ni, Y.; Ma, X.; Bao, Y.; Liu, J.; Huang, F.; Hu, C.; Xie, G.; Zhao, A.; Jia, W.; et al. Branched-chain and aromatic amino acid profiles and diabetes risk in Chinese populations. *Sci. Rep.* **2016**, *6*, 20594. [CrossRef]
28. Semba, R.D.; Gonzalez-Freire, M.; Moaddel, R.; Sun, K.; Fabbri, E.; Zhang, P.; Carlson, O.D.; Khadeer, M.; Chia, C.W.; Salem, N.; et al. Altered Plasma Amino Acids and Lipids Associated With Abnormal Glucose Metabolism and Insulin Resistance in Older Adults. *J. Clin. Endocrinol. Metab.* **2018**, *103*, 3331–3339. [CrossRef]
29. Adachi, Y.; Ono, N.; Imaizumi, A.; Muramatsu, T.; Andou, T.; Shimodaira, Y.; Nagao, K.; Kageyama, Y.; Mori, M.; Noguchi, Y.; et al. Plasma Amino Acid Profile in Severely Frail Elderly Patients in Japan. *Int. J. Gerontol.* **2018**, *12*, 290–293. [CrossRef]
30. Kochlik, B.; Stuetz, W.; Pérès, K.; Féart, C.; Tegner, J.; Rodriguez-Mañas, L.; Grune, T.; Weber, D. Associations of Plasma 3-Methylhistidine with Frailty Status in French Cohorts of the FRAILOMIC Initiative. *J. Clin. Med.* **2019**, *8*, 1010. [CrossRef]
31. Lustgarten, M.S.; Price, L.L.; Chale, A.; Phillips, E.M.; Fielding, R.A. Branched chain amino acids are associated with muscle mass in functionally limited older adults. *J. Gerontol. A Biol. Sci. Med. Sci.* **2014**, *69*, 717–724. [CrossRef] [PubMed]
32. Moaddel, R.; Fabbri, E.; Khadeer, M.A.; Carlson, O.D.; Gonzalez-Freire, M.; Zhang, P.; Semba, R.D.; Ferrucci, L. Plasma Biomarkers of Poor Muscle Quality in Older Men and Women from the Baltimore Longitudinal Study of Aging. *J. Gerontol. A Biol. Sci. Med. Sci.* **2016**, *71*, 1266–1272. [CrossRef] [PubMed]
33. Rodríguez-Mañas, L.; Bayer, A.J.; Kelly, M.; Zeyfang, A.; Izquierdo, M.; Laosa, O.; Hardman, T.C.; Sinclair, A.J.; Moreira, S.; Cook, J.; et al. An evaluation of the effectiveness of a multi-modal intervention in frail and pre-frail older people with type 2 diabetes—the MID-Frail study: Study protocol for a randomised controlled trial. *Trials* **2014**, *15*, 34. [CrossRef] [PubMed]
34. Rodriguez-Mañas, L.; Laosa, O.; Vellas, B.; Paolisso, G.; Topinkova, E.; Oliva-Moreno, J.; Bourdel-Marchasson, I.; Izquierdo, M.; Hood, K.; Zeyfang, A.; et al. Effectiveness of a multimodal intervention in functionally impaired older people with type 2 diabetes mellitus. *J. Cachexia. Sarcopenia Muscle* **2019**. [CrossRef]
35. Fried, L.P.; Tangen, C.M.; Walston, J.; Newman, A.B.; Hirsch, C.; Gottdiener, J.; Seeman, T.; Tracy, R.; Kop, W.J.; Burke, G.; et al. Frailty in older adults: Evidence for a phenotype. *J. Gerontol. A Biol. Sci. Med. Sci.* **2001**, *56*, M146–M156. [CrossRef] [PubMed]
36. Folstein, M.F.; Folstein, S.E.; McHugh, P.R. "Mini-mental state". A practical method for grading the cognitive state of patients for the clinician. *J. Psychiatr. Res.* **1975**, *12*, 189–198. [CrossRef]
37. Mahoney, F.I.; Barthel, D.W. Functional Evaluation: The barthel index. *Md. State Med. J.* **1965**, *14*, 61–65.
38. Ståhle, L.; Wold, S. Partial least squares analysis with cross-validation for the two-class problem: A Monte Carlo study. *J. Chemom.* **1987**, *1*, 185–196. [CrossRef]
39. Westerhuis, J.A.; Hoefsloot, H.C.J.; Smit, S.; Vis, D.J.; Smilde, A.K.; van Velzen, E.J.J.; van Duijnhoven, J.P.M.; van Dorsten, F.A. Assessment of PLSDA cross validation. *Metabolomics* **2008**, *4*, 81–89. [CrossRef]
40. Smit, S.; van Breemen, M.J.; Hoefsloot, H.C.J.; Smilde, A.K.; Aerts, J.M.F.G.; de Koster, C.G. Assessing the statistical validity of proteomics based biomarkers. *Anal. Chim. Acta* **2007**, *592*, 210–217. [CrossRef]
41. Marzetti, E.; Landi, F.; Marini, F.; Cesari, M.; Buford, T.W.; Manini, T.M.; Onder, G.; Pahor, M.; Bernabei, R.; Leeuwenburgh, C.; et al. Patterns of Circulating Inflammatory Biomarkers in Older Persons with Varying Levels of Physical Performance: A Partial Least Squares-Discriminant Analysis Approach. *Front. Med.* **2014**, *1*, 27. [CrossRef] [PubMed]
42. Chen, R.; Snyder, M. Promise of Personalized Omics to Precision Medicine. *Wiley Interdiscip. Rev. Syst. Biol. Med.* **2013**, *5*, 73. [CrossRef] [PubMed]
43. Loscalzo, J.; Barabasi, A.-L. Systems biology and the future of medicine. *Wiley Interdiscip. Rev. Syst. Biol. Med.* **2011**, *3*, 619–627. [CrossRef] [PubMed]
44. Guijas, C.; Montenegro-Burke, J.R.; Warth, B.; Spilker, M.E.; Siuzdak, G. Metabolomics activity screening for identifying metabolites that modulate phenotype. *Nat. Biotechnol.* **2018**, *36*, 316–320. [CrossRef] [PubMed]
45. Karczewski, K.J.; Snyder, M.P. Integrative omics for health and disease. *Nat. Rev. Genet.* **2018**, *19*, 299–310. [CrossRef] [PubMed]

46. Wishart, D.S. Metabolomics for Investigating Physiological and Pathophysiological Processes. *Physiol. Rev.* **2019**, *99*, 1819–1875. [CrossRef] [PubMed]
47. Johnson, P.; Perry, S.V. Biological activity and the 3-methylhistidine content of actin and myosin. *Biochem. J.* **1970**, *119*, 293–298. [CrossRef]
48. Asatoor, A.M.; Armstrong, M.D. 3-methylhistidine, a component of actin. *Biochem. Biophys. Res. Commun.* **1967**, *26*, 168–174. [CrossRef]
49. Sheffield-Moore, M.; Dillon, E.L.; Randolph, K.M.; Casperson, S.L.; White, G.R.; Jennings, K.; Rathmacher, J.; Schuette, S.; Janghorbani, M.; Urban, R.J.; et al. Isotopic decay of urinary or plasma 3-methylhistidine as a potential biomarker of pathologic skeletal muscle loss. *J. Cachexia. Sarcopenia Muscle* **2014**, *5*, 19–25. [CrossRef]
50. Marchesini, G.; Forlani, G.; Zoli, M.; Vannini, P.; Pisi, E. Muscle protein breakdown in uncontrolled diabetes as assessed by urinary 3-methylhistidine excretion. *Diabetologia* **1982**, *23*, 456–458. [CrossRef]
51. Wagenmakers, A.J. Protein and amino acid metabolism in human muscle. *Adv. Exp. Med. Biol.* **1998**, *441*, 307–319. [PubMed]
52. Jang, C.; Hui, S.; Zeng, X.; Cowan, A.J.; Wang, L.; Chen, L.; Morscher, R.J.; Reyes, J.; Frezza, C.; Hwang, H.Y.; et al. Metabolite Exchange between Mammalian Organs Quantified in Pigs. *Cell Metab.* **2019**, *30*, 594–606.e3. [CrossRef] [PubMed]
53. Gancheva, S.; Jelenik, T.; Álvarez-Hernández, E.; Roden, M. Interorgan Metabolic Crosstalk in Human Insulin Resistance. *Physiol. Rev.* **2018**, *98*, 1371–1415. [CrossRef] [PubMed]
54. Jagoe, R.T.; Engelen, M.P.K.J. Muscle wasting and changes in muscle protein metabolism in chronic obstructive pulmonary disease. *Eur. Respir. J.* **2003**, *22*, 52s–63s. [CrossRef] [PubMed]
55. Ilaiwy, A.; Quintana, M.T.; Bain, J.R.; Muehlbauer, M.J.; Brown, D.I.; Stansfield, W.E.; Willis, M.S. Cessation of biomechanical stretch model of C2C12 cells models myocyte atrophy and anaplerotic changes in metabolism using non-targeted metabolomics analysis. *Int. J. Biochem. Cell Biol.* **2016**, *79*, 80–92. [CrossRef]
56. Lu, Y.; Wang, Y.; Liang, X.; Zou, L.; Ong, C.N.; Yuan, J.M.; Koh, W.P.; Pan, A. Serum amino acids in association with prevalent and incident type 2 diabetes in a Chinese population. *Metabolites* **2019**, *9*, 14. [CrossRef]
57. Seibert, R.; Abbasi, F.; Hantash, F.M.; Caulfield, M.P.; Reaven, G.; Kim, S.H. Relationship between insulin resistance and amino acids in women and men. *Physiol. Rep.* **2015**, *3*, e12392. [CrossRef]
58. Cheng, S.; Rhee, E.P.; Larson, M.G.; Lewis, G.D.; McCabe, E.L.; Shen, D.; Palma, M.J.; Roberts, L.D.; Dejam, A.; Souza, A.L.; et al. Metabolite profiling identifies pathways associated with metabolic risk in humans. *Circulation* **2012**, *125*, 2222–2231. [CrossRef]
59. Wu, G.; Morris, S.M. Arginine metabolism: Nitric oxide and beyond. *Biochem. J.* **1998**, *336*, 1–17. [CrossRef]
60. Mangoni, A.A.; Rodionov, R.N.; Mcevoy, M.; Zinellu, A.; Carru, C.; Sotgia, S. New horizons in arginine metabolism, ageing and chronic disease states. *Age Ageing* **2019**, *48*, 776–782. [CrossRef]
61. Cao, Y.-F.; Li, J.; Zhang, Z.; Liu, J.; Sun, X.-Y.; Feng, X.-F.; Luo, H.-H.; Yang, W.; Li, S.-N.; Yang, X.; et al. Plasma Levels of Amino Acids Related to Urea Cycle and Risk of Type 2 Diabetes Mellitus in Chinese Adults. *Front. Endocrinol.* **2019**, *10*, 50. [CrossRef] [PubMed]
62. Ducker, G.S.; Rabinowitz, J.D. One-Carbon Metabolism in Health and Disease. *Cell Metab.* **2017**, *25*, 27–42. [CrossRef] [PubMed]
63. Koutros, S.; Meyer, T.E.; Fox, S.D.; Issaq, H.J.; Veenstra, T.D.; Huang, W.Y.; Yu, K.; Albanes, D.; Chu, L.W.; Andriole, G.; et al. Prospective evaluation of serum sarcosine and risk of prostate cancer in the prostate, lung, colorectal and ovarian cancer screening trial. *Carcinogenesis* **2013**, *34*, 2281–2285. [CrossRef] [PubMed]
64. De Vogel, S.; Ulvik, A.; Meyer, K.; Ueland, P.M.; Nygård, O.; Vollset, S.E.; Tell, G.S.; Gregory, J.F.; Tretli, S.; Bjørge, T. Sarcosine and other metabolites along the choline oxidation pathway in relation to prostate cancer—A large nested case-control study within the JANUS cohort in Norway. *Int. J. Cancer* **2014**, *134*, 197–206. [CrossRef] [PubMed]
65. Hasokawa, M.; Shinohara, M.; Tsugawa, H.; Bamba, T.; Fukusaki, E.; Nishiumi, S.; Nishimura, K.; Yoshida, M.; Ishida, T.; Hirata, K.; et al. Identification of biomarkers of stent restenosis with serum metabolomic profiling using gas chromatography/mass spectrometry. *Circ. J.* **2012**, *76*, 1864–1873. [CrossRef]
66. Tsai, C.H.; Huang, H.C.; Liu, B.L.; Li, C.I.; Lu, M.K.; Chen, X.; Tsai, M.C.; Yang, Y.W.; Lane, H.Y. Activation of N-methyl-D-aspartate receptor glycine site temporally ameliorates neuropsychiatric symptoms of Parkinson's disease with dementia. *Psychiatry Clin. Neurosci.* **2014**, *68*, 692–700. [CrossRef]

67. Walters, R.O.; Arias, E.; Diaz, A.; Burgos, E.S.; Guan, F.; Tiano, S.; Mao, K.; Green, C.L.; Qiu, Y.; Shah, H.; et al. Sarcosine Is Uniquely Modulated by Aging and Dietary Restriction in Rodents and Humans. *Cell Rep.* **2018**, *25*, 663–676. [CrossRef]
68. Svingen, G.F.T.; Schartum-Hansen, H.; Pedersen, E.R.; Ueland, P.M.; Tell, G.S.; Mellgren, G.; Njølstad, P.R.; Seifert, R.; Strand, E.; Karlsson, T.; et al. Prospective associations of systemic and urinary choline metabolites with incident type 2 diabetes. *Clin. Chem.* **2016**, *62*, 755–765. [CrossRef]
69. van der Veen, J.N.; Kennelly, J.P.; Wan, S.; Vance, J.E.; Vance, D.E.; Jacobs, R.L. The critical role of phosphatidylcholine and phosphatidylethanolamine metabolism in health and disease. *Biochim. Biophys. Acta Biomembr.* **2017**, *1859*, 1558–1572. [CrossRef]
70. Funai, K.; Lodhi, I.J.; Spears, L.D.; Yin, L.; Song, H.; Klein, S.; Semenkovich, C.F. Skeletal muscle phospholipid metabolism regulates insulin sensitivity and contractile function. *Diabetes* **2016**, *65*, 358–370. [CrossRef]
71. Rockenfeller, P.; Koska, M.; Pietrocola, F.; Minois, N.; Knittelfelder, O.; Sica, V.; Franz, J.; Carmona-Gutierrez, D.; Kroemer, G.; Madeo, F. Phosphatidylethanolamine positively regulates autophagy and longevity. *Cell Death Differ.* **2015**, *22*, 499–508. [CrossRef] [PubMed]
72. Le Floc'h, N.; Otten, W.; Merlot, E. Tryptophan metabolism, from nutrition to potential therapeutic applications. *Amino Acids* **2011**, *41*, 1195–1205. [CrossRef] [PubMed]
73. Marcos-Pérez, D.; Sánchez-Flores, M.; Maseda, A.; Lorenzo-López, L.; Millán-Calenti, J.C.; Strasser, B.; Gostner, J.M.; Fuchs, D.; Pásaro, E.; Valdiglesias, V.; et al. Frailty Status in Older Adults Is Related to Alterations in Indoleamine 2,3-Dioxygenase 1 and Guanosine Triphosphate Cyclohydrolase I Enzymatic Pathways. *J. Am. Med. Dir. Assoc.* **2017**, *18*, 1049–1057. [CrossRef] [PubMed]
74. Chen, T.; Zheng, X.; Ma, X.; Bao, Y.; Ni, Y.; Hu, C.; Rajani, C.; Huang, F.; Zhao, A.; Jiia, W.; et al. Tryptophan Predicts the Risk for Future Type 2 Diabetes. *PLoS ONE* **2016**, *11*, e0162192. [CrossRef] [PubMed]
75. Yu, E.; Papandreou, C.; Ruiz-Canela, M.; Guasch-Ferre, M.; Clish, C.B.; Dennis, C.; Liang, L.; Corella, D.; Fitó, M.; Razquin, C.; et al. Association of tryptophan metabolites with incident type 2 diabetes in the PREDIMED trial: A case–cohort study. *Clin. Chem.* **2018**, *64*, 1211–1220. [CrossRef]
76. Huxtable, R.J. Physiological actions of taurine. *Physiol. Rev.* **1992**, *72*, 101–163. [CrossRef]
77. Lambert, I.H.; Kristensen, D.M.; Holm, J.B.; Mortensen, O.H. Physiological role of taurine—From organism to organelle. *Acta Physiol.* **2015**, *213*, 191–212. [CrossRef]
78. De Luca, G.; Calpona, P.R.; Caponetti, A.; Romano, G.; Di Benedetto, A.; Cucinotta, D.; Di Giorgio, R.M. Taurine and osmoregulation: Platelet taurine content, uptake, and release in type 2 diabetic patients. *Metabolism* **2001**, *50*, 60–64. [CrossRef]
79. Franconi, F.A.; Bennardini, F.R.; Giuseppe, A.; Miceli, S.M.; Ciuti, M.; Mian, M. Plasma and platelet taurine are reduced in subjects with mellitus: Effects of taurine. *Am. J. Clin. Nutr.* **1995**, *61*, 1115–1119. [CrossRef]
80. Ito, T.; Schaffer, S.W.; Azuma, J. The potential usefulness of taurine on diabetes mellitus and its complications. *Amino Acids* **2012**, *42*, 1529–1539. [CrossRef]
81. Scicchitano, B.M.; Sica, G. The Beneficial Effects of Taurine to Counteract Sarcopenia. *Curr. Protein Pept. Sci.* **2018**, *19*, 673–680. [CrossRef] [PubMed]
82. Schmidt, J.A.; Rinaldi, S.; Scalbert, A.; Ferrari, P.; Achaintre, D.; Gunter, M.J.; Appleby, P.N.; Key, T.J.; Travis, R.C. Plasma concentrations and intakes of amino acids in male meat-eaters, fish-eaters, vegetarians and vegans: A cross-sectional analysis in the EPIC-Oxford cohort. *Eur. J. Clin. Nutr.* **2016**, *70*, 306–312. [CrossRef] [PubMed]

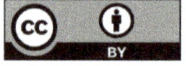

© 2020 by the authors. Licensee MDPI, Basel, Switzerland. This article is an open access article distributed under the terms and conditions of the Creative Commons Attribution (CC BY) license (http://creativecommons.org/licenses/by/4.0/).

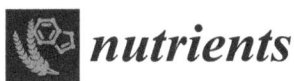

Article

Gut Microbial, Inflammatory and Metabolic Signatures in Older People with Physical Frailty and Sarcopenia: Results from the BIOSPHERE Study

Anna Picca [1,2], Francesca Romana Ponziani [2], Riccardo Calvani [1,2,*], Federico Marini [3], Alessandra Biancolillo [3,4], Hélio José Coelho-Júnior [5], Jacopo Gervasoni [1,2], Aniello Primiano [1,2], Lorenza Putignani [6], Federica Del Chierico [7], Sofia Reddel [7], Antonio Gasbarrini [1,2], Francesco Landi [1,2], Roberto Bernabei [1,2,*] and Emanuele Marzetti [1,2]

[1] Institute of Internal Medicine and Geriatrics, Università Cattolica del Sacro Cuore, 00168 Rome, Italy; anna.picca1@gmail.com (A.P.); jacopo.gervasoni@policlinicogemelli.it (J.G.); aniello.primiano@unicatt.it (A.P.); antonio.gasbarrini@unicatt.it (A.G.); francesco.landi@unicatt.it (F.L.); emanuele.marzetti@policlinicogemelli.it (E.M.)
[2] Fondazione Policlinico Universitario "Agostino Gemelli" IRCCS, 00168 Rome, Italy; francesca.ponziani@gmail.com
[3] Department of Chemistry, Sapienza Università di Roma, 00185 Rome, Italy; federico.marini@uniroma1.it (F.M.); alessandra.biancolillo@univaq.it (A.B.)
[4] Department of Physical and Chemical Sciences, University of L'Aquila, 67100 Coppito, Italy
[5] Applied Kinesiology Laboratory–LCA, School of Physical Education, University of Campinas, 13.083-851 Campinas-SP, Brazil; coelhojunior@hotmail.com.br
[6] Unit of Parasitology and Unit of Human Microbiome, Bambino Gesù Children's Hospital IRCCS, 00168 Rome, Italy; lorenza.putignani@opbg.net
[7] Unit of Human Microbiome, Bambino Gesù Children's Hospital IRCCS, 00168 Rome, Italy; federica.delchierico@opbg.net (F.D.C.); sofia.reddel@opbg.net (S.R.)
* Correspondence: riccardo.calvani@gmail.com (R.C.); roberto.bernabei@unicatt.it (R.B.); Tel.: +39-(06)-3015-5559 (R.C.); +39-(06)-3015-4859 (R.B.); Fax: +39-(06)-3051-911 (R.C. & R.B.)

Received: 30 November 2019; Accepted: 23 December 2019; Published: 26 December 2019

Abstract: Physical frailty and sarcopenia (PF&S) share multisystem derangements, including variations in circulating amino acids and chronic low-grade inflammation. Gut microbiota balances inflammatory responses in several conditions and according to nutritional status. Therefore, an altered gut-muscle crosstalk has been hypothesized in PF&S. We analyzed the gut microbial taxa, systemic inflammation, and metabolic characteristics of older adults with and without PF&S. An innovative multi-marker analytical approach was applied to explore the classification performance of potential biomarkers for PF&S. Thirty-five community dwellers aged 70+, 18 with PF&S, and 17 nonPF&S controls were enrolled. Sequential and Orthogonalized Covariance Selection (SO-CovSel), a multi-platform regression method developed to handle highly correlated variables, was applied. The SO-CovSel model with the best prediction ability using the smallest number of variables was built using seven mediators. The model correctly classified 91.7% participants with PF&S and 87.5% nonPF&S controls. Compared with the latter group, PF&S participants showed higher serum concentrations of aspartic acid, lower circulating levels of concentrations of threonine and macrophage inflammatory protein 1α, increased abundance of *Oscillospira* and *Ruminococcus* microbial taxa, and decreased abundance of Barnesiellaceae and Christensenellaceae. Future investigations are warranted to determine whether these biomediators are involved in PF&S pathophysiology and may, therefore, provide new targets for interventions.

Keywords: aging; muscle; amino acids; metabolism; systemic inflammation; profiling; biomarkers; multi-marker; physical performance; gut microbiota

1. Introduction

Sarcopenia, the progressive age-related decline in muscle mass and strength/function, is a major determinant of negative health-related outcomes, including disability, loss of independence, institutionalization, and mortality [1,2].

When focusing on the physical domain, sarcopenia shows remarkable clinical overlap with frailty, a geriatric "multidimensional syndrome characterized by decreased reserve and diminished resistance to stressors", often envisioned as a pre-disability condition [3]. As such, sarcopenia can be considered to be the biological substratum for the development of physical frailty (PF) and the pathophysiologic foundation of adverse PF-related health outcomes [4,5].

Due to the described commonalities, the two conditions have recently been merged into a new entity (i.e., PF & sarcopenia—PF&S) [6] that was operationalized in the context of the "Sarcopenia and Physical fRailty IN older people: multi-componenT Treatment strategies" (SPRINTT) project [7,8].

Multisystem derangements contribute to muscle loss and may ultimately lead to the development of PF&S [9]. Anabolic resistance, chronic low-grade inflammation, and oxidative stress are advocated among the factors contributing to PF&S [10,11]. These mechanisms are enhanced in the setting of physical inactivity and poor nutrition [12,13]. In this scenario, multi-component interventions encompassing physical activity and adapted nutrition are pillars for the prevention of adverse outcomes associated with PF&S [14].

As recently shown by our group, older adults with PF&S are commonly overweight or obese [15], a feature that has been incorporated in the concept of sarcopenic obesity [16]. Compelling evidence indicates that excessive adiposity contributes to physical frailty and functional limitations in advanced age [17,18]. Adipose tissue is metabolically active and promotes systemic inflammation and oxidative stress [19]. In addition, obesity exacerbates fat infiltration within muscles (i.e., myosteatosis), which, in turn, contributes to muscle dysfunction and physical frailty [20,21].

Gut microbiota is a major player in balancing pro- and anti-inflammatory responses in various disease conditions and in relation to nutritional status [22]. Indeed, the existence of a gut-muscle axis has been hypothesized in the context of PF&S [23]. However, the mechanisms whereby changes in gut microbes–host interactions may influence AA availability, systemic inflammation, and muscle homeostasis in PF&S are yet unexplored.

To address this research question, we used data from the "BIOmarkers associated with Sarcopenia and Physical frailty in EldeRly pErsons" (BIOSPHERE) and the Gut-Liver (GuLiver) Axis studies. BIOSPHERE was designed to determine and validate a panel of PF&S biomarkers pertaining to several pathophysiologic domains (i.e., inflammation, oxidative stress, muscle remodeling, neuromuscular junction dysfunction, and AA metabolism) through multivariate statistical modeling [10,11,24]. The GuLiver Axis study was designed to analyze the relationship among gut microbiota, inflammation, and nutritional and metabolic status in people with and without liver disease [25,26].

The availability of these well-characterized cohorts of older adults enabled us to explore the association among gut microbial profiles, systemic inflammation, and metabolic characteristics in PF&S.

2. Materials and Methods

2.1. Participants

Participants were recruited among enrollees of BIOSPHERE and GuLiver Axis studies. Both studies were approved by the Ethics Committee of the Università Cattolica del Sacro Cuore (Rome, Italy; protocol number BIOSPHERE: 8498/15; protocol number GuLiver Axis: 741). Study procedures and criteria for participant selection have been previously described [24,25].

In both studies, community-dwellers aged 70+ were recruited after signing written informed consent. The presence of PF&S was established according to the operational definition elaborated in the SPRINTT project [7,27]: (a) physical frailty, based on a summary score on the Short Physical Performance Battery (SPPB) [28] between 3 and 9; (b) low appendicular muscle mass (aLM), according to the cutpoints of the Foundation for the National Institutes of Health (FNIH) sarcopenia project [29]; and (c) absence of mobility disability (i.e., ability to complete the 400-m walk test) [30]. The present investigation involved 35 participants, 18 with PF&S, and 17 nonsarcopenic nonfrail (nonPF&S) controls. Gut microbial profiles, circulating inflammatory mediators, and serum AAs and derivatives were assessed.

2.2. Measurement of Appendicular Lean Mass by Dual X-ray Absorptiometry (DXA)

aLM was quantified through whole-body DXA scans on a Hologic Discovery A densitometer (Hologic, Inc., Bedford, MA, USA) according to the manufacturer's procedures. Criteria for low aLM were as follows: (a) aLM to body mass index (BMI) ratio (aLM$_{BMI}$) <0.789 and <0.512 in men and women; or (b) crude aLM <19.75 kg in men and <15.02 kg in women when the aLM/BMI criterion was not met [29].

2.3. Blood Sample and Stool Collection

Blood samples were collected in the morning by venipuncture of the median cubital vein after overnight fasting, using commercial collection tubes (BD Vacutainer®; Becton, Dickinson and Co., Franklin Lakes, NJ, USA). Serum separation was obtained after 30 min of clotting at room temperature and subsequent centrifugation at 1000× g for 15 min at 4 °C. The upper clear fraction (serum) was collected in 0.5 mL aliquots and stored at −80 °C until analysis.

Participants were carefully instructed on the procedures for fecal sample collection. Stool samples were collected at home in a commercial sterile, dry screw-top container. Upon collection, stool samples were delivered to the Human Microbiome Unit at the Bambino Gesù Children's Hospital (Rome, Italy) and immediately frozen at −80 °C until further processing.

2.4. Measurement of Circulating Inflammatory Mediators

A multi-marker immunoassay was used to measure circulating levels of a panel of inflammatory markers [11,25,26,31]. Briefly, a set of 27 pro- and anti-inflammatory mediators, including cytokines, chemokines, and growth factors, were assayed in duplicate in serum samples using the Bio-Plex Pro Human Cytokine 27-plex Assay kit (#M500KCAF0Y, Bio-Rad, Hercules, CA, USA) on a Bio-Plex® System with Luminex xMap Technology (Bio-Rad) (Table 1). Data acquisition was performed with the Bio-Plex Manager Software 6.1 (Bio-Rad) using instrument default settings. Optimization of standard curves across all of the assayed analytes was carried out to remove outliers. Results were obtained as concentrations (pg/mL).

Table 1. List of serum inflammatory biomarkers assayed by multiplex immunoassay.

Cytokines	IFNγ, IL1β, IL1Ra, IL2, IL4, IL5, IL6, IL7, IL8, IL9, IL10, IL12, IL13, IL15, IL17, TNF-α
Chemokines	CCL5, CCL11, IP-10, MCP-1, MIP-1α, MIP-1β
Growth factors	FGF-β, G-CSF, GM-CSF, PDGF-BB

Abbreviations: CCL, C-C motif chemokine ligand; FGF, fibroblast growth factor; G-CSF, granulocyte colony-stimulating factor; GM-CSF, granulocyte macrophage colony-stimulating factor; IFN, interferon; IL, interleukin; IL1Ra, interleukin 1 receptor agonist; IP: interferon-induced protein; MCP-1: monocyte chemoattractant protein 1; MIP: macrophage inflammatory protein; PDGFBB, platelet derived growth factor BB; TNF, tumor necrosis factor.

2.5. Determination of Circulating Amino Acids

Serum concentrations of 37 AAs and derivatives were determined by ultraperformance liquid chromatography/mass spectrometry (UPLC/MS), as described previously [10]. Briefly, 50 µL of sample was added to 100 µL 10% (w/v) sulfosalicylic acid containing an internal standard mix (50 µM) (Cambridge Isotope Laboratories, Inc., Tewksbury, MA, USA) and subsequently centrifuged at 1000× g for 15 min. The supernatant was collected, and 10 µL was mixed with 70 µL of borate buffer and

20 µL of AccQ Tag reagents (Waters Corporation, Milford, MA, USA). The mixture was subsequently heated at 55 °C for 10 min. Samples were eventually loaded onto a CORTECS UPLC C18 column 1.6 µm 2.1 × 150 mm (Waters Corporation) for chromatographic separation (ACQUITY H-Class, Waters Corporation) and eluted at a flow rate of 500 µL/min with a linear gradient (9 min) from 99:1 to 1:99 water 0.1% formic acid/acetonitrile 0.1% formic acid. Analyte detection was performed on an ACQUITY QDa single quadrupole mass spectrometer equipped with electrospray source operating in positive mode (Waters Corporation). AA controls (level 1 and level 2) manufactured by the MCA laboratory of the Queen Beatrix Hospital (Winterswijk, The Netherlands) were used to monitor the analytic process.

2.6. Gut Microbiota DNA Extraction, 16S rRNA Amplification, and Sequencing

Total genome DNA was extracted from fecal samples using the QIAmp Fast DNA Stool mini kit (Qiagen, Germany), according to the manufacturer's instructions.

The V3-V4 region of the 16S rRNA gene (~460 bp) was amplified using the primer pairs 16S_F (5′-TCG TCG GCA GCG TCA GAT GTG TAT AAG AGA CAG CCT ACG GGN GGC WGC AG-3′) and 16S_R (5′-GTC TCG TGG GCT CGG AGA TGT GTA TAA GAG ACA GGA CTA CHV GGG TAT CTA ATC C–3′), reported in the MiSeq rRNA Amplicon Sequencing protocol (Illumina, San Diego, CA, USA). Amplification reactions were set up using a 2× KAPA HiFi HotStart Ready Mix (KAPA Biosystems Inc., Wilmington, MA, USA). AMPure XP beads (Beckman Coulter Inc., Beverly, MA, USA) were employed to clean-up the DNA amplicons. To obtain a unique combination of bar-code sequences, a second amplification step was performed using the Illumina Nextera forward and reverse adaptor-primers (Illumina, San Diego, CA, USA). The final library was quantified after a clean-up step using a Quant-iT™ PicoGreen® dsDNA Assay Kit (Thermo Fisher Scientific, Waltham, MA, USA) and diluted in an equimolar concentration (4 nM).

Samples were sequenced using an Illumina MiSeqTM platform, following the manufacturer's specifications, generating 300 base-length paired-end reads. Bacterial 16S rRNA amplicon data were analyzed using a combination of the QIIME 1.9.1 software pipeline and the VSEARCH v1.1 pipeline. Fastq-join was used to merge paired-end raw sequences, followed by a split library step (QIIME). After dereplication and chimera checking (VSEARCH), reads were then clustered into operational taxonomic units (OTUs) at 97% identity. Taxonomy of each of 16S rRNA gene sequence was assigned using the UCLUST against the Greengenes 13.8 database (97% sequence similarity).

2.7. Statistical Analysis

Analyses were performed using the freely available software environment for statistical computing and graphics R statistics program (version 3.4.0). Sequential and Orthogonalized Covariance Selection (SO-CovSel) statistics were run under Matlab R2015b environment by means of in-house written functions (freely available at www.chem.uniroma1.it/romechemometrics/research/algorithms/).

Descriptive statistics were run on all data. Differences in demographic, anthropometric, clinical, functional characteristics, and inflammatory and metabolic markers between PF&S and nonPF&S participants were assessed via t-test statistics and χ^2 or Fisher exact tests, for continuous and categorical variables, respectively. All tests were two-sided, with statistical significance set at $p < 0.05$.

To compare the gut microbiota alpha diversity between PF&S and nonPF&S participants, Chao1 index was calculated on raw data and differences were assessed by Wilcoxon test.

Data were then preprocessed removing OTUs not seen more than three times in at least 20% of the samples and were normalized using a regularized logarithm transformation (rlog). Differential abundance analysis between PF&S and nonPF&S groups at the phylum, family, and genus levels was carried out using a negative binomial distribution on data normalized by "size factors", taking into account sequencing depth between samples. Differences in bacterial abundance were reported as $\log_2$ fold change ($\log_2 FC$). Only comparisons with a $\log_2 FC >$ or $< \pm 1.5$ and an adjusted (Benjamini–Hochberg method) p value < 0.05 were considered significant.

After import into MatLab, serum concentrations of inflammatory and metabolic markers and the abundance of gut microbial OTUs were organized into three matrices (Table 2), to be further processed through a multi-block approach. Given its ability to provide accurate predictions and, at the same time, to identify a parsimonious number of relevant variables (putative markers), the analysis was carried out through the recently developed SO-CovSel algorithm [32].

Table 2. Composition of the multi-block dataset used for Sequential and Orthogonalized Covariance Selection (SO-CovSel) analysis.

Data Block	Biological Pathway	Variables
Matrix 1	Inflammation	CCL5, CCL11, IFN-γ, FGF-β, G-CSF, GM-CSF, IL1β, IL1ra, IL2, IL4, IL5, IL6, IL7, IL8, IL9, IL10, IL12, IL13, IL15, IL17, IP-10, MCP-1, MIP-1α, MIP-1β, PDGF-BB, TNF-α
Matrix 2	Protein/amino acid metabolism	1-methylhistidine, 3-methylhistidine, 4-hydroxyproline, α-aminobutyric acid, β-alanine, β-aminobutyric acid, γ-aminobutyric acid, alanine, aminoadipic acid, anserine, arginine, asparagine, aspartic acid, carnosine, citrulline, cystathionine, cystine, ethanolamine, glutamic acid, glycine, histidine, isoleucine, leucine, lysine, methionine, ornithine, phenylalanine, phosphoethanolamine, phosphoserine, proline, sarcosine, serine, taurine, threonine, tryptophan, tyrosine, valine
Matrix 3	Gut microbiota	*Actinobacteria, Adlercreutzia, Aerostipes, Aerotruncus, Akkermansia, Alcaligenaceae, Atopobium, Bacteroidaceae, Bacteroides, Bacteroidetes, Barnesiellaceae, Bifidobacteriaceae, Bifidobacterium, Bilophila, Blautia, Carnobacteriaceae, Christensenella, Christensenellaceae, Clostridiaceae, Collinsella, Coprococcus, Coriobacteriaceae, Cyanobacteria, Dehalobacteriaceae, Dehalobacterium, Desulfovibrionaceae, Dethiosulfovibrionaceae, Dialister, Dorea, Eggerthella, Enterobacteriaceae, Enterococcaceae, Enterococcus, Erysipelotrichaceae, EtOH8, Eubacterium, Euryarchaeota, Faecalibacterium, Firmicutes, Granulicatella, Haemophilus, Lachnobacterium, Lachnospira, Lachnospiraceae, Lactobacillaceae, Lactobacillus, Methanobacteriaceae, Methanobrevibacter, Mogibacteriacea, Oscillospira, Parabacteroides, Paraprevotella, Paraprevotellaceae, Pasteurellaceae, Peptostreptococcaceae, Phascolarctobacterium, Porphyromonadaceae, Prevotella, Prevotellaceae, Proteobacteria, Pyramidobacter, Rikenellaceae, Roseburia, Ruminococcaceae, Ruminococcus, Ruminococcus, S24-7, Slackia, Streptococcaceae, Streptococcus, Sutterella, Synergistetes, Tenericutes, TM7, Veillonella, Veillonellaceae, Verrucomicrobia, Verrucomicrobiaceae*

SO-CovSel is a predictive method that couples variable selection (through the CovSel approach) with sequential multiblock modeling, and it can be used to deal with both quantitative and qualitative responses. According to the method, the response(s) to be predicted can be expressed as a linear combination of variables from the different blocks, as described by the following equation:

$$Y = X_1 B_1 + X_2 B_2 + X_3 B_3$$

The matrices B_1, B_2, and B_3 collect the regression coefficients relating the individual blocks to the response(s). Within the multiblock linear regression framework summarized by the previous equation, one of the main peculiarities of the SO-CovSel methods is that not all the variables from the various blocks are used as predictors, but only the most relevant ones, which are selected according to the CovSel algorithm [33]. In CovSel, the first variable is selected as the one having the maximum covariance with the response. The subsequent variables are selected according to the same criterion, but after having orthogonalized both the X and the Y with respect to the contribution of the previously selected predictors, to avoid redundancy. The other main characteristic of the SO-CovSel method, which derives from its analogy with sequential and orthogonalized partial least squares regression (SO-PLS) [34,35], is that the different blocks are sequentially modeled, after having been orthogonalized with respect to the contribution of the previous ones. This avoids scaling issues and allows evaluating whether the block adds new information or it is redundant.

Based on these considerations, for a problem involving three blocks of predictors, as the one addressed in the present study, the SO-CovSel algorithm can be schematically summarized by the following steps:

1. CovSel algorithm is used to select relevant variables and calculate a regression model between the first block and the responses

$$Y = X_{1sel}B_1 + E_1$$

2. The second block is orthogonalized with respect to the variables selected in the first block

$$X_{2orth} = \left[I - X_{1sel}\left(X_{1sel}^T X_{1sel}\right) X_{1sel}^T\right] X_2$$

3. CovSel algorithm is used to select relevant variables and calculate a regression model between the orthogonalized second block and the residuals from the first fit

$$E_1 = X_{2selorth} B_{2orth} + E_2$$

4. The third block is orthogonalized with respect to the variables selected in the first and second blocks

$$X_{3orth} = \left[I - X_{12sel}\left(X_{12sel}^T X_{12sel}\right) X_{12sel}^T\right] X_3$$

where

$$X_{12sel} = [X_{1sel} X_{2orthsel}]$$

5. CovSel algorithm is used to select relevant variables and calculate a regression model between the orthogonalized third block and the residuals from the second fit

$$E_2 = X_{3selorth} B_{3orth} + E_3$$

6. An overall prediction model is built as

$$Y = \hat{Y} + E_3 = X_{1sel}B_1 + X_{2selorth}B_{2orth} + X_{3selorth}B_{3orth} + E_3$$

where the predicted response $\hat{Y}$ is calculated as

$$\hat{Y} = X_{1sel}B_1 + X_{2selorth}B_{2orth} + X_{3selorth}B_{3orth}$$

The algorithm, described in the steps above for regression (i.e., for the prediction of a quantitative response) can easily be adapted for classification problems, such as the one addressed in the present study. Indeed, by suitably coding the response matrix Y, a classification problem can be straightforwardly turned into a regression one. In particular, for a problem involving two classes, Y is a binary coded vector that takes the value 1 for PF&S participants and 0 for nonPF&S controls. The classification is then accomplished by properly thresholding the value of the predicted response.

3. Results

3.1. Characteristics of the Study Population

Thirty-five participants were included in the study: 18 older adults with PF&S (mean age 75.5 ± 3.9 years; 56.0% women) and 17 nonPF&S controls (mean age 73.9 ± 3.2 years; 29.0% women). Clinical and demographic characteristics of study participants are presented in Table 3. Age, sex distribution, and number of co-morbid conditions and medications did not differ between groups. Participants with PF&S showed higher BMI than nonPF&S controls.

Table 3. Main characteristics of study participants according to the presence of physical frailty & sarcopenia (PF&S).

	PF&S ($n = 18$)	NonPF&S ($n = 17$)	p
Age, years (mean ± SD)	75.5 ± 3.9	73.9 ± 3.2	0.2204
Gender (female), n (%)	10 (56)	5 (29)	0.2223
BMI, kg/m^2 (mean ± SD)	32.14 ± 6.02	26.27 ± 2.55	0.0008
SPPB (mean ± SD)	7.19 ± 1.22	11.24 ± 0.97	<0.0001
aLM, kg (mean ± SD)	17.75 ± 3.17	22.50 ± 2.93	<0.0001
aLM$_{BMI}$ (mean ± SD)	0.55 ± 0.11	0.87 ± 0.15	<0.0001
Number of disease conditions * (mean ± SD)	3.2 ± 1.7	3.0 ± 2.1	0.8046
Number of medications ** (mean ± SD)	3.4 ± 1.2	2.9 ± 1.6	0.1034

Abbreviations: aLM: appendicular lean mass; BMI: body mass index; PF&S: physical frailty & sarcopenia; nonPF&S: nonphysically frail, nonsarcopenic; SD: standard deviation; SPPB: short physical performance battery. * Includes hypertension, coronary artery disease, prior stroke, peripheral vascular disease, diabetes, chronic obstructive pulmonary disease, and osteoarthritis. ** Includes prescription and over-the-counter medications.

3.2. Features of Gut Microbiota According to the Presence of PF&S

No differences in microbial alpha diversity were determined between PF&S and nonPF&S participants (Figure 1).

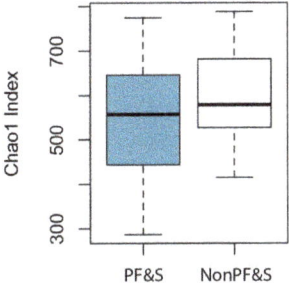

Figure 1. Chao1 index of gut microbial alpha diversity in participants with PF&S and in nonPF&S controls.

The analysis of the differential abundance of microbial taxa between PF&S and nonPF&S groups at the phylum, family, and genus levels showed an increase in Peptostreptococcaceae ($p = 0.008$ Table S1) and Bifidobacteriaceae ($p = 0.013$) at the family level and of *Dialister* ($p = 0.028$), *Pyramidobacter* ($p = 0.043$), and *Eggerthella* ($p = 0.05$) at the genus level, and a depletion in *Slackia* ($p < 0.0001$) and *Eubacterium* ($p = 0.028$) in PF&S participants (Figure 2). No significant differences in the relative abundance of intestinal bacteria phyla were found between groups.

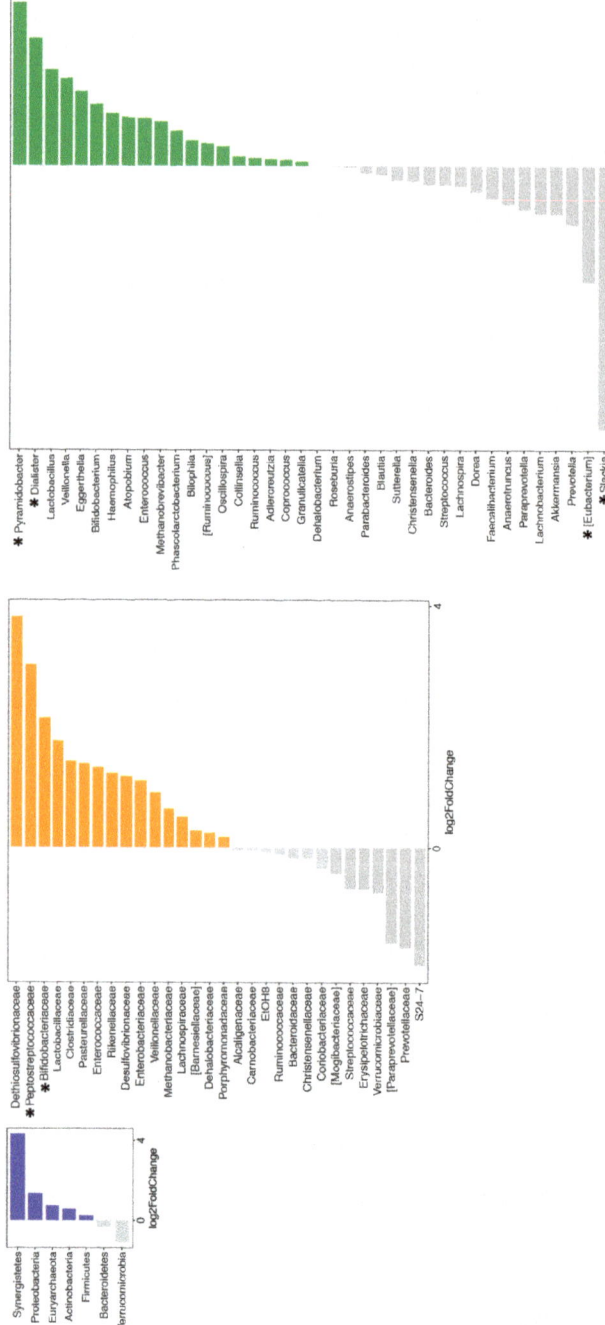

Figure 2. Comparison of gut microbiota relative abundance at the phylum (left panel, blue), family (middle panel, orange), and genus (right panel, green) levels between participants with PF&S and nonPF&S controls. Comparisons with a negative log$_2$ fold change (log2FC) are represented in grey. Only comparisons with a log2FC higher or lower than ± 1.5 and an adjusted p value < 0.05 are considered significant (*).

3.3. SO-CovSel Analysis

Serum levels of 64 biomolecules, including cytokines, chemokines, growth factors, amino acids, and derivatives, and the abundance of 77 gut microbial taxa, were assayed through multiple analytical platforms. Concentrations of serum mediators are reported in Table S2. Several SO-CovSel models were built using the multimatrix dataset. Among all of the tested models, the one that allowed the best classification of PF&S and nonPF&S participants with the smallest number of variables was selected. This latter was built using only seven analytes (Table 4).

Table 4. Levels of relevant analytes as resulted from SO-CovSel analysis.

	PF&S ($n = 18$)	nonPF&S ($n = 17$)
MIP-1α (pg/mL)	2.98 (11.04)	10.64 (11.15)
Aspartic acid (μmol/L)	26.95 (9.33)	16.10 (9.28)
Threonine (μmol/L)	109.90 (33.60)	125.80 (55.60)
Barnesiellaceae (log2FC)	0.0010 (0.007)	0.0030 (0.003)
Christensenellaceae (log2FC)	0.0004 (0.005)	0.0023 (0.004)
Oscillospira (log2FC)	0.0147 (0.227)	0.0109 (0.009)
Ruminococcus (log2FC)	0.0674 (0.091)	0.0620 (0.058)

Data are shown as median and interquartile range.

The rate of correct classification was 91.7% for PF&S participants and 87.5% for the nonPF&S group (90.0% in the whole study population), with an average area under the receiver operating characteristic (AUROC) curve very close to 1. When compared with their distributions under the null hypothesis, all of the classification figures of merit were statistically significant ($p < 0.0001$). Among the discriminant analytes selected by the SO-CovSel model, participants with PF&S showed lower levels of MIP-1β. As for the metabolic signature, the level of the aspartic acid was higher in PF&S participants, while that of threonine was higher in the nonPF&S group. Among the gut microbes contributing to the model, *Oscillospira* and *Ruminococcus* were more abundant in PF&S participants, while Barnesiellaceae *and* Christensenellaceae were higher in the nonPF&S group (Table 4).

4. Discussion

In this study, we profiled the gut microbiota and determined the levels of inflammatory and metabolic markers in older adults with and without PF&S to investigate whether PF&S is associated with specific profiles of gut microbial taxa and circulating biomolecules. We also applied an innovative multi-marker analytical approach to determine the classification performance of a set of potential biomarkers for PF&S.

Findings from the present study highlight the possibility that changes in gut microbiota composition may be associated with PF&S. Although no differences in microbial alpha diversity were found between PF&S and nonPF&S groups, results from the analysis of the differential abundance of gut microbial taxa showed increased Peptostreptococcaceae and Bifidobacteriaceae at the family level and *Dialister*, *Pyramidobacter*, and *Eggerthella* at the genus level, and depletion of *Slackia* and *Eubacterium* in participants with PF&S. The taxa involved in the association between gut microbiota and PF&S identified in the present study are in-keeping with those previously associated with frailty and biological aging [36–42].

The application of the SO-CovSel-based analytical strategy by incorporating all of the assayed variables into three different matrices allowed distinguishing participants with PF&S from nonPF&S controls by using only seven markers, among which gut microbes were the most represented (Table 4).

The existence of a gut microbiota profile associated with sarcopenia and involving changes in the abundance of health-related *Bifidobacteria* has previously been shown in rats [43]. While very little is known about a possible functional link between *Oscillospira* and PF&S, the existence of a trait for butyrate-producing bacteria *Ruminococcus* is in-keeping with previously reported associations between *Ruminococcus* abundance and frailty [40]. Indeed, *Oscillospira* represents a more enigmatic and under-studied anaerobic butyrate producer (*Clostridium* clusters IV) often associated with leanness [44], with a metabolism and physiology not fully understood [44,45]. However, the overall apparent dysbiotic shift of gut microbiota towards a greater abundance of butyrate-producing bacteria in PF&S similar to what was observed in higher functioning people may indicate a positive role for these microbes in muscle function. Indeed, butyrate, by reinforcing tight junction assembly and enhancing intestinal barrier function [46], may prevent endotoxin translocation and reduce systemic inflammation [47]. Short-chain fatty acids (SCFAs), including butyrate, also promote fatty acid oxidation, thereby improving muscle bioenergetics [48] and limiting myosteatosis [49,50]. On the other hand, reduced SCFA production may trigger insulin resistance and result in increased fatty acid deposition within the muscle. The ensuing lower muscle quality may further promote insulin resistance, feeding a vicious circle that contributes to the onset and progression of PF&S [51,52]. Whether and how *Ruminococcus* and *Oscillospira* abundance impacts muscle metabolism and function in the context of PF&S warrants further investigation. In this regard, it is noteworthy that the abundance of *Bacteroides* was increased by aerobic training in healthy older women, which was associated with improved cardiorespiratory fitness [53]. Variations in *Ruminococcus* in association with *Eubacterium* and *Eggerthella* were also identified in frail nursing-home residents compared with fit matched community-dwellers [36,37]. This finding was attributed to different dietary patterns and, in particular, to long-term protein supplementation among nursing-home residents [40]. Indeed, diet influences gut microbiota composition and functionality, which may ultimately impact skeletal muscle. While high protein intake has been endorsed as a strategy against sarcopenia [54], protein-enriched diets may shift bacterial metabolism towards AA degradation and fermentation [55]. Hence, the role of gut microbes as transducers of nutrient signaling to the host implies the need of monitoring the composition and function of gut microbiota during nutritional interventions for sarcopenia.

This view is strengthened by the presence of the AAs aspartic acid and threonine among the most relevant mediators in the SO-CovSel model.

Aspartic acid, together with asparagine and glutamic acid is among the AAs providing amino groups and ammonia for the synthesis of glutamine and alanine, whose carbon skeletons can solely be used for the de novo synthesis of Kreb's cycle intermediates and glutamine [56]. Notably, we previously showed that higher serum levels of aspartic acid, asparagine, and glutamic acid were among the descriptors of the AA signature of older persons with PF&S [10].

Threonine is an essential AA (EAA) that must be provided with the diet to meet nutritional requirements and is relevant for muscle protein turnover and overall metabolism [57]. The finding of threonine as a contributor to the SO-CovSel model in discriminating PF&S participants is in-keeping with a recent work reporting levels of several EAAs, including threonine, as inversely associated with sarcopenia in community-dwelling older adults [58]. Low plasma levels of EAAs were also found in severely frail older people [59]. These findings may be associated to malnutrition (both quantitative and qualitative), a common underlying factor of frailty and sarcopenia [60].

Finally, the relationship observed between the abundance of specific intestinal bacteria, metabolic markers, and serum levels of distinct inflammatory biomolecules suggests the existence of an additional pathway through which changes in gut microbiota may impinge on PF&S pathophysiology. A relationship among gut microbiota composition, chronic inflammation, and age-related conditions was shown in pre-clinical models [61] but not in humans. Furthermore, altered gut microbiota composition has been hypothesized to contribute to anabolic resistance and muscle wasting through promoting chronic inflammation [62,63]. Age-associated alterations in intestinal mucosa permeability (i.e., "leaky gut") and the resulting systemic absorption of bacterial products may further ignite systemic inflammation [64–66]. Although our investigation does not provide mechanistic elements to support such a hypothesis, the relevance of systemic inflammation to PF&S has previously been shown [11]. From this perspective, systemic inflammation would represent one of the effectors of the "gut-muscle axis" that has recently been proposed to contribute to the development of PF&S [23,63,67].

Hence, untangling the relationship among gut microbiota, metabolic changes and muscle homeostasis in advanced age represents a highly promising research area to devise new interventions against PF&S.

Although reporting novel findings, our study presents some limitations that need to be acknowledged. Participants with PF&S had higher BMI than controls, indicative of a sarcopenic obesity phenotype. Because this body composition profile is intrinsic to the PF&S condition [27], the relative contribution of low muscle and excessive adiposity to systemic inflammation, metabolic changes, and gut microbiota composition could not be discerned. The cross-sectional design of the present investigation does not allow inferring causality about changes in gut microbiota and the development of PF&S. Nevertheless, the presence of a gut-muscle axis actively involved in the genesis of frailty and sarcopenia is supported by other studies (reviewed in [67]). Here, for the first time, we show that specific relationships exist among gut microbiota, systemic inflammatory mediators, and metabolic alterations in older adults with PF&S. The relatively small size of the study population comprising only Caucasian people calls for a cautious interpretation of results and impedes generalization of findings to other ethnic groups. Because of the limited sample size, the possible influence of numerous factors, including diet, physical activity, co-morbid conditions, and medications, could not be taken into account in the analysis. Finally, although a fairly large number of metabolic and inflammatory biomolecules were assayed, it cannot be excluded that more robust associations between gut microbiota composition and PF&S might have been obtained through the analysis of a larger range of biomediators.

Supplementary Materials: The following are available online at http://www.mdpi.com/2072-6643/12/1/65/s1, Table S1: Differential abundance analysis of bacterial taxa at phylum, family, and genus level in participants with physical frailty and sarcopenia (PF&S) and nonPF&S. Table S2: Serum concentrations of nonsignificant inflammatory mediators, amino acids, and derivatives in participants with and without physical frailty & sarcopenia (PF&S).

Author Contributions: Conceptualization, A.P. (Anna Picca), E.M., and F.R.P.; methodology, A.P. (Aniello Primiano), F.D.C., J.G., and S.R.; software, A.B. and F.M.; validation, A.P. (Anna Picca), E.M., F.R.P., H.J.C.-J., and R.C.; formal analysis, A.B. and F.M.; investigation, A.P. (Anna Picca), E.M., and R.C.; resources, A.G., F.L., L.P., and R.B.; data curation, A.P. (Anna Picca), F.R.P., and R.C.; writing—original draft preparation, A.P. (Anna Picca) and E.M.; writing—review and editing, F.M., H.J.C.-J., J.G., and R.C.; visualization, A.P. (Aniello Primiano), F.D.C., J.G., and S.R.; supervision, A.G., F.L., L.P., and R.B.; funding acquisition, R.B. All authors have read and agreed to the published version of the manuscript.

Funding: This research was funded by Innovative Medicines Initiative-Joint Undertaking [IMI-JU #115621], Intramural Research Grants from the Università Cattolica del Sacro Cuore [D3.2 2013 and D3.2 2015], the nonprofit research foundation "Centro Studi Achille e Linda Lorenzon", Fondazione Policlinico Universitario "Agostino Gemelli" IRCCS, the Italian Ministry of Education, Universities and Research, and Coordenação de Aperfeiçoamento de Pessoal de Nível Superior (CAPES; Finance Code 001).

Acknowledgments: The authors would like to thank all participants for their involvement in this study.

Conflicts of Interest: The authors declare no conflict of interest. The funders had no role in the design of the study; in the collection, analyses, or interpretation of data; in the writing of the manuscript; or in the decision to publish the results.

References

1. Hirani, V.; Blyth, F.; Naganathan, V.; Le Couteur, D.G.; Seibel, M.J.; Waite, L.M.; Handelsman, D.J.; Cumming, R.G. Sarcopenia is associated with incident disability, institutionalization, and mortality in community-dwelling older men: The Concord Health and Ageing in Men Project. *J. Am. Med. Dir. Assoc.* **2015**, *16*, 607–613. [CrossRef] [PubMed]
2. Marzetti, E.; Calvani, R.; Tosato, M.; Cesari, M.; Di Bari, M.; Cherubini, A.; Collamati, A.; D'Angelo, E.; Pahor, M.; Bernabei, R.; et al. SPRINTT Consortium. Sarcopenia: An overview. *Aging Clin. Exp. Res.* **2017**, *29*, 11–17. [CrossRef] [PubMed]
3. Cesari, M.; Calvani, R.; Marzetti, E. Frailty in older persons. *Clin. Geriatr. Med.* **2017**, *33*, 293–303. [CrossRef] [PubMed]
4. Landi, F.; Calvani, R.; Cesari, M.; Tosato, M.; Martone, A.M.; Bernabei, R.; Onder, G.; Marzetti, E. Sarcopenia as the biological substrate of physical frailty. *Clin. Geriatr. Med.* **2015**, *31*, 367–374. [CrossRef] [PubMed]

5. Cesari, M.; Landi, F.; Vellas, B.; Bernabei, R.; Marzetti, E. Sarcopenia and physical frailty: Two sides of the same coin. *Front. Aging Neurosci.* **2014**, *6*, 192. [CrossRef]
6. Cesari, M.; Landi, F.; Calvani, R.; Cherubini, A.; Di Bari, M.; Kortebein, P.; Del Signore, S.; Le Lain, R.; Vellas, B.; Pahor, M.; et al. SPRINTT Consortium. Rationale for a preliminary operational definition of physical frailty and sarcopenia in the SPRINTT trial. *Aging Clin. Exp. Res.* **2017**, *29*, 81–88. [CrossRef]
7. Marzetti, E.; Calvani, R.; Landi, F.; Hoogendijk, E.O.; Fougère, B.; Vellas, B.; Pahor, M.; Bernabei, R.; Cesari, M. SPRINTT Consortium. Innovative Medicines Initiative: The SPRINTT project. *J. Frailty Aging* **2015**, *4*, 207–208. [CrossRef]
8. Calvani, R.; Marini, F.; Cesari, M.; Tosato, M.; Anker, S.D.; von Haehling, S.; Miller, R.R.; Bernabei, R.; Landi, F.; Marzetti, E. SPRINTT consortium. Biomarkers for physical frailty and sarcopenia: State of the science and future developments. *J. Cachexia Sarcopenia Muscle* **2015**, *6*, 278–286. [CrossRef]
9. Picca, A.; Calvani, R.; Bossola, M.; Allocca, E.; Menghi, A.; Pesce, V.; Lezza, A.M.S.; Bernabei, R.; Landi, F.; Marzetti, E. Update on mitochondria and muscle aging: All wrong roads lead to sarcopenia. *Biol. Chem.* **2018**, *399*, 421–436. [CrossRef]
10. Calvani, R.; Picca, A.; Marini, F.; Biancolillo, A.; Gervasoni, J.; Persichilli, S.; Primiano, A.; Coelho-Junior, H.J.; Bossola, M.; Urbani, A.; et al. A distinct pattern of circulating amino acids characterizes older persons with physical frailty and sarcopenia: Results from the BIOSPHERE study. *Nutrients* **2018**, *10*, 1691. [CrossRef]
11. Marzetti, E.; Picca, A.; Marini, F.; Biancolillo, A.; Coelho-Junior, H.J.; Gervasoni, J.; Bossola, M.; Cesari, M.; Onder, G.; Landi, F.; et al. Inflammatory signatures in older persons with physical frailty and sarcopenia: The frailty "cytokinome" at its core. *Exp. Gerontol.* **2019**, *122*, 129–138. [CrossRef] [PubMed]
12. Landi, F.; Calvani, R.; Tosato, M.; Martone, A.M.; Ortolani, E.; Savera, G.; Sisto, A.; Marzetti, E. Anorexia of aging: Risk factors, consequences, and potential treatments. *Nutrients* **2016**, *8*, 69. [CrossRef] [PubMed]
13. Landi, F.; Calvani, R.; Tosato, M.; Martone, A.M.; Ortolani, E.; Savera, G.; D'Angelo, E.; Sisto, A.; Marzetti, E. Protein intake and muscle health in old age: From biological plausibility to clinical evidence. *Nutrients* **2016**, *8*, 295. [CrossRef] [PubMed]
14. Landi, F.; Cesari, M.; Calvani, R.; Cherubini, A.; Di Bari, M.; Bejuit, R.; Mshid, J.; Andrieu, S.; Sinclair, A.J.; Sieber, C.C.; et al. SPRINTT Consortium. The "Sarcopenia and Physical fRailty IN older people: Multi-componenT Treatment strategies" (SPRINTT) randomized controlled trial: Design and methods. *Aging Clin. Exp. Res.* **2017**, *29*, 89–100. [CrossRef]
15. Chen, H.; Rejeski, W.J.; Gill, T.M.; Guralnik, J.; King, A.C.; Newman, A.; Blair, S.N.; Conroy, D.; Liu, C.; Manini, T.M.; et al. LIFE Study. A comparison of self-report indices of major mobility disability to failure on the 400-m walk test: The LIFE study. *J. Gerontol. A Biol. Sci. Med. Sci.* **2018**, *73*, 513–518. [CrossRef]
16. Roubenoff, R. Sarcopenic obesity: Does muscle loss cause fat gain? Lessons from rheumatoid arthritis and osteoarthritis. *Ann. N. Y. Acad. Sci.* **2006**, *904*, 553–557. [CrossRef]
17. Binkley, N.; Krueger, D.; Buehring, B. What's in a name revisited: Should osteoporosis and sarcopenia be considered components of "dysmobility syndrome?". *Osteoporos. Int.* **2013**, *24*, 2955–2959. [CrossRef]
18. Porter Starr, K.N.; McDonald, S.R.; Bales, C.W. Obesity and physical frailty in older adults: A scoping review of lifestyle intervention trials. *J. Am. Med. Dir. Assoc.* **2014**, *15*, 240–250. [CrossRef]
19. Hulsegge, G.; Herber-Gast, G.-C.M.; Spijkerman, A.M.W.; Susan, H.; Picavet, J.; van der Schouw, Y.T.; Bakker, S.J.L.; Gansevoort, R.T.; Dollé, M.E.T.; Smit, H.A.; et al. Obesity and age-related changes in markers of oxidative stress and inflammation across four generations. *Obesity* **2016**, *24*, 1389–1396. [CrossRef]
20. Goodpaster, B.H.; Carlson, C.L.; Visser, M.; Kelley, D.E.; Scherzinger, A.; Harris, T.B.; Stamm, E.; Newman, A.B. Attenuation of skeletal muscle and strength in the elderly: The health ABC study. *J. Appl. Physiol.* **2001**, *90*, 2157–2165. [CrossRef]
21. Visser, M.; Goodpaster, B.H.; Kritchevsky, S.B.; Newman, A.B.; Nevitt, M.; Rubin, S.M.; Simonsick, E.M.; Harris, T.B. Muscle mass, muscle strength, and muscle fat infiltration as predictors of incident mobility limitations in well-functioning older persons. *J. Gerontol. A Biol. Sci. Med. Sci.* **2005**, *60*, 324–333. [CrossRef] [PubMed]
22. O'Connor, E.M. The role of gut microbiota in nutritional status. *Curr. Opin. Clin. Nutr. Metab. Care* **2013**, *16*, 509–516. [CrossRef] [PubMed]
23. Picca, A.; Fanelli, F.; Calvani, R.; Mulè, G.; Pesce, V.; Sisto, A.; Pantanelli, C.; Bernabei, R.; Landi, F.; Marzetti, E. Gut dysbiosis and muscle aging: Searching for novel targets against sarcopenia. *Mediat. Inflamm.* **2018**, *2018*. [CrossRef] [PubMed]

24. Calvani, R.; Picca, A.; Marini, F.; Biancolillo, A.; Cesari, M.; Pesce, V.; Lezza, A.M.S.; Bossola, M.; Leeuwenburgh, C.; Bernabei, R.; et al. The "BIOmarkers associated with Sarcopenia and PHysical frailty in EldeRly pErsons" (BIOSPHERE) study: Rationale, design and methods. *Eur. J. Intern. Med.* **2018**, *56*, 19–25. [CrossRef]
25. Ponziani, F.R.; Putignani, L.; Paroni Sterbini, F.; Petito, V.; Picca, A.; Del Chierico, F.; Reddel, S.; Calvani, R.; Marzetti, E.; Sanguinetti, M.; et al. Influence of hepatitis C virus eradication with direct-acting antivirals on the gut microbiota in patients with cirrhosis. *Aliment. Pharmacol. Ther.* **2018**, *48*, 1301–1311. [CrossRef]
26. Ponziani, F.R.; Bhoori, S.; Castelli, C.; Putignani, L.; Rivoltini, L.; Del Chierico, F.; Sanguinetti, M.; Morelli, D.; Paroni Sterbini, F.; Petito, V.; et al. Hepatocellular carcinoma is associated with gut microbiota profile and inflammation in nonalcoholic fatty liver disease. *Hepatology* **2019**, *69*, 107–120. [CrossRef]
27. Marzetti, E.; Cesari, M.; Calvani, R.; Msihid, J.; Tosato, M.; Rodriguez-Mañas, L.; Lattanzio, F.; Cherubini, A.; Bejuit, R.; Di Bari, M.; et al. SPRINTT Consortium. The "Sarcopenia and Physical fRailty IN older people: Multi-componenT Treatment strategies" (SPRINTT) randomized controlled trial: Case finding, screening and characteristics of eligible participants. *Exp. Gerontol.* **2018**, *113*, 48–57. [CrossRef]
28. Guralnik, J.M.; Simonsick, E.M.; Ferrucci, L.; Glynn, R.J.; Berkman, L.F.; Blazer, D.G.; Scherr, P.A.; Wallace, R.B. A short physical performance battery assessing lower extremity function: Association with self-reported disability and prediction of mortality and nursing home admission. *J. Gerontol.* **1994**, *49*, M85–M94. [CrossRef]
29. Studenski, S.A.; Peters, K.W.; Alley, D.E.; Cawthon, P.M.; McLean, R.R.; Harris, T.B.; Ferrucci, L.; Guralnik, J.M.; Fragala, M.S.; Kenny, A.M.; et al. The FNIH sarcopenia project: Rationale, study description, conference recommendations, and final estimates. *J. Gerontol. A Biol. Sci. Med. Sci.* **2014**, *69*, 547–558. [CrossRef]
30. Newman, A.B.; Simonsick, E.M.; Naydeck, B.L.; Boudreau, R.M.; Kritchevsky, S.B.; Nevitt, M.C.; Pahor, M.; Satterfield, S.; Brach, J.S.; Studenski, S.A.; et al. Association of long-distance corridor walk performance with mortality, cardiovascular disease, mobility limitation, and disability. *JAMA* **2006**, *295*, 2018–2026. [CrossRef]
31. Picca, A.; Guerra, F.; Calvani, R.; Bucci, C.; Lo Monaco, M.R.; Bentivoglio, A.R.; Landi, F.; Bernabei, R.; Marzetti, E. Mitochondrial-derived vesicles as candidate biomarkers in Parkinson's disease: Rationale, design and methods of the EXosomes in PArkiNson Disease (EXPAND) study. *Int. J. Mol. Sci.* **2019**, *20*, 2373. [CrossRef] [PubMed]
32. Biancolillo, A.; Marini, F.; Roger, J. SO-CovSel: A novel method for variable selection in a multiblock framework. *J. Chemom.* **2019**, e3120. [CrossRef]
33. Roger, J.M.; Palagos, B.; Bertrand, D.; Fernandez-Ahumada, E. CovSel: Variable selection for highly multivariate and multi-response calibration. Application to IR spectroscopy. *Chemom. Intell. Lab. Syst.* **2011**, *106*, 216–223. [CrossRef]
34. Naes, T.; Tomic, O.; Mevik, B.-H.; Martens, H. Path modelling by sequential PLS regression. *J. Chemom.* **2011**, *25*, 28–40. [CrossRef]
35. Biancolillo, A.; Naes, T. The Sequential and Orthogonalized PLS Regression for Multiblock Regression: Theory, Examples, and Extensions. In *Data Fusion Methodology and Applications*; Cocchi, M., Ed.; Elsevier: Oxford, UK, 2019; Volume 31, pp. 157–177.
36. Claesson, M.J.; Jeffery, I.B.; Conde, S.; Power, S.E.; O'connor, E.M.; Cusack, S.; Harris, H.M.B.; Coakley, M.; Lakshminarayanan, B.; O'sullivan, O.; et al. Gut microbiota composition correlates with diet and health in the elderly. *Nature* **2012**, *488*, 178–184. [CrossRef]
37. Jackson, M.A.; Jackson, M.; Jeffery, I.B.; Beaumont, M.; Bell, J.T.; Clark, A.G.; Ley, R.E.; O'Toole, P.W.; Spector, T.D.; Steves, C.J. Signatures of early frailty in the gut microbiota. *Genome Med.* **2016**, *8*, 8. [CrossRef]
38. Maffei, V.J.; Kim, S.; Blanchard, E.; Luo, M.; Jazwinski, S.M.; Taylor, C.M.; Welsh, D.A. Biological Aging and the Human Gut Microbiota. *J. Gerontol. A Biol. Sci. Med. Sci.* **2017**, *72*, 1474–1482. [CrossRef]
39. Ticinesi, A.; Milani, C.; Lauretani, F.; Nouvenne, A.; Mancabelli, L.; Lugli, G.A.; Turroni, F.; Duranti, S.; Mangifesta, M.; Viappiani, A.; et al. Gut microbiota composition is associated with polypharmacy in elderly hospitalized patients. *Sci. Rep.* **2017**, *7*, 11102. [CrossRef]
40. Haran, J.P.; Bucci, V.; Dutta, P.; Ward, D.; McCormick, B. The nursing home elder microbiome stability and associations with age, frailty, nutrition and physical location. *J. Med. Microbiol.* **2018**, *67*, 40–51. [CrossRef]
41. Verdi, S.; Jackson, M.A.; Beaumont, M.; Bowyer, R.C.E.; Bell, J.T.; Spector, T.D.; Steves, C.J. An investigation into physical frailty as a link between the gut microbiome and cognitive health. *Front. Aging Neurosci.* **2018**, *10*, 398. [CrossRef]

42. Ogawa, T.; Hirose, Y.; Honda-Ogawa, M.; Sugimoto, M.; Sasaki, S.; Kibi, M.; Kawabata, S.; Ikebe, K.; Maeda, Y. Composition of salivary microbiota in elderly subjects. *Sci. Rep.* **2018**, *8*, 414. [CrossRef] [PubMed]
43. Siddharth, J.; Chakrabarti, A.; Pannérec, A.; Karaz, S.; Morin-Rivron, D.; Masoodi, M.; Feige, J.N.; Parkinson, S.J. Aging and sarcopenia associate with specific interactions between gut microbes, serum biomarkers and host physiology in rats. *Aging* **2017**, *9*, 1698–1720. [CrossRef] [PubMed]
44. Gophna, U.; Konikoff, T.; Nielsen, H.B. Oscillospira and related bacteria—From metagenomic species to metabolic features. *Environ. Microbiol.* **2017**, *19*, 835–841. [CrossRef] [PubMed]
45. Konikoff, T.; Gophna, U. Oscillospira: A central, enigmatic component of the human gut microbiota. *Trends Microbiol.* **2016**, *24*, 523–524. [CrossRef] [PubMed]
46. Peng, L.; Li, Z.-R.; Green, R.S.; Holzman, I.R.; Lin, J. Butyrate enhances the intestinal barrier by facilitating tight junction assembly via activation of AMP-activated protein kinase in Caco-2 cell monolayers. *J. Nutr.* **2009**, *139*, 1619–1625. [CrossRef] [PubMed]
47. Cox, M.A.; Jackson, J.; Stanton, M.; Rojas-Triana, A.; Bober, L.; Laverty, M.; Yang, X.; Zhu, F.; Liu, J.; Wang, S.; et al. Short-chain fatty acids act as antiinflammatory mediators by regulating prostaglandin E2 and cytokines. *World J. Gastroenterol.* **2009**, *15*, 5549–5557. [CrossRef]
48. Saint-Georges-Chaumet, Y.; Edeas, M. Microbiota-mitochondria inter-talk: Consequence for microbiota-host interaction. *Pathog. Dis.* **2016**, *74*, ftv096. [CrossRef]
49. Hénique, C.; Mansouri, A.; Vavrova, E.; Lenoir, V.; Ferry, A.; Esnous, C.; Ramond, E.; Girard, J.; Bouillaud, F.; Prip-Buus, C.; et al. Increasing mitochondrial muscle fatty acid oxidation induces skeletal muscle remodeling toward an oxidative phenotype. *FASEB J.* **2015**, *29*, 2473–2483. [CrossRef]
50. Gumucio, J.P.; Qasawa, A.H.; Ferrara, P.J.; Malik, A.N.; Funai, K.; McDonagh, B.; Mendias, C.L. Reduced mitochondrial lipid oxidation leads to fat accumulation in myosteatosis. *FASEB J.* **2019**, *33*, 7863–7881. [CrossRef]
51. Poggiogalle, E.; Lubrano, C.; Gnessi, L.; Mariani, S.; Di Martino, M.; Catalano, C.; Lenzi, A.; Donini, L.M. The decline in muscle strength and muscle quality in relation to metabolic derangements in adult women with obesity. *Clin. Nutr.* **2019**, *38*, 2430–2435. [CrossRef]
52. Sachs, S.; Zarini, S.; Kahn, D.E.; Harrison, K.A.; Perreault, L.; Phang, T.; Newsom, S.A.; Strauss, A.; Kerege, A.; Schoen, J.A.; et al. Intermuscular adipose tissue directly modulates skeletal muscle insulin sensitivity in humans. *Am. J. Physiol. Endocrinol. Metab.* **2019**, *316*, E866–E879. [CrossRef] [PubMed]
53. Morita, E.; Yokoyama, H.; Imai, D.; Takeda, R.; Ota, A.; Kawai, E.; Hisada, T.; Emoto, M.; Suzuki, Y.; Okazaki, K. Aerobic exercise training with brisk walking increases intestinal bacteroides in healthy elderly women. *Nutrients* **2019**, *11*, 868. [CrossRef] [PubMed]
54. Landi, F.; Calvani, R.; Tosato, M.; Martone, A.M.; Picca, A.; Ortolani, E.; Savera, G.; Salini, S.; Ramaschi, M.; Bernabei, R.; et al. Animal-derived protein consumption is associated with muscle mass and strength in community-dwellers: Results from the Milan EXPO survey. *J. Nutr. Health Aging* **2017**, *21*, 1050–1056. [CrossRef] [PubMed]
55. Beaumont, M.; Portune, K.J.; Steuer, N.; Lan, A.; Cerrudo, V.; Audebert, M.; Dumont, F.; Mancano, G.; Khodorova, N.; Andriamihaja, M.; et al. Quantity and source of dietary protein influence metabolite production by gut microbiota and rectal mucosa gene expression: A randomized, parallel, double-blind trial in overweight humans. *Am. J. Clin. Nutr.* **2017**, *106*, 1005–1019. [CrossRef] [PubMed]
56. Wagenmakers, A.J.M. Protein and amino acid metabolism in human muscle. *Adv. Exp. Med. Biol.* **1998**, *441*, 307–319. [CrossRef]
57. Wu, G. Amino acids: Metabolism, functions, and nutrition. *Amino Acids* **2009**, *37*, 1–17. [CrossRef]
58. Lu, Y.; Karagounis, L.G.; Ng, T.P.; Carre, C.; Narang, V.; Wong, G.; Ying Tan, C.T.; Zin Nyunt, M.S.; Gao, Q.; Abel, B.; et al. Systemic and metabolic signature of sarcopenia in community-dwelling older adults. *J. Gerontol. A Biol. Sci. Med. Sci.* **2019**. [CrossRef]
59. Adachi, Y.; Ono, N.; Imaizumi, A.; Muramatsu, T.; Andou, T.; Shimodaira, Y.; Nagao, K.; Kageyama, Y.; Mori, M.; Noguchi, Y.; et al. Plasma amino acid profile in severely frail elderly patients in Japan. *Int. J. Gerontol.* **2018**, *12*, 290–293. [CrossRef]
60. Cruz-Jentoft, A.J.; Kiesswetter, E.; Drey, M.; Sieber, C.C. Nutrition, frailty, and sarcopenia. *Aging Clin. Exp. Res.* **2017**, *29*, 43–48. [CrossRef]

61. Thevaranjan, N.; Puchta, A.; Schulz, C.; Naidoo, A.; Szamosi, J.C.; Verschoor, C.P.; Loukov, D.; Schenck, L.P.; Jury, J.; Foley, K.P.; et al. Age-associated microbial dysbiosis promotes intestinal permeability, systemic inflammation, and macrophage dysfunction. *Cell Host Microbe* **2017**, *21*, 455–466. [CrossRef]
62. Grosicki, G.J.; Fielding, R.A.; Lustgarten, M.S. Gut microbiota contribute to age-related changes in skeletal muscle size, composition, and function: Biological basis for a gut-muscle axis. *Calcif. Tissue Int.* **2018**, *102*, 433–442. [CrossRef] [PubMed]
63. Ticinesi, A.; Lauretani, F.; Milani, C.; Nouvenne, A.; Tana, C.; Del Rio, D.; Maggio, M.; Ventura, M.; Meschi, T. Aging gut microbiota at the cross-road between nutrition, physical frailty, and sarcopenia: Is there a gut–muscle axis? *Nutrients* **2017**, *9*, 1303. [CrossRef] [PubMed]
64. Ferrucci, L.; Fabbri, E. Inflammageing: Chronic inflammation in ageing, cardiovascular disease, and frailty. *Nat. Rev. Cardiol.* **2018**, *15*, 505–522. [CrossRef] [PubMed]
65. Sovran, B.; Hugenholtz, F.; Elderman, M.; Van Beek, A.A.; Graversen, K.; Huijskes, M.; Boekschoten, M.V.; Savelkoul, H.F.J.; De Vos, P.; Dekker, J.; et al. Age-associated impairment of the mucus barrier function is associated with profound changes in microbiota and immunity. *Sci. Rep.* **2019**, *9*, 1437. [CrossRef]
66. Ticinesi, A.; Lauretani, F.; Tana, C.; Nouvenne, A.; Ridolo, E.; Meschi, T. Exercise and immune system as modulators of intestinal microbiome: Implications for the gut-muscle axis hypothesis. *Exerc. Immunol. Rev.* **2019**, *25*, 84–95.
67. Ticinesi, A.; Nouvenne, A.; Cerundolo, N.; Catania, P.; Prati, B.; Tana, C.; Meschi, T. Gut microbiota, muscle mass and function in aging: A focus on physical frailty and sarcopenia. *Nutrients* **2019**, *11*, 1633. [CrossRef]

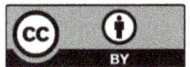

© 2019 by the authors. Licensee MDPI, Basel, Switzerland. This article is an open access article distributed under the terms and conditions of the Creative Commons Attribution (CC BY) license (http://creativecommons.org/licenses/by/4.0/).

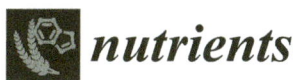

Communication

Dietary Protein and Physical Activity Interventions to Support Muscle Maintenance in End-Stage Renal Disease Patients on Hemodialysis

Floris K. Hendriks [1,2], Joey S.J. Smeets [1], Frank M. van der Sande [3], Jeroen P. Kooman [2,3] and Luc J.C. van Loon [1,*]

1. Department of Human Biology, NUTRIM School of Nutrition and Translational Research in Metabolism, Maastricht University Medical Centre+, P.O. Box 616, 6200 MD Maastricht, The Netherlands; f.hendriks@maastrichtuniversity.nl (F.K.H.); joey.smeets@maastrichtuniversity.nl (J.S.J.S.)
2. Department of Internal Medicine, NUTRIM School of Nutrition and Translational Research in Metabolism, Maastricht University Medical Centre+, P.O. Box 616, 6200 MD Maastricht, The Netherlands; jeroen.kooman@mumc.nl
3. Division of Nephrology, Department of Internal Medicine, Maastricht University Medical Centre+, P.O. Box 5800, 6202 AZ Maastricht, The Netherlands; f.vander.sande@mumc.nl
* Correspondence: L.vanLoon@maastrichtuniversity.nl; Tel.: +(31)-43-3881397

Received: 30 October 2019; Accepted: 3 December 2019; Published: 5 December 2019

Abstract: End-stage renal disease patients have insufficient renal clearance capacity left to adequately excrete metabolic waste products. Hemodialysis (HD) is often employed to partially replace renal clearance in these patients. However, skeletal muscle mass and strength start to decline at an accelerated rate after initiation of chronic HD therapy. An essential anabolic stimulus to allow muscle maintenance is dietary protein ingestion. Chronic HD patients generally fail to achieve recommended protein intake levels, in particular on dialysis days. Besides a low protein intake on dialysis days, the protein equivalent of a meal is extracted from the circulation during HD. Apart from protein ingestion, physical activity is essential to allow muscle maintenance. Unfortunately, most chronic HD patients have a sedentary lifestyle. Yet, physical activity and nutritional interventions to support muscle maintenance are generally not implemented in routine patient care. To support muscle maintenance in chronic HD patients, quantity and timing of protein intake should be optimized, in particular throughout dialysis days. Furthermore, implementing physical activity either during or between HD sessions may improve the muscle protein synthetic response to protein ingestion. A well-orchestrated combination of physical activity and nutritional interventions will be instrumental to preserve muscle mass in chronic HD patients.

Keywords: muscle wasting; exercise; nutrition; kidney disease

1. Introduction

Chronic kidney disease (CKD) is currently a public health problem with a global prevalence of 10% and the cause of approximately 33 million disability-adjusted life-years worldwide [1,2]. Development and progression of CKD are associated with the age-related decline in renal function, especially in individuals with hypertension and diabetes mellitus [3–5]. Therefore, the rapid ageing of our population is expected to further increase prevalence of CKD and its progression to end-stage renal disease (ESRD) [6,7]. The glomerular filtration rate in ESRD patients is below 15 mL/min/1.73 m^2 and insufficient to adequately remove metabolic waste products and fluids from the body [8,9]. Due to the accumulation of metabolic waste products in their body, ESRD patients experience phenotypic changes that resemble the ageing process, with a progressive loss of skeletal muscle mass and strength [10].

To prevent lethal consequences of metabolic waste product accumulation in ESRD patients, hemodialysis (HD) can be used to partially replace renal solute removal [11]. Over the past decades, survival of patients undergoing HD has improved substantially [12,13]. However, prevention of the adverse effects of HD on body composition has made less progression. After initiation of chronic hemodialysis (CHD) therapy, the age-related loss of skeletal muscle mass and strength accelerates and patients typically develop impairments in physical function [14–17]. Protein-energy wasting, a severe state of malnutrition, is observed in 28%–54% of CHD patients [18,19]. Loss of skeletal muscle mass and strength predisposes CHD patients to frailty and substantially reduces their quality of life [20]. Furthermore, the decline in skeletal muscle mass and strength is associated with higher hospitalization and mortality rates in CHD patients [20–22]. As the duration of CHD treatment is associated with its detrimental effects on body composition, the improved survival rate of CHD patients will generate new challenges for healthcare [14]. This emphasizes the need to understand and counteract skeletal muscle mass and strength loss in CHD patients.

2. Muscle Maintenance

Skeletal muscle mass is regulated through a dynamic balance between continuous synthesis and breakdown of muscle proteins. The muscle protein pool has shown to possess a turnover rate of 1%–2% per day, allowing skeletal muscle tissue to adapt to circumstances such as changes in physical activity pattern (e.g., muscle hypertrophy following resistance-type exercise training) [23]. Ingesting several protein-containing meals throughout the day results in a sinusoidal pattern of subsequent increases and decreases in skeletal muscle protein synthesis and breakdown rates [24]. Skeletal muscle protein synthesis rates are high during post-prandial periods and low during post-absorptive periods, whilst skeletal muscle protein breakdown rates follow a reverse pattern. Muscle maintenance is achieved when skeletal muscle protein synthesis rates equal skeletal muscle protein breakdown rates over a given period.

Protein ingestion is an essential requirement to maintain skeletal muscle mass. After consumption, dietary protein is absorbed as amino acids in the intestine, with a large fraction being subsequently released into the circulation [25]. The release of amino acids into the circulation following protein ingestion elevates plasma amino acid concentrations for a post-prandial period of up to 5 h [26]. These circulating plasma amino acids serve as precursors for de novo synthesis of muscle protein [27]. However, amino acids are more than simply building blocks for muscle protein synthesis, as they can function as signaling molecules. The post-prandial increase in plasma essential amino acid concentrations, and leucine in particular, stimulates anabolic signaling through several molecular pathways, such as the mammalian target of rapamycin complex 1 (mTORC1) pathway [28,29]. This post-prandial anabolic signaling increases skeletal muscle protein synthesis rates and inhibits proteolysis, allowing net muscle protein accretion [27].

Muscle loss can be attributed both to an increase in muscle protein breakdown as well as to a decline in muscle protein synthesis rates. Previous work has reported increased muscle proteolysis in CHD patients due to inflammation, metabolic acidosis, and the dialysis procedure itself [30–33]. Furthermore, it has been suggested that the muscle protein synthetic response to feeding is impaired in patients with CKD [34]. Whereas a maximal post-prandial muscle protein synthetic response has been reported after ingesting up to 20 g of a high-quality protein in healthy young adults, a lesser response has been observed in older individuals [27,35,36]. More recently, van Vliet et al. were unable to detect a measurable increase in skeletal muscle protein synthesis rates in CHD patients following ingestion of a meal containing 20 g protein [37]. The latter suggests that CHD patients suffer from a blunted muscle protein synthetic response to feeding, a phenomenon that has been coined anabolic resistance. In healthy elderly individuals, it has been shown that the anabolic resistance of skeletal muscle tissue can be overcome through ingesting a greater amount of protein (at least 30 g of a high-quality protein) [38] and/or performing a bout of resistance-type exercise prior to feeding [39]. When tailored specific to CHD patients, these anabolic strategies may prove essential to attenuate or even prevent the accelerated loss of skeletal muscle mass and strength in ESRD patients undergoing HD.

3. Dietary Protein Intake in ESRD Patients on HD

For healthy young adults, the recommended dietary protein intake to achieve a net balance between muscle protein synthesis and breakdown rates has been set at 0.8 g protein/kg body weight/day by the World Health Organization [40,41]. This level of protein intake may not be sufficient to support muscle maintenance in CHD patients. According to the National Kidney Foundation K/DOQI Clinical Practice Guidelines, these patients are recommended to ingest >1.2 g protein/kg body weight/day [42–45]. However, CHD patients generally do not meet this recommended level of protein intake. Previous studies in this population have observed a dietary protein intake of 0.9–1.0 g protein/kg body weight/day [46–51]. Especially on dialysis days, factors such as time constraints and reduced appetite make it difficult for patients to consume ample dietary protein [52]. As a result, dietary protein intake in CHD patients has been reported to be ~0.8 g protein/kg body weight on dialysis days compared to ~1.0 g protein/kg body weight on non-dialysis days [50].

In addition to low protein intake, another factor compromises plasma amino acid availability on dialysis days. During HD, both metabolic waste products as well as circulating amino acids are able to diffuse through the semipermeable dialysis membrane [11]. The diffusion into the dialysate results in a considerable extraction of circulating amino acids throughout HD [30,53–56]. We have recently shown that during a single HD session, ~12 g amino acids are extracted from the circulation in CHD patients who ingest their habitual diet during HD [57]. This amount equals the quantity of amino acids that is released into the circulation following ingestion of a typical meal (containing 20–25 g protein). Loss of circulating amino acids causes a significant decline of plasma amino acid concentrations throughout HD [55,57]. Moreover, Ikizler et al. showed that in fasting CHD patients, plasma amino acid concentrations remain low for at least 2 h after cessation of HD [30]. The HD-induced decline in plasma amino acid concentrations has been shown to cause substantial catabolism of skeletal muscle tissue in fasted CHD patients [58,59]. The continuous extraction of amino acids throughout HD stimulates skeletal muscle tissue to release amino acids into the circulation [60,61]. This homeostatic process attenuates the decline in plasma amino acid concentrations and may prevent subsequent detrimental effects on organs that are necessary to sustain life [62]. In addition, the decline in plasma amino acid concentrations reduces the availability of precursors for de novo synthesis of muscle proteins during and following HD. To allow a muscle protein synthetic response during this period, the extraction of circulating amino acids should be compensated for through amino acid and/or protein administration.

Provision of protein-rich nutrition during HD is often recommended to increase dietary protein intake on dialysis days [63–66]. Ingestion of 40–60 g protein has been shown to prevent the HD-induced decline in plasma amino acid concentrations in multiple studies [58,59,67,68]. Furthermore, Pupim et al. demonstrated that ingestion of 57 g protein resulted in a positive forearm amino acid balance throughout HD [58]. Thus, HD-associated skeletal muscle catabolism may be prevented through ingestion of sufficient protein during HD. Several studies have also observed long-term beneficial effects of protein supplementation during HD, such as an increase in lean body mass, improvement in physical function, and decrease in mortality [69–71]. However, data from our lab [57] and others [56,67] indicate that protein ingestion during HD is also accompanied by an increase in amino acid extraction, presumably due to a higher subsequent plasma-dialysate diffusion gradient (Figure 1). Due to this extraction following protein ingestion during HD, less amino acids become available to stimulate muscle protein synthesis rates and serve as precursors for de novo synthesis of muscle protein. Considering the anabolic resistance of skeletal muscle tissue that is also present in this population, CHD patients will need to ingest well above 20 g high-quality protein during HD to allow a post-prandial increase in skeletal muscle protein synthesis and an inhibition of proteolysis.

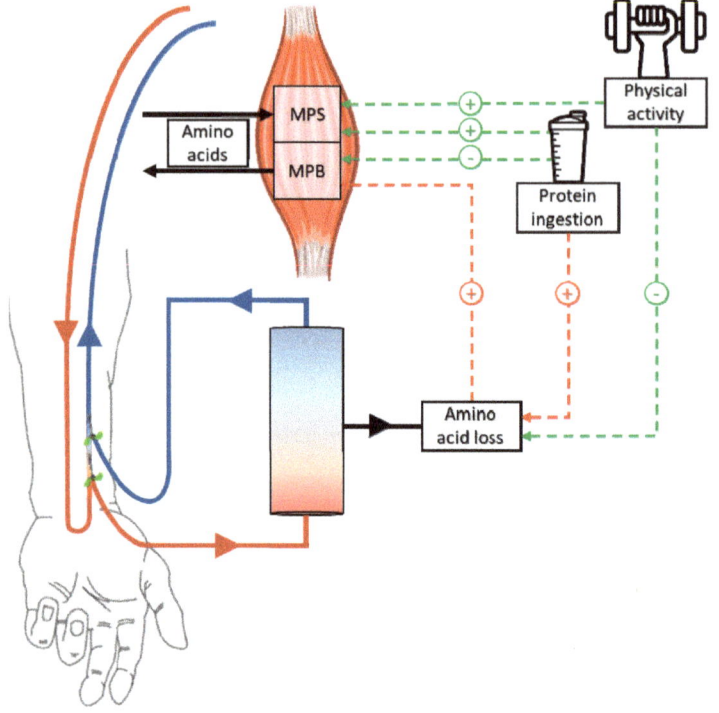

Figure 1. Conceptual overview of the effects of hemodialysis, protein ingestion, and physical activity on the muscle protein synthetic and proteolytic response. The extraction of amino acids during hemodialysis (HD) stimulates muscle protein breakdown (MPB) rates due to decreased plasma amino acid concentrations. Protein ingestion can maintain, or even increase, plasma amino acid concentrations throughout HD, which increases muscle protein synthesis (MPS) rates, while it may attenuate the HD-induced increase in MPB rates. However, elevated plasma amino acid concentrations also increase the amount of amino acids that are extracted during HD. Physical activity before or during HD may increase the use of plasma amino acids for de novo MPS, and thereby reduce the amount of amino acids that are extracted from the circulation during HD. Dashed lines in green represent processes that support muscle maintenance, whereas dashed lines in red represent processes that compromise muscle maintenance.

However, high quality (animal-derived) protein is rich in phosphorous [72]. In CHD patients, an increased dietary protein intake may lead to hyperphosphatemia or the need for phosphate binders. Furthermore, it has been suggested that an increased dietary protein intake in CHD patients provides more uremic toxin precursors and leads to higher uremic solute concentrations between HD sessions [73]. Recently, our laboratory has shown that the ingestion of branched-chain ketoacids, which contain no phosphorous or nitrogen, significantly stimulates skeletal muscle protein synthesis rates in healthy elderly individuals [74]. Ketoacid supplementation in CKD patients has been shown to reduce the generation of toxic metabolic waste products, while maintaining a good nutritional status [75]. However, it remains to be established whether ketoacid supplementation could support muscle maintenance in CHD patients.

4. Physical Activity in ESRD Patients on HD

Another key component for muscle maintenance is physical activity. Physical activity and exercise stimulate skeletal muscle protein synthesis rates, with post-absorptive muscle protein synthesis rates being elevated for up to 24 or even 48 h [76,77]. Furthermore, physical activity performed prior to food intake augments the post-prandial muscle protein synthetic response to feeding [78–81]. In contrast, a decline in physical activity reduces the muscle protein synthetic response to feeding [82–84]. In other words, whereas physical activity makes skeletal muscle tissue more sensitive to the anabolic properties of amino acids, muscle disuse leads to anabolic resistance of skeletal muscle tissue [85]. In support, daily exercise has been shown to increase skeletal muscle protein synthesis rates throughout the day [86], while a decline in physical activity has been shown to lower daily muscle protein synthesis rates [87]. Consequently, ample physical activity has been associated with a reduced age-related loss of muscle mass and strength [88,89], whereas a decline in the level of physical activity (e.g., during bed rest or limb immobilization) has been shown to induce a rapid decline in muscle mass and strength [90,91].

According to the Physical Activity Guidelines for Americans, patients with chronic diseases should follow the key physical activity guidelines for healthy adults to achieve substantial health benefits [92]. These guidelines recommend patients to perform at least 150–300 min per week of moderate-intensity aerobic exercise, 75–150 min of vigorous-intensity aerobic exercise per week, or an equivalent combination of both. In addition, muscle-strengthening activities that involve all major muscle groups should be performed at least twice per week. However, these guidelines do not contain specific recommendations for CHD patients. The Renal Association Clinical Practice Guideline on Hemodialysis recommends that all CHD patients without contraindication should perform at least 30 min of supervised moderate-intensity exercise during every dialysis session [93]. In addition, the guideline states that CHD patients should be encouraged to undertake physical activity on non-dialysis days. In line with this recommendation, it has recently been suggested that mortality rates are reduced in CHD patients who perform at least 4000 steps on non-dialysis days [94].

However, CHD patients typically adopt a sedentary lifestyle and spend less time being physically active than healthy adults [95,96]. In the United States, almost 50% of CHD patients perform exercise once or less than once per week [96]. A HD session represents a long (3–4 h) sedentary period, which often hinders CHD patients to engage in physical activity and, as such, dialysis treatments contribute to the lower physical activity levels [97,98]. Gomes et al. observed that CHD patients took 4362 ± 2084 and 7007 ± 3437 steps on dialysis and non-dialysis days, respectively, compared to 8792 ± 2870 steps taken by age-matched healthy controls [98]. The low habitual physical activity level in these patients is another key factor responsible for the accelerated loss of muscle mass and strength in CHD patients [17]. Interventions in CHD patients targeted to preserve or even increase muscle mass should not only provide nutritional support but also increase physical activity levels to maximize their impact.

5. Interventions to Support Muscle Maintenance in ESRD Patients on HD

Physical activity interventions for CHD patients may implement exercise during HD (intradialytic) or between HD sessions (interdialytic). A recent meta-analysis by Clarckson et al. reported no differences in the efficacy of intradialytic when compared with interdialytic exercise on improvements of physical function in CHD patients [99]. Due to exercise intolerance, CHD patients typically show low adherence and poor compliance to long-term unsupervised physical activity intervention programs [100]. HD sessions represent an opportunity to integrate supervised physical activity in the weekly routine of CHD patients. Intradialytic physical activity is considered safe and shows greater adherence rates than interdialytic physical activity [100–102]. Furthermore, supervision of intradialytic exercise sessions provides the opportunity to prescribe a patient-specific and progressive exercise program. Physical activity during HD has some limitations compared to interdialytic physical activity, such as constrains regarding exercise intensity and upper limb exercises. On the other hand, intradialytic physical activity provides distraction for CHD patients during their treatment and has been shown to improve their quality of life [101]. Therefore, we would advocate the implementation of an intradialytic exercise program in lifestyle interventions designed for (sedentary) CHD patients.

In addition to timing, the type of exercise is an important determinant of its potential to support muscle maintenance. Resistance-type exercise training is considered most potent to augment muscle mass and strength. In healthy adults, resistance-type exercise training has been shown to induce a robust increase in both skeletal muscle mass as well as strength [103–105]. Furthermore, resistance-type exercise also sensitizes skeletal muscle tissue to the anabolic properties of amino acids and, as such, increases the post-prandial muscle protein synthetic response to feeding [78,79,81]. In support, it has been reported that a single bout of resistance-type exercise performed prior to HD increases amino acid uptake by muscle tissue following intradialytic protein ingestion [106]. Intradialytic resistance-type exercise programs have shown to increase skeletal muscle strength, thereby improving physical function outcome measures such as the 6-min walk test [99,107–110]. In a systematic review of nine trials that assessed progressive resistance-type exercise training in ESRD patients on HD, Chan and Cheema concluded that resistance-type exercise training can effectively induce regional skeletal muscle hypertrophy [111]. However, due to inconsistent results of previous studies [69,112–118], it remains unclear whether resistance-type exercise can increase skeletal muscle mass on a whole-body level in CHD patients.

Protein ingestion during recovery from resistance-type exercise is required to achieve a positive net protein balance and, as such, to allow net muscle protein accretion [76]. Due to practical matters, the majority of studies that assessed the impact of resistance-type exercise training in CHD patients implemented their training sessions before or during HD [119]. As circulating amino acids are extracted during HD, recovery from those exercise sessions typically occurred during conditions of reduced amino acid availability. This may have attenuated the anabolic effects of the exercise training programs. Furthermore, the combination of amino acid extraction during HD and the anabolic resistance of skeletal muscle tissue in CHD patients likely increases the amount of protein that is required following intradialytic resistance-type exercise. We suggest that at least 30 g protein should be provided to CHD patients during recovery from resistance-type exercise performed immediately prior or during HD to allow a muscle protein synthetic response.

Besides protein ingestion during recovery from exercise, it has been advocated that every main meal (breakfast, lunch, and dinner) should contain 20 g high-quality protein to optimally stimulate muscle protein synthesis rates throughout the day [120,121]. We suggest that CHD patients should ingest well above 20 g high-quality protein per main meal to compensate for the blunted muscle protein synthetic response to feeding, recognizing that additional measures to prevent hyperphosphatemia might be necessary. In addition, ingesting a protein-rich snack prior to sleep, especially on training days, may further support muscle mass maintenance [24]. Though the impact of these nutritional strategies has not been assessed in CHD patients, they would likely be supplemental in the prevention of protein malnutrition in this population. Effectiveness of any nutritional intervention largely depends on long-term adherence and compliance. However, adherence to dietary interventions in CHD patients is often poor due to barriers such as dialysis time, motivation, and lack of social support [122]. Therefore, CHD patients should be advised on protein options that are easy to prepare, convenient to consume, and have an acceptable taste.

A well-orchestrated lifestyle intervention program combining exercise and nutritional interventions for CHD patients is required to attenuate or even prevent the loss of muscle mass, strength, and functional capacity in this population. For such a multimodal interventional approach to be effective, a (more) personalized supervision of CHD patients provided by a team of healthcare specialists with physical activity and nutritional expertise is required. A close collaboration between nephrologists, physical therapists, and dietitians in both research and clinical care will be essential to improve the health and well-being of the growing number of CHD patients.

6. Conclusions

The gradual loss of skeletal muscle mass in CHD patients accelerates after initiation of intermittent HD treatment. Muscle protein breakdown rates in CHD patients are increased, while muscle protein synthesis rates fail to match this increase due to insufficient protein ingestion, amino acid extraction during HD, and the prevalence of anabolic resistance. Protein intake of CHD patients should be increased on dialysis days to compensate for extraction of circulating amino acids during HD and to compensate for the blunted muscle protein synthetic response to feeding in these patients. Implementing structured physical activity in the daily routine of CHD patients represents a feasible strategy to increase the skeletal muscle protein synthetic response to protein ingestion and, as such, to alleviate anabolic resistance. More insight in the impact of protein ingestion and exercise in CHD patients on both dialysis as well as non-dialysis days is required to develop more effective nutritional and exercise intervention programs that can attenuate or even prevent muscle loss in CHD patients.

Author Contributions: Writing—original draft preparation, F.K.H. and L.J.C.v.L.; writing—review and editing, J.S.J.S., F.M.v.d.S., and J.P.K., All authors read and approved the final manuscript.

Funding: This work was supported by a grant from the NUTRIM NWO Graduate Programme.

Conflicts of Interest: The authors declare no conflicts of interest. The funders had no role in the writing of the manuscript or in the decision to publish.

References

1. Mortality, G.B.D. Catrgory: Causes of Death. Global, regional, and national life expectancy, all-cause mortality, and cause-specific mortality for 249 causes of death, 1980–2015: A systematic analysis for the Global Burden of Disease Study 2015. *Lancet* **2016**, *388*, 1459–1544. [CrossRef]
2. Dalys, G.B.D.; Collaborators, H.; Murray, C.J.; Barber, R.M.; Foreman, K.J.; Abbasoglu Ozgoren, A.; Abd-Allah, F.; Abera, S.F.; Aboyans, V.; Abraham, J.P.; et al. Global, regional, and national disability-adjusted life years (DALYs) for 306 diseases and injuries and healthy life expectancy (HALE) for 188 countries, 1990-2013: Quantifying the epidemiological transition. *Lancet* **2015**, *386*, 2145–2191. [CrossRef]
3. Gansevoort, R.T.; Correa-Rotter, R.; Hemmelgarn, B.R.; Jafar, T.H.; Heerspink, H.J.L.; Mann, J.F.; Matsushita, K.; Wen, C.P. Chronic kidney disease and cardiovascular risk: Epidemiology, mechanisms, and prevention. *Lancet* **2013**, *382*, 339–352. [CrossRef]
4. Hill, N.R.; Fatoba, S.T.; Oke, J.L.; Hirst, J.A.; O'Callaghan, C.A.; Lasserson, D.S.; Hobbs, F.D. Global Prevalence of Chronic Kidney Disease-A Systematic Review and Meta-Analysis. *PLoS ONE* **2016**, *11*, e0158765. [CrossRef] [PubMed]
5. Webster, A.C.; Nagler, E.V.; Morton, R.L.; Masson, P. Chronic Kidney Disease. *Lancet* **2017**, *389*, 1238–1252. [CrossRef]
6. Van Oostrom, S.H.; Gijsen, R.; Stirbu, I.; Korevaar, J.C.; Schellevis, F.G.; Picavet, H.S.; Hoeymans, N. Time Trends in Prevalence of Chronic Diseases and Multimorbidity Not Only due to Aging: Data from General Practices and Health Surveys. *PLoS ONE* **2016**, *11*, e0160264. [CrossRef]
7. Tonelli, M.; Riella, M. Chronic kidney disease and the ageing population. *Nephron Clin. Pract.* **2014**, *128*, 319–322. [CrossRef]
8. Levey, A.S.; Eckardt, K.U.; Tsukamoto, Y.; Levin, A.; Coresh, J.; Rossert, J.; De Zeeuw, D.; Hostetter, T.H.; Lameire, N.; Eknoyan, G. Definition and classification of chronic kidney disease: A position statement from Kidney Disease: Improving Global Outcomes (KDIGO). *Kidney Int.* **2005**, *67*, 2089–2100. [CrossRef]
9. Agarwal, R. Defining end-stage renal disease in clinical trials: A framework for adjudication. *Nephrol. Dial. Transplant.* **2016**, *31*, 864–867. [CrossRef]
10. Kooman, J.P.; Kotanko, P.; Schols, A.M.; Shiels, P.G.; Stenvinkel, P. Chronic kidney disease and premature ageing. *Nat. Rev. Nephrol.* **2014**, *10*, 732–742. [CrossRef]
11. Himmelfarb, J.; Ikizler, T.A. Hemodialysis. *N. Engl. J. Med.* **2010**, *363*, 1833–1845. [CrossRef] [PubMed]
12. Fleming, G.M. Renal replacement therapy review. *Organogenesis* **2014**, *7*, 2–12. [CrossRef] [PubMed]
13. Marshall, M.R.; Polkinghorne, K.R.; Kerr, P.G.; Agar, J.W.; Hawley, C.M.; McDonald, S.P. Temporal Changes in Mortality Risk by Dialysis Modality in the Australian and New Zealand Dialysis Population. *Am. J. Kidney Dis.* **2015**, *66*, 489–498. [CrossRef] [PubMed]
14. Marcelli, D.; Brand, K.; Ponce, P.; Milkowski, A.; Marelli, C.; Ok, E.; Merello Godino, J.I.; Gurevich, K.; Jirka, T.; Rosenberger, J.; et al. Longitudinal Changes in Body Composition in Patients After Initiation of Hemodialysis Therapy: Results from an International Cohort. *J. Ren. Nutr.* **2016**, *26*, 72–80. [CrossRef] [PubMed]

15. Spiegel, B.M.; Melmed, G.; Robbins, S.; Esrailian, E. Biomarkers and health-related quality of life in end-stage renal disease: A systematic review. *Clin. J. Am. Soc. Nephrol.* **2008**, *3*, 1759–1768. [CrossRef]
16. Kurella Tamura, M.; Covinsky, K.E.; Chertow, G.M.; Yaffe, K.; Landefeld, C.S.; McCulloch, C.E. Functional status of elderly adults before and after initiation of dialysis. *N. Engl. J. Med.* **2009**, *361*, 1539–1547. [CrossRef]
17. Johansen, K.L.; Shubert, T.; Doyle, J.; Soher, B.; Sakkas, G.K.; Kent-Braun, J.A. Muscle atrophy in patients receiving hemodialysis: Effects on muscle strength, muscle quality, and physical function. *Kidney Int.* **2003**, *63*, 291–297. [CrossRef]
18. Carrero, J.J.; Thomas, F.; Nagy, K.; Arogundade, F.; Avesani, C.M.; Chan, M.; Chmielewski, M.; Cordeiro, A.C.; Espinosa-Cuevas, A.; Fiaccadori, E.; et al. Global Prevalence of Protein-Energy Wasting in Kidney Disease: A Meta-analysis of Contemporary Observational Studies From the International Society of Renal Nutrition and Metabolism. *J. Ren. Nutr.* **2018**, *28*, 380–392. [CrossRef]
19. Fouque, D.; Kalantar-Zadeh, K.; Kopple, J.; Cano, N.; Chauveau, P.; Cuppari, L.; Franch, H.; Guarnieri, G.; Ikizler, T.A.; Kaysen, G.; et al. A proposed nomenclature and diagnostic criteria for protein-energy wasting in acute and chronic kidney disease. *Kidney Int.* **2008**, *73*, 391–398. [CrossRef]
20. Broers, N.J.; Usvyat, L.A.; Kooman, J.P.; van der Sande, F.M.; Lacson, E., Jr.; Kotanko, P.; Maddux, F.W. Quality of Life in Dialysis Patients: A Retrospective Cohort Study. *Nephron* **2015**, *130*, 105–112. [CrossRef]
21. Isoyama, N.; Qureshi, A.R.; Avesani, C.M.; Lindholm, B.; Barany, P.; Heimburger, O.; Cederholm, T.; Stenvinkel, P.; Carrero, J.J. Comparative associations of muscle mass and muscle strength with mortality in dialysis patients. *Clin. J. Am. Soc. Nephrol.* **2014**, *9*, 1720–1728. [CrossRef] [PubMed]
22. Borges, M.C.; Vogt, B.P.; Martin, L.C.; Caramori, J.C. Malnutrition Inflammation Score cut-off predicting mortality in maintenance hemodialysis patients. *Clin. Nutr. ESPEN* **2017**, *17*, 63–67. [CrossRef] [PubMed]
23. Mamerow, M.M.; Mettler, J.A.; English, K.L.; Casperson, S.L.; Arentson-Lantz, E.; Sheffield-Moore, M.; Layman, D.K.; Paddon-Jones, D. Dietary protein distribution positively influences 24-h muscle protein synthesis in healthy adults. *J. Nutr.* **2014**, *144*, 876–880. [CrossRef] [PubMed]
24. Trommelen, J.; van Loon, L.J. Pre-Sleep Protein Ingestion to Improve the Skeletal Muscle Adaptive Response to Exercise Training. *Nutrients* **2016**, *8*, 763. [CrossRef] [PubMed]
25. Groen, B.B.; Horstman, A.M.; Hamer, H.M.; de Haan, M.; van Kranenburg, J.; Bierau, J.; Poeze, M.; Wodzig, W.K.; Rasmussen, B.B.; van Loon, L.J. Post-Prandial Protein Handling: You Are What You Just Ate. *PLoS ONE* **2015**, *10*, e0141582. [CrossRef] [PubMed]
26. Kouw, I.W.; Gorissen, S.H.; Burd, N.A.; Cermak, N.M.; Gijsen, A.P.; van Kranenburg, J.; van Loon, L.J. Postprandial Protein Handling Is Not Impaired in Type 2 Diabetes Patients When Compared with Normoglycemic Controls. *J. Clin. Endocrinol. Metab.* **2015**, *100*, 3103–3111. [CrossRef]
27. Wall, B.T.; Gorissen, S.H.; Pennings, B.; Koopman, R.; Groen, B.B.; Verdijk, L.B.; van Loon, L.J. Aging Is Accompanied by a Blunted Muscle Protein Synthetic Response to Protein Ingestion. *PLoS ONE* **2015**, *10*, e0140903. [CrossRef]
28. Bohe, J.; Low, A.; Wolfe, R.R.; Rennie, M.J. Human muscle protein synthesis is modulated by extracellular, not intramuscular amino acid availability: A dose-response study. *J. Physiol.* **2003**, *552*, 315–324. [CrossRef]
29. Rieu, I.; Balage, M.; Sornet, C.; Giraudet, C.; Pujos, E.; Grizard, J.; Mosoni, L.; Dardevet, D. Leucine supplementation improves muscle protein synthesis in elderly men independently of hyperaminoacidaemia. *J. Physiol.* **2006**, *575*, 305–315. [CrossRef]
30. Ikizler, T.A.; Pupim, L.B.; Brouillette, J.R.; Levenhagen, D.K.; Farmer, K.; Hakim, R.M.; Flakoll, P.J. Hemodialysis stimulates muscle and whole body protein loss and alters substrate oxidation. *Am. J. Physiol. Endocrinol. Metab.* **2002**, *282*, E107–E116. [CrossRef]
31. Wang, X.H.; Mitch, W.E. Mechanisms of muscle wasting in chronic kidney disease. *Nat. Rev. Nephrol.* **2014**, *10*, 504–516. [CrossRef] [PubMed]
32. Kooman, J.P.; Dekker, M.J.; Usvyat, L.A.; Kotanko, P.; van der Sande, F.M.; Schalkwijk, C.G.; Shiels, P.G.; Stenvinkel, P. Inflammation and premature aging in advanced chronic kidney disease. *Am. J. Physiol. Ren. Physiol.* **2017**, *313*, F938–F950. [CrossRef] [PubMed]
33. Lofberg, E.; Gutierrez, A.; Anderstam, B.; Wernerman, J.; Bergstrom, J.; Price, S.R.; Mitch, W.E.; Alvestrand, A. Effect of bicarbonate on muscle protein in patients receiving hemodialysis. *Am. J. Kidney Dis.* **2006**, *48*, 419–429. [CrossRef] [PubMed]
34. Garibotto, G. Muscle amino acid metabolism and the control of muscle protein turnover in patients with chronic renal failure. *Nutrition* **1999**, *15*, 145–155. [CrossRef]

35. Cuthbertson, D.; Smith, K.; Babraj, J.; Leese, G.; Waddell, T.; Atherton, P.; Wackerhage, H.; Taylor, P.M.; Rennie, M.J. Anabolic signaling deficits underlie amino acid resistance of wasting, aging muscle. *FASEB J.* **2005**, *19*, 422–424. [CrossRef]
36. Morton, R.W.; McGlory, C.; Phillips, S.M. Nutritional interventions to augment resistance training-induced skeletal muscle hypertrophy. *Front. Physiol.* **2015**, *6*, 245. [CrossRef]
37. Van Vliet, S.; Skinner, S.K.; Beals, J.W.; Pagni, B.A.; Fang, H.Y.; Ulanov, A.V.; Li, Z.; Paluska, S.A.; Mazzulla, M.; West, D.W.D.; et al. Dysregulated Handling of Dietary Protein and Muscle Protein Synthesis After Mixed-Meal Ingestion in Maintenance Hemodialysis Patients. *Kidney Int. Rep.* **2018**, *3*, 1403–1415. [CrossRef]
38. Pennings, B.; Groen, B.; de Lange, A.; Gijsen, A.P.; Zorenc, A.H.; Senden, J.M.; van Loon, L.J. Amino acid absorption and subsequent muscle protein accretion following graded intakes of whey protein in elderly men. *Am. J. Physiol. Endocrinol. Metab.* **2012**, *302*, E992–E999. [CrossRef]
39. Yang, Y.; Breen, L.; Burd, N.A.; Hector, A.J.; Churchward-Venne, T.A.; Josse, A.R.; Tarnopolsky, M.A.; Phillips, S.M. Resistance exercise enhances myofibrillar protein synthesis with graded intakes of whey protein in older men. *Br. J. Nutr.* **2012**, *108*, 1780–1788. [CrossRef]
40. World Health Organization; Food and Agriculture Organization of the United Nations; United Nations University. *Protein and Amino Acid Requirements in Human Nutrition*; World Health Organization: Geneva, Switzerland, 2007.
41. Rand, W.M.; Pellett, P.L.; Young, V.R. Meta-analysis of nitrogen balance studies for estimating protein requirements in healthy adults. *Am. J. Clin. Nutr.* **2003**, *77*, 109–127. [CrossRef] [PubMed]
42. Borah, M.F.; Schoenfeld, P.Y.; Gotch, F.A.; Sargent, J.A.; Wolfson, M.; Humphreys, M.H. Nitrogen balance during intermittent dialysis therapy of uremia. *Kidney Int.* **1978**, *14*, 491–500. [CrossRef] [PubMed]
43. Rao, M.; Sharma, M.; Juneja, R.; Jacob, S.; Jacob, C.K. Calculated nitrogen balance in hemodialysis patients: Influence of protein intake. *Kidney Int.* **2000**, *58*, 336–345. [CrossRef] [PubMed]
44. Kopple, J.D. National Kidney Foundation K/DOQI Clinical Practice Guidelines for Nutrition in Chronic Renal Failure. *Am. J. Kidney Dis.* **2001**, *37*, S66–S70. [CrossRef] [PubMed]
45. Fouque, D.; Vennegoor, M.; ter Wee, P.; Wanner, C.; Basci, A.; Canaud, B.; Haage, P.; Konner, K.; Kooman, J.; Martin-Malo, A.; et al. EBPG guideline on nutrition. *Nephrol. Dial. Transplant.* **2007**, *22* (Suppl. 2), ii45–ii87. [CrossRef]
46. Burrowes, J.D.; Larive, B.; Cockram, D.B.; Dwyer, J.; Kusek, J.W.; McLeroy, S.; Poole, D.; Rocco, M.V.; Hemodialysis Study, G. Effects of dietary intake, appetite, and eating habits on dialysis and non-dialysis treatment days in hemodialysis patients: Cross-sectional results from the HEMO study. *J. Ren. Nutr.* **2003**, *13*, 191–198. [CrossRef]
47. Kalantar-Zadeh, K.; Kopple, J.D.; Deepak, S.; Block, D.; Block, G. Food intake characteristics of hemodialysis patients as obtained by food frequency questionnaire. *J. Ren. Nutr.* **2002**, *12*, 17–31. [CrossRef]
48. Lorenzo, V.; de Bonis, E.; Rufino, M.; Hernandez, D.; Rebollo, S.G.; Rodriguez, A.P.; Torres, A. Caloric rather than protein deficiency predominates in stable chronic haemodialysis patients. *Nephrol. Dial. Transplant.* **1995**, *10*, 1885–1889.
49. Wolfson, M.; Strong, C.J.; Minturn, D.; Gray, D.K.; Kopple, J.D. Nutritional status and lymphocyte function in maintenance hemodialysis patients. *Am. J. Clin. Nutr.* **1984**, *39*, 547–555. [CrossRef]
50. Martins, A.M.; Dias Rodrigues, J.C.; de Oliveira Santin, F.G.; Barbosa Brito Fdos, S.; Bello Moreira, A.S.; Lourenco, R.A.; Avesani, C.M. Food intake assessment of elderly patients on hemodialysis. *J. Ren. Nutr.* **2015**, *25*, 321–326. [CrossRef]
51. Bossola, M.; Leo, A.; Viola, A.; Carlomagno, G.; Monteburini, T.; Cenerelli, S.; Santarelli, S.; Boggi, R.; Miggiano, G.; Vulpio, C.; et al. Dietary intake of macronutrients and fiber in Mediterranean patients on chronic hemodialysis. *J. Nephrol.* **2013**, *26*, 912–918. [CrossRef] [PubMed]
52. Clark-Cutaia, M.N.; Sevick, M.A.; Thurheimer-Cacciotti, J.; Hoffman, L.A.; Snetselaar, L.; Burke, L.E.; Zickmund, S.L. Perceived Barriers to Adherence to Hemodialysis Dietary Recommendations. *Clin. Nurs. Res.* **2018**. [CrossRef] [PubMed]
53. Alp Ikizler, T.; Flakoll, P.J.; Parker, R.A.; Hakim, R.M. Amino acid and albumin losses during hemodialysis. *Kidney Int.* **1994**, *46*, 830–837. [CrossRef] [PubMed]
54. Yokomatsu, A.; Fujikawa, T.; Toya, Y.; Shino-Kakimoto, M.; Itoh, Y.; Mitsuhashi, H.; Tamura, K.; Hirawa, N.; Yasuda, G.; Umemura, S. Loss of amino acids into dialysate during hemodialysis using hydrophilic and

nonhydrophilic polyester-polymer alloy and polyacrylonitrile membrane dialyzers. *Ther. Apher. Dial.* **2014**, *18*, 340–346. [CrossRef]
55. Navarro, J.F.; Marcen, R.; Teruel, J.L.; Martin del Rio, R.; Gamez, C.; Mora, C.; Ortuno, J. Effect of different membranes on amino-acid losses during haemodialysis. *Nephrol. Dial. Transplant.* **1998**, *13*, 113–117. [CrossRef]
56. Wolfson, M.; Jones, M.R.; Kopple, J.D. Amino acid losses during hemodialysis with infusion of amino acids and glucose. *Kidney Int.* **1982**, *21*, 500–506. [CrossRef]
57. Hendriks, F.K.; Smeets, J.S.J.; Broers, N.J.H.; Van Kranenburg, J.M.X.; Sande, F.M.; Kooman, J.P.; Van Loon, L.J.C. Amino acid loss during hemodialysis in end-stage renal disease patients. *Clin. Nutr.* **2018**, *37*, S96. [CrossRef]
58. Pupim, L.B.; Majchrzak, K.M.; Flakoll, P.J.; Ikizler, T.A. Intradialytic oral nutrition improves protein homeostasis in chronic hemodialysis patients with deranged nutritional status. *J. Am. Soc. Nephrol.* **2006**, *17*, 3149–3157. [CrossRef]
59. Pupim, L.B.; Flakoll, P.J.; Brouillette, J.R.; Levenhagen, D.K.; Hakim, R.M.; Ikizler, T.A. Intradialytic parenteral nutrition improves protein and energy homeostasis in chronic hemodialysis patients. *J. Clin. Investig.* **2002**, *110*, 483–492. [CrossRef]
60. Frontera, W.R.; Ochala, J. Skeletal muscle: A brief review of structure and function. *Calcif. Tissue Int.* **2015**, *96*, 183–195. [CrossRef]
61. Raj, D.S.; Adeniyi, O.; Dominic, E.A.; Boivin, M.A.; McClelland, S.; Tzamaloukas, A.H.; Morgan, N.; Gonzales, L.; Wolfe, R.; Ferrando, A. Amino acid repletion does not decrease muscle protein catabolism during hemodialysis. *Am. J. Physiol. Endocrinol. Metab.* **2007**, *292*, E1534–E1542. [CrossRef] [PubMed]
62. Lim, V.S.; Ikizler, T.A.; Raj, D.S.; Flanigan, M.J. Does hemodialysis increase protein breakdown? Dissociation between whole-body amino acid turnover and regional muscle kinetics. *J. Am. Soc. Nephrol.* **2005**, *16*, 862–868. [CrossRef] [PubMed]
63. Ikizler, T.A.; Cano, N.J.; Franch, H.; Fouque, D.; Himmelfarb, J.; Kalantar-Zadeh, K.; Kuhlmann, M.K.; Stenvinkel, P.; TerWee, P.; Teta, D.; et al. Prevention and treatment of protein energy wasting in chronic kidney disease patients: A consensus statement by the International Society of Renal Nutrition and Metabolism. *Kidney Int.* **2013**, *84*, 1096–1107. [CrossRef] [PubMed]
64. Kalantar-Zadeh, K.; Ikizler, T.A. Let them eat during dialysis: An overlooked opportunity to improve outcomes in maintenance hemodialysis patients. *J. Ren. Nutr.* **2013**, *23*, 157–163. [CrossRef]
65. Kistler, B.M.; Benner, D.; Burrowes, J.D.; Campbell, K.L.; Fouque, D.; Garibotto, G.; Kopple, J.D.; Kovesdy, C.P.; Rhee, C.M.; Steiber, A.; et al. Eating During Hemodialysis Treatment: A Consensus Statement from the International Society of Renal Nutrition and Metabolism. *J. Ren. Nutr.* **2018**, *28*, 4–12. [CrossRef] [PubMed]
66. Sabatino, A.; Regolisti, G.; Karupaiah, T.; Sahathevan, S.; Sadu Singh, B.K.; Khor, B.H.; Salhab, N.; Karavetian, M.; Cupisti, A.; Fiaccadori, E. Protein-energy wasting and nutritional supplementation in patients with end-stage renal disease on hemodialysis. *Clin. Nutr.* **2017**, *36*, 663–671. [CrossRef]
67. Veeneman, J.M.; Kingma, H.A.; Boer, T.S.; Stellaard, F.; De Jong, P.E.; Reijngoud, D.J.; Huisman, R.M. Protein intake during hemodialysis maintains a positive whole body protein balance in chronic hemodialysis patients. *Am. J. Physiol. Endocrinol. Metab.* **2003**, *284*, E954–E965. [CrossRef]
68. Sundell, M.B.; Cavanaugh, K.L.; Wu, P.; Shintani, A.; Hakim, R.M.; Ikizler, T.A. Oral protein supplementation alone improves anabolism in a dose-dependent manner in chronic hemodialysis patients. *J. Ren. Nutr.* **2009**, *19*, 412–421. [CrossRef]
69. Dong, J.; Sundell, M.B.; Pupim, L.B.; Wu, P.; Shintani, A.; Ikizler, T.A. The effect of resistance exercise to augment long-term benefits of intradialytic oral nutritional supplementation in chronic hemodialysis patients. *J. Ren. Nutr.* **2011**, *21*, 149–159. [CrossRef]
70. Weiner, D.E.; Tighiouart, H.; Ladik, V.; Meyer, K.B.; Zager, P.G.; Johnson, D.S. Oral intradialytic nutritional supplement use and mortality in hemodialysis patients. *Am. J. Kidney Dis.* **2014**, *63*, 276–285. [CrossRef]
71. Tomayko, E.J.; Kistler, B.M.; Fitschen, P.J.; Wilund, K.R. Intradialytic protein supplementation reduces inflammation and improves physical function in maintenance hemodialysis patients. *J. Ren. Nutr.* **2015**, *25*, 276–283. [CrossRef] [PubMed]
72. Kalantar-Zadeh, K.; Gutekunst, L.; Mehrotra, R.; Kovesdy, C.P.; Bross, R.; Shinaberger, C.S.; Noori, N.; Hirschberg, R.; Benner, D.; Nissenson, A.R.; et al. Understanding sources of dietary phosphorus in the

treatment of patients with chronic kidney disease. *Clin. J. Am. Soc. Nephrol.* **2010**, *5*, 519–530. [CrossRef] [PubMed]

73. Eloot, S.; Van Biesen, W.; Glorieux, G.; Neirynck, N.; Dhondt, A.; Vanholder, R. Does the adequacy parameter Kt/V (urea) reflect uremic toxin concentrations in hemodialysis patients? *PLoS ONE* **2013**, *8*, e76838. [CrossRef] [PubMed]

74. Fuchs, C.J.; Hermans, W.J.H.; Holwerda, A.M.; Smeets, J.S.J.; Senden, J.M.; van Kranenburg, J.; Gijsen, A.P.; Wodzig, W.K.H.W.; Schierbeek, H.; Verdijk, L.B.; et al. Branched-chain amino acid and branched-chain ketoacid ingestion increases muscle protein synthesis rates in vivo in older adults: A double-blind, randomized trial. *Am. J. Clin. Nutr.* **2019**, *110*, 862–872. [CrossRef] [PubMed]

75. Shah, A.P.; Kalantar-Zadeh, K.; Kopple, J.D. Is there a role for ketoacid supplements in the management of CKD? *Am. J. Kidney Dis.* **2015**, *65*, 659–673. [CrossRef] [PubMed]

76. Phillips, S.M.; Tipton, K.D.; Aarsland, A.; Wolf, S.E.; Wolfe, R.R. Mixed muscle protein synthesis and breakdown after resistance exercise in humans. *Am. J. Physiol.* **1997**, *273*, E99–E107. [CrossRef]

77. Biolo, G.; Maggi, S.P.; Williams, B.D.; Tipton, K.D.; Wolfe, R.R. Increased rates of muscle protein turnover and amino acid transport after resistance exercise in humans. *Am. J. Physiol.* **1995**, *268*, E514–E520. [CrossRef]

78. Burd, N.A.; West, D.W.; Moore, D.R.; Atherton, P.J.; Staples, A.W.; Prior, T.; Tang, J.E.; Rennie, M.J.; Baker, S.K.; Phillips, S.M. Enhanced amino acid sensitivity of myofibrillar protein synthesis persists for up to 24 h after resistance exercise in young men. *J. Nutr.* **2011**, *141*, 568–573. [CrossRef]

79. Trommelen, J.; Holwerda, A.M.; Kouw, I.W.; Langer, H.; Halson, S.L.; Rollo, I.; Verdijk, L.B.; LJ, V.A.N.L. Resistance Exercise Augments Postprandial Overnight Muscle Protein Synthesis Rates. *Med. Sci. Sports Exerc.* **2016**, *48*, 2517–2525. [CrossRef]

80. Pennings, B.; Koopman, R.; Beelen, M.; Senden, J.M.; Saris, W.H.; van Loon, L.J. Exercising before protein intake allows for greater use of dietary protein-derived amino acids for de novo muscle protein synthesis in both young and elderly men. *Am. J. Clin. Nutr.* **2011**, *93*, 322–331. [CrossRef]

81. Holwerda, A.M.; Kouw, I.W.; Trommelen, J.; Halson, S.L.; Wodzig, W.K.; Verdijk, L.B.; van Loon, L.J. Physical Activity Performed in the Evening Increases the Overnight Muscle Protein Synthetic Response to Presleep Protein Ingestion in Older Men. *J. Nutr.* **2016**, *146*, 1307–1314. [CrossRef] [PubMed]

82. Glover, E.I.; Phillips, S.M.; Oates, B.R.; Tang, J.E.; Tarnopolsky, M.A.; Selby, A.; Smith, K.; Rennie, M.J. Immobilization induces anabolic resistance in human myofibrillar protein synthesis with low and high dose amino acid infusion. *J. Physiol.* **2008**, *586*, 6049–6061. [CrossRef] [PubMed]

83. Wall, B.T.; Dirks, M.L.; Snijders, T.; van Dijk, J.W.; Fritsch, M.; Verdijk, L.B.; van Loon, L.J. Short-term muscle disuse lowers myofibrillar protein synthesis rates and induces anabolic resistance to protein ingestion. *Am. J. Physiol. Endocrinol. Metab.* **2016**, *310*, E137–E147. [CrossRef] [PubMed]

84. Breen, L.; Stokes, K.A.; Churchward-Venne, T.A.; Moore, D.R.; Baker, S.K.; Smith, K.; Atherton, P.J.; Phillips, S.M. Two weeks of reduced activity decreases leg lean mass and induces "anabolic resistance" of myofibrillar protein synthesis in healthy elderly. *J. Clin. Endocrinol. Metab.* **2013**, *98*, 2604–2612. [CrossRef] [PubMed]

85. Dideriksen, K.; Reitelseder, S.; Holm, L. Influence of amino acids, dietary protein, and physical activity on muscle mass development in humans. *Nutrients* **2013**, *5*, 852–876. [CrossRef] [PubMed]

86. Holwerda, A.M.; Paulussen, K.J.M.; Overkamp, M.; Smeets, J.S.J.; Gijsen, A.P.; Goessens, J.P.B.; Verdijk, L.B.; van Loon, L.J.C. Daily resistance-type exercise stimulates muscle protein synthesis in vivo in young men. *J. Appl. Physiol. (1985)* **2018**, *124*, 66–75. [CrossRef] [PubMed]

87. Shad, B.J.; Thompson, J.L.; Holwerda, A.M.; Stocks, B.; Elhassan, Y.S.; Philp, A.; LJC, V.A.N.L.; Wallis, G.A. One Week of Step Reduction Lowers Myofibrillar Protein Synthesis Rates in Young Men. *Med. Sci. Sports Exerc.* **2019**, *51*, 2125–2134. [CrossRef]

88. Peterson, M.J.; Giuliani, C.; Morey, M.C.; Pieper, C.F.; Evenson, K.R.; Mercer, V.; Cohen, H.J.; Visser, M.; Brach, J.S.; Kritchevsky, S.B.; et al. Physical activity as a preventative factor for frailty: The health, aging, and body composition study. *J. Gerontol. Ser. A Biol. Sci. Med. Sci.* **2009**, *64*, 61–68. [CrossRef]

89. Zampieri, S.; Pietrangelo, L.; Loefler, S.; Fruhmann, H.; Vogelauer, M.; Burggraf, S.; Pond, A.; Grim-Stieger, M.; Cvecka, J.; Sedliak, M.; et al. Lifelong physical exercise delays age-associated skeletal muscle decline. *J. Gerontol. Ser. A Biol. Sci. Med. Sci.* **2015**, *70*, 163–173. [CrossRef]

90. Dirks, M.L.; Wall, B.T.; van de Valk, B.; Holloway, T.M.; Holloway, G.P.; Chabowski, A.; Goossens, G.H.; van Loon, L.J. One Week of Bed Rest Leads to Substantial Muscle Atrophy and Induces Whole-Body Insulin Resistance in the Absence of Skeletal Muscle Lipid Accumulation. *Diabetes* **2016**, *65*, 2862–2875. [CrossRef]
91. Dirks, M.L.; Wall, B.T.; Nilwik, R.; Weerts, D.H.; Verdijk, L.B.; van Loon, L.J. Skeletal muscle disuse atrophy is not attenuated by dietary protein supplementation in healthy older men. *J. Nutr.* **2014**, *144*, 1196–1203. [CrossRef] [PubMed]
92. Piercy, K.L.; Troiano, R.P.; Ballard, R.M.; Carlson, S.A.; Fulton, J.E.; Galuska, D.A.; George, S.M.; Olson, R.D. The Physical Activity Guidelines for Americans. *JAMA* **2018**, *320*, 2020–2028. [CrossRef] [PubMed]
93. Ashby, D.; Borman, N.; Burton, J.; Corbett, R.; Davenport, A.; Farrington, K.; Flowers, K.; Fotheringham, J.; Andrea Fox, R.N.; Franklin, G.; et al. Renal Association Clinical Practice Guideline on Haemodialysis. *BMC Nephrol.* **2019**, *20*, 379. [CrossRef] [PubMed]
94. Matsuzawa, R.; Roshanravan, B.; Shimoda, T.; Mamorita, N.; Yoneki, K.; Harada, M.; Watanabe, T.; Yoshida, A.; Takeuchi, Y.; Matsunaga, A. Physical Activity Dose for Hemodialysis Patients: Where to Begin? Results from a Prospective Cohort Study. *J. Ren. Nutr.* **2018**, *28*, 45–53. [CrossRef]
95. Broers, N.J.H.; Martens, R.J.H.; Cornelis, T.; van der Sande, F.M.; Diederen, N.M.P.; Hermans, M.M.H.; Wirtz, J.; Stifft, F.; Konings, C.; Dejagere, T.; et al. Physical Activity in End-Stage Renal Disease Patients: The Effects of Starting Dialysis in the First 6 Months after the Transition Period. *Nephron* **2017**, *137*, 47–56. [CrossRef]
96. Tentori, F.; Elder, S.J.; Thumma, J.; Pisoni, R.L.; Bommer, J.; Fissell, R.B.; Fukuhara, S.; Jadoul, M.; Keen, M.L.; Saran, R.; et al. Physical exercise among participants in the Dialysis Outcomes and Practice Patterns Study (DOPPS): Correlates and associated outcomes. *Nephrol. Dial. Transpl.* **2010**, *25*, 3050–3062. [CrossRef]
97. Da Costa Rosa, C.S.; Nishimoto, D.Y.; Freitas Junior, I.F.; Ciolac, E.G.; Monteiro, H.L. Factors Associated with Levels of Physical Activity in Chronic Kidney Disease Patients Undergoing Hemodialysis: The Role of Dialysis Versus Nondialysis Day. *J. Phys. Act. Health* **2017**, *14*, 726–732. [CrossRef]
98. Gomes, E.P.; Reboredo, M.M.; Carvalho, E.V.; Teixeira, D.R.; Carvalho, L.F.; Filho, G.F.; de Oliveira, J.C.; Sanders-Pinheiro, H.; Chebli, J.M.; de Paula, R.B.; et al. Physical Activity in Hemodialysis Patients Measured by Triaxial Accelerometer. *Biomed. Res. Int.* **2015**, *2015*, 645645. [CrossRef] [PubMed]
99. Clarkson, M.J.; Bennett, P.N.; Fraser, S.F.; Warmington, S.A. Exercise interventions for improving objective physical function in patients with end-stage kidney disease on dialysis: A systematic review and meta-analysis. *Am. J. Physiol. Ren. Physiol.* **2019**, *316*, F856–F872. [CrossRef]
100. Koh, K.P.; Fassett, R.G.; Sharman, J.E.; Coombes, J.S.; Williams, A.D. Effect of intradialytic versus home-based aerobic exercise training on physical function and vascular parameters in hemodialysis patients: A randomized pilot study. *Am. J. Kidney Dis.* **2010**, *55*, 88–99. [CrossRef]
101. Salhab, N.; Karavetian, M.; Kooman, J.; Fiaccadori, E.; El Khoury, C.F. Effects of intradialytic aerobic exercise on hemodialysis patients: A systematic review and meta-analysis. *J. Nephrol.* **2019**. [CrossRef] [PubMed]
102. Anding, K.; Bar, T.; Trojniak-Hennig, J.; Kuchinke, S.; Krause, R.; Rost, J.M.; Halle, M. A structured exercise programme during haemodialysis for patients with chronic kidney disease: Clinical benefit and long-term adherence. *BMJ Open* **2015**, *5*, e008709. [CrossRef] [PubMed]
103. Campbell, W.W.; Crim, M.C.; Young, V.R.; Evans, W.J. Increased energy requirements and changes in body composition with resistance training in older adults. *Am. J. Clin. Nutr.* **1994**, *60*, 167–175. [CrossRef] [PubMed]
104. Churchward-Venne, T.A.; Tieland, M.; Verdijk, L.B.; Leenders, M.; Dirks, M.L.; de Groot, L.C.; van Loon, L.J. There Are No Nonresponders to Resistance-Type Exercise Training in Older Men and Women. *J. Am. Med. Dir. Assoc.* **2015**, *16*, 400–411. [CrossRef]
105. Snijders, T.; Leenders, M.; de Groot, L.; van Loon, L.J.C.; Verdijk, L.B. Muscle mass and strength gains following 6months of resistance type exercise training are only partly preserved within one year with autonomous exercise continuation in older adults. *Exp. Gerontol.* **2019**, *121*, 71–78. [CrossRef]
106. Majchrzak, K.M.; Pupim, L.B.; Flakoll, P.J.; Ikizler, T.A. Resistance exercise augments the acute anabolic effects of intradialytic oral nutritional supplementation. *Nephrol. Dial. Transplant.* **2008**, *23*, 1362–1369. [CrossRef]
107. Bessa, B.; de Oliveira Leal, V.; Moraes, C.; Barboza, J.; Fouque, D.; Mafra, D. Resistance training in hemodialysis patients: A review. *Rehabil. Nurs.* **2015**, *40*, 111–126. [CrossRef]
108. Saitoh, M.; Ogawa, M.; Dos Santos, M.R.; Kondo, H.; Suga, K.; Itoh, H.; Tabata, Y. Effects of Intradialytic Resistance Exercise on Protein Energy Wasting, Physical Performance and Physical Activity in Ambulatory

Patients on Dialysis: A Single-Center Preliminary Study in a Japanese Dialysis Facility. *Ther. Apher. Dial.* **2016**, *20*, 632–638. [CrossRef]

109. Gomes Neto, M.; de Lacerda, F.F.R.; Lopes, A.A.; Martinez, B.P.; Saquetto, M.B. Intradialytic exercise training modalities on physical functioning and health-related quality of life in patients undergoing maintenance hemodialysis: Systematic review and meta-analysis. *Clin. Rehabil.* **2018**, *32*, 1189–1202. [CrossRef]

110. Salhab, N.; Alrukhaimi, M.; Kooman, J.; Fiaccadori, E.; Aljubori, H.; Rizk, R.; Karavetian, M. Effect of Intradialytic Exercise on Hyperphosphatemia and Malnutrition. *Nutrients* **2019**, *11*, 2464. [CrossRef]

111. Chan, D.; Cheema, B.S. Progressive Resistance Training in End-Stage Renal Disease: Systematic Review. *Am. J. Nephrol.* **2016**, *44*, 32–45. [CrossRef] [PubMed]

112. Cheema, B.; Abas, H.; Smith, B.; O'Sullivan, A.; Chan, M.; Patwardhan, A.; Kelly, J.; Gillin, A.; Pang, G.; Lloyd, B.; et al. Progressive exercise for anabolism in kidney disease (PEAK): A randomized, controlled trial of resistance training during hemodialysis. *J. Am. Soc. Nephrol.* **2007**, *18*, 1594–1601. [CrossRef] [PubMed]

113. Kopple, J.D.; Wang, H.; Casaburi, R.; Fournier, M.; Lewis, M.I.; Taylor, W.; Storer, T.W. Exercise in maintenance hemodialysis patients induces transcriptional changes in genes favoring anabolic muscle. *J. Am. Soc. Nephrol.* **2007**, *18*, 2975–2986. [CrossRef] [PubMed]

114. Kirkman, D.L.; Mullins, P.; Junglee, N.A.; Kumwenda, M.; Jibani, M.M.; Macdonald, J.H. Anabolic exercise in haemodialysis patients: A randomised controlled pilot study. *J. Cachexia Sarcopenia Muscle* **2014**, *5*, 199–207. [CrossRef]

115. Van den Ham, E.C.; Kooman, J.P.; Schols, A.M.; Nieman, F.H.; Does, J.D.; Akkermans, M.A.; Janssen, P.P.; Gosker, H.R.; Ward, K.A.; MacDonald, J.H.; et al. The functional, metabolic, and anabolic responses to exercise training in renal transplant and hemodialysis patients. *Transplantation* **2007**, *83*, 1059–1068. [CrossRef]

116. Martin-Alemany, G.; Valdez-Ortiz, R.; Olvera-Soto, G.; Gomez-Guerrero, I.; Aguire-Esquivel, G.; Cantu-Quintanilla, G.; Lopez-Alvarenga, J.C.; Miranda-Alatriste, P.; Espinosa-Cuevas, A. The effects of resistance exercise and oral nutritional supplementation during hemodialysis on indicators of nutritional status and quality of life. *Nephrol. Dial. Transplant.* **2016**, *31*, 1712–1720. [CrossRef]

117. Molsted, S.; Harrison, A.P.; Eidemak, I.; Andersen, J.L. The effects of high-load strength training with protein- or nonprotein-containing nutritional supplementation in patients undergoing dialysis. *J. Ren. Nutr.* **2013**, *23*, 132–140. [CrossRef]

118. Martin-Alemany, G.; Espinosa-Cuevas, M.L.A.; Perez-Navarro, M.; Wilund, K.R.; Miranda-Alatriste, P.; Cortes-Perez, M.; Garcia-Villalobos, G.; Gomez-Guerrero, I.; Cantu-Quintanilla, G.; Ramirez-Mendoza, M.; et al. Effect of Oral Nutritional Supplementation With and Without Exercise on Nutritional Status and Physical Function of Adult Hemodialysis Patients: A Parallel Controlled Clinical Trial (AVANTE-HEMO Study). *J. Ren. Nutr.* **2019**. [CrossRef]

119. Molsted, S.; Bjorkman, A.S.D.; Lundstrom, L.H. Effects of strength training to patients undergoing dialysis: A systematic review. *Dan. Med. J.* **2019**, *66*, A5526.

120. Witard, O.C.; Wardle, S.L.; Macnaughton, L.S.; Hodgson, A.B.; Tipton, K.D. Protein Considerations for Optimising Skeletal Muscle Mass in Healthy Young and Older Adults. *Nutrients* **2016**, *8*, 181. [CrossRef]

121. Trommelen, J.; Betz, M.W.; van Loon, L.J.C. The Muscle Protein Synthetic Response to Meal Ingestion Following Resistance-Type Exercise. *Sports Med.* **2019**, *49*, 185–197. [CrossRef] [PubMed]

122. Oquendo, L.G.; Asencio, J.M.M.; de Las Nieves, C.B. Contributing factors for therapeutic diet adherence in patients receiving haemodialysis treatment: An integrative review. *J. Clin. Nurs.* **2017**, *26*, 3893–3905. [CrossRef] [PubMed]

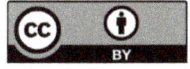

© 2019 by the authors. Licensee MDPI, Basel, Switzerland. This article is an open access article distributed under the terms and conditions of the Creative Commons Attribution (CC BY) license (http://creativecommons.org/licenses/by/4.0/).

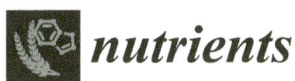

Article

Malnutrition as a Strong Predictor of the Onset of Sarcopenia

Charlotte Beaudart [1,*], Dolores Sanchez-Rodriguez [1,2,†], Médéa Locquet [1,†], Jean-Yves Reginster [1,3], Laetitia Lengelé [1] and Olivier Bruyère [1]

[1] WHO Collaborating Centre for Public Health Aspects of Musculoskeletal Health and Aging, Division of Public Health, Epidemiology and Health Economics, University of Liège, CHU—Sart Tilman, Quartier Hôpital, Avenue Hippocrate 13 (Bât. B23), 4000 Liège, Belgium; dolores.sanchez@uliege.be (D.S.-R.); medea.locquet@uliege.be (M.L.); jyr.ch@bluewin.ch (J.-Y.R.); llengele@uliege.be (L.L.); olivier.bruyere@uliege.be (O.B.)
[2] Geriatrics Department, Parc de Salut Mar Rehabilitation Research Group, Hospital del Mar Medical Research Institute (IMIM), Universitat Pompeu Fabra, 08002 Barcelona, Spain
[3] Chair for Biomarkers of Chronic Diseases, Biochemistry Department, College of Science, King Saud University, Riyadh 11451, Saudi Arabia
* Correspondence: c.beaudart@uliege.be; Tel.: +32-43-66-3230
† Dolores Sanchez-Rodriguez and Médéa Locquet share the second authorship of the manuscript.

Received: 28 October 2019; Accepted: 20 November 2019; Published: 27 November 2019

Abstract: This study aims to explore the association between malnutrition diagnosed according to both the Global Leadership Initiative of Malnutrition (GLIM) and the European Society of Clinical Nutrition and Metabolism (ESPEN) criteria and the onset of sarcopenia/severe sarcopenia, diagnosed according to the European Working Group on Sarcopenia in Older People 2 (EWGSOP2) criterion, in the sarcopenia and physical impairment with advancing age (SarcoPhAge) cohort during a four-year follow-up. Adjusted Cox-regression and Kaplan-Meier curves were performed. Among the 534 community-dwelling participants recruited in the SarcoPhAge study, 510 were free from sarcopenia at baseline, of whom 336 had complete data (186 women and 150 men, mean age of 72.5 ± 5.8 years) to apply the GLIM and ESPEN criteria. A significantly higher risk of developing sarcopenia/severe sarcopenia during the four-year follow-up based on the GLIM [sarcopenia: Adjusted hazard ratio (HR) = 3.23 (95% confidence interval (CI) 1.73–6.05); severe sarcopenia: Adjusted HR = 2.87 (95% CI 1.25–6.56)] and ESPEN [sarcopenia: Adjusted HR = 4.28 (95% CI 1.86–9.86); severe sarcopenia: Adjusted HR = 3.86 (95% CI 1.29–11.54)] criteria was observed. Kaplan-Meier curves confirmed this relationship (log rank $p < 0.001$ for all). These results highlighted the importance of malnutrition since it has been shown to be associated with an approximately fourfold higher risk of developing sarcopenia/severe sarcopenia during a four-year follow-up.

Keywords: sarcopenia; EWGSOP2; malnutrition; GLIM; SarcoPhAge

1. Introduction

Malnutrition is a major cause of adverse health consequences, such as impaired physical function [1], hospitalization [2], and mortality [3,4] in older people. One of the most prominent features of malnutrition is that it is a reversible disease, and a wide variety of effective therapeutic approaches are available and adaptable to the different etiologies and patient requirements [5,6].

In 2016, the World Health Organization launched the World Report on Ageing and Health, an action plan to promote initiatives towards a better ageing process [7]. The European Society of Clinical Nutrition and Metabolism (ESPEN) followed the WHO's strategy, revisited the concepts of malnutrition and nutrition-related diseases. ESPEN developed malnutrition criteria [8] and guidelines on the definition and terminology of clinical nutrition [9] which unified the terminology to be used in malnutrition and nutrition-related diseases, i.e., sarcopenia, frailty, cachexia/disease-related malnutrition, and starvation-related underweight [8], and organized them as a conceptual tree of nutritional disorders [9]. The ESPEN approach is a two-tier process: In the first step, patients are identified as being at risk of malnutrition by any validated screening tool; in the second step, malnutrition is defined by a combination of weight loss, low body mass index, and low muscle mass [8].

The efforts by the WHO and ESPEN to shed light on malnutrition and nutrition-related diseases have been followed by the largest societies of clinical nutrition and metabolism. In the malnutrition field, the Global Leadership Initiative on Malnutrition (GLIM) [10] launched the GLIM criteria, the first international definition of malnutrition [11]; in the sarcopenia field, the European Working Group on Sarcopenia in Older People has published the revised European consensus on definition and diagnosis (EWGSOP2) [12], which updates the most widely acknowledged previous definition.

The GLIM criteria are a three-step approach, first, patients are identified by any validated screening tool, and second, they are diagnosed for presence of, at least, one phenotypic (weight loss, low body mass index, and low muscle mass) and one etiologic criteria (reduced food intake or assimilation or disease burden and inflammation). A third step is severity grading, which is based on the phenotypic criteria. The EWGSOP2 consensus follows this same three-step approach, first, screening by SARC-F questionnaire, and second, patients are diagnosed in presence of low muscle strength and low muscle mass. The third step is severity grading, based on the impairment of physical performance. The GLIM and EWGSOP2 criteria are harmonized definitions that share muscle mass as a criterion to enhance the comparability of studies [13], and sarcopenia has loss of muscle function as its most highlighted differential feature [14].

Nutritional intake is one of the most important modulators in human health, and an inadequate balance between intake and expenditure is the main cause of malnutrition [14] and nutrition-related diseases [13,15]. The association between a poor balanced diet with reduced micro and macronutrients and the presence of sarcopenia at baseline in community-dwelling older people has been recently described by our research group [16]. Likewise, malnutrition must be decisive for the onset of sarcopenia. However, the prospective associations between the two diseases remain unknown, and the incidence of sarcopenia in longitudinal studies is truly unexplored.

Our research group has followed the call to action launched by the GLIM and ESPEN to shed light on the overlap between malnutrition and nutrition-related diseases [10]. Our objective is to assess the relationship between baseline malnutrition according to the GLIM and the ESPEN criteria and the incidence of sarcopenia and severe sarcopenia in the sarcopenia and physical impairment with advancing age (SarcoPhAge) cohort during a four-year follow-up.

2. Materials and Methods

This was a prospective, descriptive study cohort. The Strengthening the Reporting of Observational Studies in Epidemiology (STROBE) statement was followed [17].

2.1. Population

Participants from the SarcoPhAge cohort were included in this study. The protocol of the SarcoPhAge study has been detailed elsewhere [18]. Briefly, the SarcoPhAge cohort is a Belgian population-based cohort developed in Liège (Belgium) involving 534 community-dwelling participants 65 years of age and older. Participants were recruited in 2013 from press advertisements and general, geriatric, osteoporosis, rehabilitation, and rheumatology outpatient clinics and were followed up each year (T0/baseline and T1, T2, T3, T4, corresponding, respectively, to one year, two years, three years, and four years of follow-up) with a clinical examination and questionnaires. No specific exclusion criteria related to health or demographic characteristics were applied, except for the exclusion of individuals with an amputated limb or with a BMI above 50 kg/m^2. Written informed consent was provided by participants, and the study was approved by the ethics committee of our institution (reference 2012/277).

The outcome measure was the incidence of sarcopenia/severe sarcopenia measured annually, i.e., the number of new cases each year, which were cumulated.

2.2. Data Collection

2.2.1. Malnutrition Diagnosis

Malnutrition was diagnosed at baseline (T0) according to the two most updated definitions of malnutrition: The ESPEN [8] and the GLIM criteria [19].

The ESPEN criteria [8] propose two ways to diagnose malnutrition. Alternative one: Body mass index (BMI) <18.5 kg/m^2. Alternative two: Unintentional weight loss combined with a low age-related BMI (<20 kg/m^2 in <70 years or <22 kg/m^2 in ≥70 years) or low fat-free mass index (FFMI) (<17 kg/m^2 in men and <15 kg/m^2 in women).

The GLIM criteria [19] require at least one phenotypic criterion and one etiological criterion, as summarized in Table 1.

Table 1. Summary of phenotypic and etiological criteria of the Global Leadership Initiative on Malnutrition (GLIM) definition.

Phenotypic	
Weight loss	A weight loss >4.5 kg in the past year was reported and used as a threshold [20]. Unintentional weight loss was obtained by clinical interview at baseline.
BMI	BMI (kg/m^2) was considered reduced if <20 kg/m^2 or <22 kg/m^2 in participants younger and older than 70 years, respectively [19].
Reduced muscle mass	FFMI <17 kg/m^2 in men and <15 kg/m^2 in women or ALMI <7 kg/m^2 in men and <5.5 kg/m^2 in women was used as a threshold [12,19].
Etiological	
Reduced food intake or assimilation	The first Mini-nutritional Assessment- Short Form (MNA-SF) [21] item was used to determine reduced food intake: "Has food intake declined over the past 3 months due to loss of appetite, digestive problems, chewing or swallowing difficulties?" Severe and moderate decreases were considered positive answers [21]. Chronic gastrointestinal conditions that adversely impact food assimilation or absorption of nutrients were also considered.
Disease burden and inflammation	Interleukin-6 (IL-6) and insulin-like growth factor 1 (IGF-1) were selected as biomarkers to assess inflammation, following recommendations by the Targeting Aging Biomarkers Workgroup for the selection of blood-based biomarkers for geroscience-guided clinical trials [22]. Quartiles for IGF-1 and IL-6 in our own data were calculated in both sexes, and the lowest quartile was considered as a sex-specific threshold: IGF-1 ≤88 ng/mL in men and ≤82 ng/mL in women and IL-6 >3.84 pg/mL in men and >2.99 pg/mL in women [23]. The number of diseases was recorded; disease burden was not assessed.

2.2.2. Sarcopenia Diagnosis

For sarcopenia diagnosis, we applied the latest criteria published by the EWGSOP, the EWGSOP2 criteria [12]. A complete diagnosis of sarcopenia was performed at baseline and at each time of follow-up (T1, T2, T3, and T4). The incidence of sarcopenia was thereby measured.

Confirmed sarcopenia was considered when participants presented both of the following:

(1) Low muscle strength (expressed in kg). Muscle strength was measured with a handgrip hand-held dynamometer (Saehan Corporation, MSD Europe Bvba, Brussels, Belgium) calibrated at the beginning of the study and at each year of follow-up for 10, 40, and 90 kg. We followed standardized procedures by asking participants to squeeze as hard as possible three times per hand. The highest value of the six measurements was considered in our analyses (Southampton protocol) [24]. Low muscle strength is defined as <27 kg in men and <16 kg in women [12].

(2) Low muscle mass. Muscle mass was measured with a dual X-ray absorptiometer (Hologic Discovery A, USA), which was calibrated daily. Fat-free mass and appendicular lean mass, obtained from whole-body DXA scans, were divided by height squared (kg/m^2) to obtain the fat-free mass index and appendicular lean mass index (ALMI) values, respectively. A low muscle mass is defined as FFMI <17 kg/m^2 in men and <15 kg/m^2 in women or ALMI <7 kg/m^2 in men and <5.5 kg/m^2 in women.

Moreover, if a person also presented low physical performance (measured by the Short Physical Performance Battery test [24] through the assessment of balance, walking speed, and the chair stand test with ≤8 points as the threshold, or measured by a 4 m gait speed test with <0.8 m/s as the threshold), that person was considered to have "severe sarcopenia". Physical performance was measured following the standardized assessment recommended by the European Society for Clinical and Economic Aspects of Osteoporosis, Osteoarthritis, and Musculoskeletal Diseases (ESCEO) [25].

2.3. Covariates

During the annual follow-up of the SarcoPhAge participants, a large number of covariates were also collected. Among these variables, we recorded the number of comorbidities that the participants were affected by and the number of drugs consumed, self-reported by each individual; the cognitive status, assessed by the mini-mental state examination (MMSE) [26]; the participants functional limitations in instrumental activities of daily living (IADLs), measured with the Lawton scale [27]; as well as the physical activity level, self-reported as the time spent in different physical activities in the past seven days based on the Minnesota Leisure Time Activity Questionnaire below, an established cut-off based on sex [28].

2.4. Statistical Analysis

The normality of the variables was checked by examining the histogram, the quantile–quantile plot, the Shapiro–Wilk test, and the difference between the mean and the median values. Quantitative variables following a Gaussian distribution were expressed as the mean ± standard deviation; quantitative variables not following a Gaussian distribution were expressed as the median (25th percentile–75th percentile). Qualitative variables were described by absolute and relative (%) frequencies.

First, the number of participants diagnosed with sarcopenia according to the EWGSOP2 criteria was measured. We excluded those participants from our database to allow us to measure the incidence of sarcopenia from a sample of participants free from the disease.

Second, the number of participants diagnosed with malnutrition according to either GLIM or ESPEN criteria was measured. To assess agreement between the criteria, we reported the Cohen kappa coefficient and its 95% confidence interval (CI) (overall concordance rate). Participants' baseline characteristics were compared between those diagnosed with malnutrition with either the ESPEN criteria or the GLIM criteria and those not diagnosed with malnutrition through a Student's t test for quantitative variables that followed a normal distribution, the Mann-Whitney U test for quantitative variables that did not follow a normal distribution, and a χ^2 test for qualitative or binary variables.

Third, the incidence of sarcopenia and severe sarcopenia was measured each year, i.e., number of new cases each year, which were cumulated. For both the ESPEN and GLIM definitions of malnutrition, the incidence of sarcopenia/severe sarcopenia was measured in each group (malnourished versus well-nourished) and compared using a χ^2 test. Since survival data were available (months of follow-up), we also applied the Cox proportional hazards model, giving the hazard ratio (HR) and 95% CI to measure the risk of developing sarcopenia/severe sarcopenia across four years of follow-up according to the baseline nutritional status. A crude HR as well as an adjusted HR were calculated, taking into account covariates that could potentially impact on muscle health and nutritional status: Sex, age, the number of concomitant diseases, the number of drugs, cognitive status, and the level of physical activity [18,29–32]. To avoid over adjustment with sarcopenia, we chose not to include BMI as a covariate. Survival curves were evaluated using the Kaplan-Meier method to explore the influence of malnutrition on the risk of developing sarcopenia/severe sarcopenia. Log-rank tests were performed.

Data were processed using the SPSS Statistics 24 (IBM Corporation, Armonk, NY, USA) software package. All results were considered statistically significant at the 5% critical level.

3. Results

3.1. Population and Diagnosis of Malnutrition

Of the 534 older adults included in the SarcoPhAge study, 510 were free from sarcopenia, as diagnosed with the EWGSOP2 definition, and they constituted our baseline population. Of those 510 participants, 416 were interviewed throughout the four-year follow-up period (94 individuals were either lost to follow-up, refused to participate, were unable to continue the study, or were dead) (Figure 1).

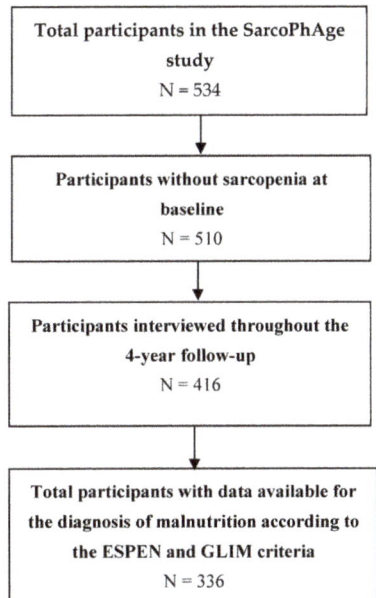

Figure 1. Flow chart of the study. European Society of Clinical Nutrition and Metabolism (ESPEN) and sarcopenia and physical impairment with advancing age (SarcoPhAge).

Finally, only 336 participants had the blood samples available that were needed to assess inflammation for the diagnosis of malnutrition according to the GLIM criteria. Our final study population at baseline was therefore composed of 336 participants (Figure 1), 55.4% women, aged 72.5 ± 5.8 years with a mean of four concomitant diseases per participant and a mean of 5.6 daily consumed drugs per participant. The population was free from cognitive disorders, with an MMSE mean score of 28.3 ± 1.8 points out of 30 (Table 2).

Table 2. Baseline characteristics of participants in the SarcoPhAge study ($n = 336$).

	Studied Sample ($n = 336$)	Malnutrition According to the ESPEN Criteria			Malnutrition According to the GLIM Criteria		
		Yes ($n = 19$)	No ($n = 317$)	p-Value	Yes ($n = 59$)	No ($n = 277$)	p-Value
Age, years	72.5 ± 5.8	71.9 ± 7.1	72.6 ± 5.7	0.62	72.0 ± 6.3	72.6 ± 5.7	0.44
Sex, women	186 (55.4%)	13 (68.4%)	173 (54.6%)	0.24	39 (66.1%)	147 (53.1%)	0.07
Number of concomitant diseases per participant	4.1 ± 2.4	5.0 ± 2.8	4.1 ± 2.4	0.09	4.9 ± 2.4	3.9 ± 2.4	0.005
Number of drugs per participant	5.6 ± 3.4	5.9 ± 3.5	5.6 ± 3.4	0.64	6.0 ± 3.3	5.6 ± 3.4	0.29
MMSE, /30 points	28.3 ± 1.8	27.9 ± 1.4	28.3 ± 1.9	0.41	28.0 ± 2.1	28.3 ± 1.7	0.14
Body mass index, kg/m^2	27.1 ± 4.6	20.9 ± 0.7	27.4 ± 0.2	<0.001	24.0 ± 4.0	27.7 ± 4.5	<0.001
Lean mass total, kg							
Men	56.5 ± 8.7	44.8 ± 4.0	57.0 ± 8.6	0.001	48.7 ± 8.1	57.7 ± 8.2	<0.001
Women	39.0 ± 5.8	35.1 ± 3.5	39.3 ± 5.9	0.013	36.1 ± 4.8	39.7 ± 5.8	0.001
ALMI, kg/m^2							
Men	8.1 ± 1.0	6.6 ± 0.7	8.1 ± 1.0	0.001	7.1 ± 1.0	8.2 ± 1.0	<0.001
Women	6.1 ± 1.0	5.3 ± 0.5	6.2 ± 1.0	0.003	5.6 ± 0.7	6.3 ± 1.0	<0.001
Muscle strength (kg)							
Men	40.4 ± 8.3	25.8 ± 7.9	41.0 ± 7.7	<0.001	35.7 ± 11.3	41.1 ± 7.5	0.006
Women	22.6 ± 6.9	23.3 ± 6.3	22.5 ± 7.0	0.69	21.7 ± 4.9	22.8 ± 7.3	0.36
Gait speed, m/s	1.02 ± 0.27	1.10 ± 0.30	1.01 ± 0.27	0.21	1.00 ± 0.30	1.03 ± 0.26	0.53
SPPB, /12 points	9.7 ± 2.0	10.2 ± 2.3	9.7 ± 1.9	0.27	9.3 ± 2.5	9.8 ± 1.8	0.08
Chair stand test, s	13.7 ± 5.2	13.6 ± 7.3	13.7 ± 5.0	0.95	14.4 ± 6.1	13.5 ± 5.0	0.26
IADL Lawton							
/5 for men	4.6 ± 1.2	3.8 ± 1.8	4.6 ± 1.2	0.09	4.2 ± 1.7	4.7 ± 1.1	0.08
/8 for women	7.6 ± 1.0	7.3 ± 1.4	7.6 ± 1.0	0.32	7.4 ± 1.3	7.6 ± 0.9	0.24
Level of physical activity, kcal/day	745.7 (270–1523.2)	840 (106–1470)	742 (270–1554)	0.57	935 (150–1470)	735 (270–1568)	0.53

Malnutrition, according to the ESPEN criteria, was present in 19 individuals (5.65%) and, according to the GLIM criteria, was present in 59 individuals (17.6%). Agreement between both definitions was low, with a Cohen kappa coefficient of 0.30 (95% CI 0.16–0.43). Once diagnosed with either the ESPEN or the GLIM criteria, malnourished participants presented a significantly lower BMI, a lower amount of lean mass, and ALMI as well as a lower muscle strength (the latest being applicable for male participants only) than well-nourished individuals (all p-values < 0.05). Participants diagnosed with malnutrition using the GLIM criteria also presented a higher number of concomitant diseases than well-nourished participants ($p = 0.005$). No other significant differences between groups were observed for the collected characteristics of the population.

3.2. Incidence of Sarcopenia

From baseline to four years of follow-up, 46 new cases of sarcopenia (13.7%) and 26 new cases of severe sarcopenia (7.74%) were reported. In participants diagnosed with malnutrition at baseline, regardless of the criteria used for the diagnosis, the incidence of sarcopenia was significantly higher than that in well-nourished individuals (Table 3). Among the 19 individuals with malnutrition according to the ESPEN criteria, seven (36.8%) developed sarcopenia throughout the four-year follow-up period, compared to 12.3% in the group of well-nourished participants. After adjusting for age, sex, the number of concomitant diseases, the number of drugs consumed, cognitive status, and the level of physical activity, an HR of 4.28 (95% CI 1.86–9.86) was found, revealing that malnourished participants, according to the ESPEN criteria, had a 4.28-fold higher risk of becoming sarcopenic within four years. The HR for severe sarcopenia was 3.86 (95% CI 1.29–11.54). Among the 59 individuals with malnutrition according to the GLIM criteria, 16 (27.1%) developed sarcopenia, compared to 10.8% among well-nourished participants ($p = 0.001$). An adjusted HR of 3.23 (95% CI 1.73–6.05) was found for the association with sarcopenia and of 2.87 (95% CI 1.25–6.56) for the association with severe sarcopenia.

Figure 2 depicts the analysis of the four-year incidence of sarcopenia and severe sarcopenia for participants with baseline malnutrition according to the GLIM and ESPEN criteria. Still, confirmed with Kaplan-Meier analyses, a significant impact of malnutrition on the onset of sarcopenia and severe sarcopenia was found, regardless of the definition used for malnutrition (log rank $p < 0.001$ for all Kaplan-Meier curves) (Figure 2A–D).

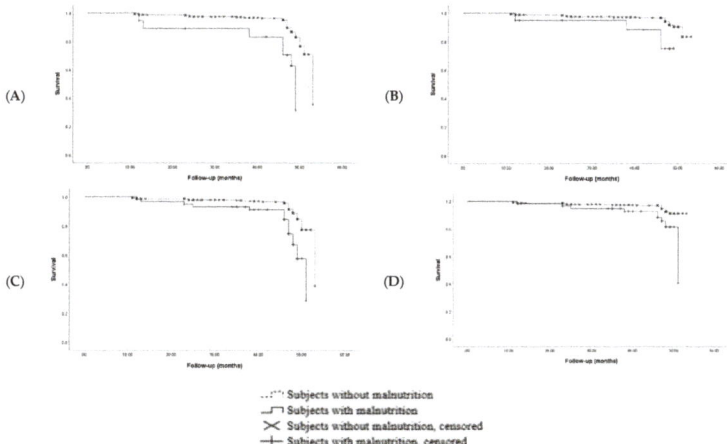

Figure 2. (**A**) Incidence of sarcopenia in participants with or without malnutrition according to the ESPEN criteria; (**B**) incidence of severe sarcopenia in participants with or without malnutrition according to the ESPEN criteria; (**C**) incidence of sarcopenia in participants with or without malnutrition according to the GLIM criteria; and (**D**) incidence of severe sarcopenia in participants with or without malnutrition according to the GLIM criteria.

Table 3. Relationship between malnutrition at baseline and the incidence of sarcopenia and severe sarcopenia during a four-year follow-up period (n = 336).

	Analysis Performed According to the ESPEN Criteria				
	Occurrence of Sarcopenia		p-Value	Crude HR (95% CI)	Adjusted HR (95% CI) *
Malnutrition status	No incident sarcopenia (n = 290)	Incident sarcopenia (n = 46)			
Well nourished	278 (95.9%)	39 (84.8%)	0.005	3.91 (1.73–8.81)	4.28 (1.86–9.86)
Malnourished	12 (4.1%)	7 (15.2%)			
	Occurrence of severe sarcopenia		p-Value	Crude HR (95% CI)	Adjusted HR (95% CI) *
Malnutrition status	No incident severe sarcopenia (n = 310)	Incident severe sarcopenia (n = 26)			
Well nourished	295 (95.2%)	22 (84.6%)	0.035	3.54 (1.21–10.34)	3.86 (1.29–11.54)
Malnourished	15 (4.8%)	4 (15.4%)			
	Analysis performed according to the GLIM criteria				
	Occurrence of sarcopenia		p-Value	Crude HR (95% CI)	Adjusted HR (95% CI) *
Malnutrition status	No incident sarcopenia (n = 290)	Incident sarcopenia (n = 46)			
Well nourished	247 (85.2%)	30 (65.2%)	0.001	3.22 (1.74–5.94)	3.23 (1.73–6.05)
Malnourished	43 (14.8%)	16 (34.8%)			
	Occurrence of severe sarcopenia		p-Value	Crude HR (95% CI)	Adjusted HR (95% CI) *
Malnutrition status	No incident severe sarcopenia (n = 310)	Incident severe sarcopenia (n = 26)			
Well nourished	260 (83.9)	17 (65.4)	0.021	2.90 (1.29–6.53)	2.87 (1.25–6.56)
Malnourished	50 (16.1)	9 (34.6)			

* Covariates: Age, sex, the number of concomitant diseases per participant, the number of drugs per participant, cognitive status, the level of physical activity.

4. Discussion

Our study had the objective to explore the association between malnutrition diagnosed according to both GLIM and ESPEN criteria and the onset of sarcopenia and severe sarcopenia. Using the SarcoPhAge study population, we found an approximately fourfold higher risk of developing sarcopenia in patients meeting the ESPEN criteria and a threefold higher risk in patients meeting the GLIM criteria during a four-year follow-up, and this association was independent of the number of concomitant diseases, the number of drugs, cognitive status, and the level of physical activity at baseline.

The prevalence of malnutrition at baseline in our sample cohort of community-dwelling older people by using the GLIM criteria (17.6%) was three times higher than the prevalence obtained by applying the ESPEN criteria (5.65%), a prevalence that might serve as a reference in community-dwelling older populations in the absence of previous reference values. This is consistent with previous studies: A prevalence of malnutrition according to the ESPEN criteria of 7.3% and with a higher mortality risk (adjusted HR = 4.4 (95% CI: 1.7–11.3)) during a seven-year follow-up period in the EPIDOS-Toulouse study was found [4]. A study conducted in advanced cancer patients assessed the prevalence of malnutrition according to the GLIM criteria (by using FFMI to measure reduced muscle mass) and the association with mortality; a prevalence of 72.2% and an odds ratio of 1.87 (95% CI 1.01–3.48, $p = 0.047$) for six-month mortality were found [33]. In hospitalized patients with hematological malignancy, the prevalence of malnutrition according to the GLIM criteria was 25.8%, and the one-year mortality risk HR was 2.39 (1.36–4.20, $p = 0.002$) [34]. In outpatients with liver disease under evaluation for liver transplantation, the prevalence of malnutrition according to the GLIM criteria was 25% [35]. The high prevalence and the strong relationship with clinical adverse consequences observed for the GLIM criteria might be due to the criteria that form the definition, as all of them are important predictors of poor prognosis and unintentional weight loss [36].

Regarding the incidence of sarcopenia, 13.7% of the participants in the SarcoPhAge cohort study developed sarcopenia during the four-year follow-up period, and 7.7% developed severe sarcopenia, with a significantly higher incidence in malnourished individuals. In our study, the ESPEN criteria seemed to be slightly more related to the incidence of sarcopenia than the new GLIM criteria. The links between malnutrition and sarcopenia have already been explored in several cross-sectional studies: In older patients with advanced chronic disease (Stages 3b–5) by using the malnutrition inflammation score (MIS) for the diagnosis of malnutrition and the EWGSOP2 for the diagnosis of sarcopenia [37], in older patients with chronic pulmonary disease by using the ESPEN [38] and the EWGSOP2 [38] criteria, and in older people discharged from post-acute care by using the ESPEN and the EWGSOP criteria [39]. However, the cross-sectional study design did not allow the authors to establish cause-effect relationships. Unfortunately, there are few longitudinal studies on malnutrition and sarcopenia that allow us to compare our findings. The multicenter prospective Gruppo Lavoro Italiano Sarcopenia—Trattamento e Nutrizione (GLISTEN) study provided an incidence of sarcopenia in hospitalized older people in acute care during a hospital stay, with 15% of new cases of sarcopenia during hospitalization (10 days) [40]. The GLISTEN study did not assess the potential impact of malnutrition on the onset of sarcopenia but highlighted that a higher incidence seemed related to ADL disability and the length of bed rest. Moreover, they highlighted a decreased probability of developing sarcopenia in patients with a higher BMI and higher skeletal muscle index [40]. Our results indicated that malnutrition seems to be one of the risk factors for sarcopenia, but the onset of sarcopenia is more than likely multifactorial, with other factors, such as sedentary lifestyle, inflammatory biomarkers, and poor balanced nutrition, that should be investigated in longitudinal cohort studies for their role as risk factors.

The role of malnutrition in the onset of sarcopenia identified in our study could partially be explained by the fact that some nutritional factors, such as protein, vitamin D/calcium, and the acid–base balance of the diet, play an important role in maintaining muscle mass [41] and, consequently, muscle strength and physical performance. This overlap between malnutrition and sarcopenia is observed throughout their management. Indeed, the treatment of sarcopenia is based on a combined intervention of nutritional therapies and resistance training, with a higher influence of the second one, particularly high-intensity resistance training (i.e., 80% 1-Repetition Maximum) to gain maximal strength or low-intensity resistance training (≤50% 1 RM) to induce strength gains [42]. The therapeutic interventions for malnutrition have been recently revisited and updated in the ESPEN guidelines of clinical nutrition and hydration in geriatrics [6] and are mostly based on food fortification [6], which is more feasible to be administered in older people than the recommended management of sarcopenia [42,43]. Our findings might be of interest in the development of early therapeutic interventions targeted at individuals who meet malnutrition criteria but are free from sarcopenia at baseline [43,44] in relation to the concept of "impactability", a term used in public health management strategies "to identify patients who are most likely to benefit from a therapeutic intervention" [45]. The placebo-controlled design of those eventual trials might present ethical issues, as malnutrition should be treated once diagnosed [6]. Very recently, considering the closer overlap between sarcopenia and malnutrition, a new clinical syndrome proposal was made, those of malnutrition sarcopenia syndrome (MSS) [46].

Strengths and Limitations

The assessment of sarcopenia and malnutrition, according to the most updated definitions, should be highlighted as a novelty and strength of our study. Indeed, a recent review of nutrition and sarcopenia screening tools highlighted the lack of standardization and use of validated and highly recognized tools to diagnose both malnutrition and sarcopenia [46]. In our study, we did not apply the screening part of both definitions. Screening could be very useful in clinic research to avoid a full diagnosis in participants for whom the screening revealed a low risk of malnutrition. However, since we had a dataset with all participants, we had sufficient data to directly apply the diagnostic criteria for our whole population.

A limitation of the study is that we measured only the causal relationship between malnutrition and sarcopenia in the sense of malnutrition being a risk factor for sarcopenia. Assessing the incidence of malnutrition in individuals with sarcopenia at baseline during the four-year longitudinal follow-up is an interesting topic for further research to better interpret the knowledge derived from our current findings and to complete the current knowledge about the pathophysiology of sarcopenia throughout the lifespan [13]. In the same vein, the dynamic aspect of malnutrition could also be considered with an analysis that does not only focus on the baseline prevalence of malnutrition but that also takes into account the incidence or the new-onset of malnutrition as a risk factor for sarcopenia. Unfortunately, in the present study, we did not have the sufficient materials to measure the malnutrition according to both criteria at each time of data collection. There was also a potential selection bias linked to cohort studies, as volunteers might present better health status than the general population. Our results are therefore non-representative of the population of interest and could not be generalized to other populations. Because our people with sarcopenia were probably in better health than the "true" population of people with sarcopenia, the association measured in our study could have been somewhat underestimated. Finally, the fact that we used an existing dataset for these analyses implies, first, that we could have missed some important covariates that could explain the incidence of sarcopenia outside of malnutrition and, second, that no power size has been calculated. However, even with a low prevalence of malnutrition in our sample ($n = 19$ for ESPEN, $n = 59$ for GLIM), a significant relationship with the incidence of sarcopenia has already been found. We can then assume that a larger sample size and a larger number of malnourished individuals will result in an even more important difference.

5. Conclusions

In conclusion, malnutrition was found to be a strong predictor of sarcopenia and severe sarcopenia during a four-year follow-up. Our research suggests that both the ESPEN and GLIM criteria might be early indicators to identify those individuals free from the disease that might develop sarcopenia in the upcoming years and to shed light on the physiopathology of sarcopenia throughout the lifespan.

Author Contributions: Conceptualization, C.B., O.B., and J.-Y.R.; Methodology, C.B.; Software, M.L.; Validation, D.S.-R., M.L., and C.B.; Formal analysis, M.L.; Investigation, C.B., D.S.-R., and M.L.; Resources, O.B. and J.-Y.R.; Data Curation, C.B., M.L. and L.L.; Writing—Original Draft Preparation, C.B., L.L. and D.S.-R.; Writing—Review & Editing, C.B., D.S.-R., and M.L.; Supervision, O.B.

Funding: M.L. is supported by a fellowship from the FNRS (Fonds National de la Recherche Scientifique de Belgium—FRSFNRS—http://www.frs-fnrs.be).

Acknowledgments: We would like to thank all participants from the SarcoPhAge study for their collaboration.

Conflicts of Interest: The authors declare no conflict of interest. The funders had no role in the design of the study; in the collection, analyses, or interpretation of data; in the writing of the manuscript; or in the decision to publish the results.

References

1. Sánchez-Rodríguez, D.; Annweiler, C.; Ronquillo-Moreno, N.; Vázquez-Ibar, O.; Escalada, F.; Duran, X.; Muniesa, J.M.; Marco, E. Prognostic Value of the ESPEN Consensus and Guidelines for Malnutrition: Prediction of Post-Discharge Clinical Outcomes in Older Inpatients. *Nutr. Clin. Pract.* **2019**, *34*, 304–312. [CrossRef]
2. Sanz-París, A.; Gómez-Candela, C.; Martín-Palmero, Á.; García-Almeida, J.M.; Burgos-Pelaez, R.; Matía-Martin, P.; Arbones-Mainar, J.M. Application of the new ESPEN definition of malnutrition in geriatric diabetic patients during hospitalization: A multicentric study. *Clin. Nutr.* **2016**, *35*, 1564–1567. [CrossRef]
3. Jiang, J.; Hu, X.; Chen, J.; Wang, H.; Zhang, L.; Dong, B.; Yang, M. Predicting long-term mortality in hospitalized elderly patients using the new ESPEN definition. *Sci. Rep.* **2017**, *7*, 4067. [CrossRef]
4. Sánchez-Rodríguez, D.; Marco, E.; Schott, A.-M.; Rolland, Y.; Blain, H.; Vázquez-Ibar, O.; Escalada, F.; Duran, X.; Muniesa, J.M.; Annweiler, C. Malnutrition according to ESPEN definition predicts long-term mortality in general older population: Findings from the EPIDOS study-Toulouse cohort. *Clin. Nutr.* **2018**, *38*, 2652–2658. [CrossRef]
5. Muscaritoli, M.; Krznarić, Z.; Singer, P.; Barazzoni, R.; Cederholm, T.; Golay, A.; Van Gossum, A.; Kennedy, N.; Kreymann, G.; Laviano, A.; et al. Effectiveness and efficacy of nutritional therapy: A systematic review following Cochrane methodology. *Clin. Nutr.* **2017**, *36*, 939–957. [CrossRef]
6. Volkert, D.; Beck, A.M.; Cederholmm, T.; Cruz-Jentoft, A.; Goisser, S.; Hooper, L.; Kiesswetter, E.; Maggio, M.; Raynaud-Simon, A.; Sieber, C.C.; et al. ESPEN guideline on clinical nutrition and hydration in geriatrics. *Clin. Nutr.* **2019**, *38*, 10–47. [CrossRef]
7. Beard, J.R.; Officer, A.; Araujo de Carvalho, I.; Sadana, R.; Margriet Pot, A.; Michel, J.; Lloyd-Sherlock, P.; Epping-Jordan, J.E.; GMEEG, P.; Mahanani, W.R.; et al. The World report on ageing and health: A policy framework for healthy ageing. *Lancet* **2016**, *387*, 2145–2154. [CrossRef]
8. Cederholm, T.; Bosaeus, I.; Barazzoni, R.; Bauer, J.; Van Gossum, A.; Klek, S.; Muscaritoli, M.; Nyulasi, I.; Ockenga, J.; Schneider, S.M.; et al. Diagnostic criteria for malnutrition—An ESPEN Consensus Statement. *Clin. Nutr.* **2015**, *34*, 335–340. [CrossRef]
9. Cederholm, T.; Barazzoni, R.; Austin, P.; Ballmer, P.; Biolo, G.; Bischoff, S.C.; Compher, C.; Correia, I.; Higashiguchi, T.; Holst, M.; et al. ESPEN guidelines on definitions and terminology of clinical nutrition. *Clin. Nutr.* **2017**, *36*, 49–64. [CrossRef]
10. Cederholm, T.; Jensen, G.L. To create a consensus on malnutrition diagnostic criteria: A report from the Global Leadership Initiative on Malnutrition (GLIM) meeting at the ESPEN Congress 2016. *Clin. Nutr.* **2017**, *36*, 7–10. [CrossRef]
11. Cederholm, T.; Jensen, G.; Correia, M.; Gonzalez, M.; Fukushima, R.; Higashiguchi, T.; Baptista, G.; Barazzoni, R.; Blaauw, R.; Coats, A.; et al. GLIM criteria for the diagnosis of malnutrition—A consensus report from the global clinical nutrition community. *J. Cachex Sarcopenia Muscle* **2019**, *10*, 207–217. [CrossRef]
12. Cruz-Jentoft, A.J.; Bahat, G.; Bauer, J.; Boirie, Y.; Bruyère, O.; Cederholm, T.; Cooper, C.; Landi, F.; Rolland, Y.; Sayer, A.A.; et al. Sarcopenia: Revised European consensus on definition and diagnosis. *Age Ageing* **2019**, *48*, 601. [CrossRef]
13. Cruz-Jentoft, A.J.; Sayer, A.A. Sarcopenia. *Lancet* **2019**, *393*, 2636–2646. [CrossRef]
14. Sieber, C.C. Malnutrition and sarcopenia. *Aging Clin. Exp. Res.* **2019**, *31*, 793–798. [CrossRef]

15. Mohseni, R.; Aliakbar, S.; Abdollahi, A.; Yekaninejad, M.S.; Maghbooli, Z.; Mirzaei, K. Relationship between major dietary patterns and sarcopenia among menopausal women. *Aging Clin. Exp. Res.* **2017**, *29*, 1241–1248. [CrossRef]
16. Beaudart, C.; Locquet, M.; Touvier, M.; Reginster, J.-Y.; Bruyère, O. Association between dietary nutrient intake and sarcopenia in the SarcoPhAge study. *Aging Clin. Exp. Res.* **2019**, *31*, 815–824. [CrossRef]
17. von Elm, E.; Altman, D.G.; Egger, M.; Pocock, S.J.; Gøtzsche, P.C.; Vandenbroucke, J.P.; Initiative, S. The Strengthening the Reporting of Observational Studies in Epidemiology (STROBE) statement: Guidelines for reporting observational studies. *Lancet (Lond. Engl.)* **2007**, *370*, 453–457. [CrossRef]
18. Beaudart, C.; Reginster, J.; Petermans, J.; Gillain, S.; Quabron, A.; Locquet, M.; Slomian, J.; Buckinx, F.; Bruyere, O. Quality of life and physical components linked to sarcopenia: The SarcoPhAge study. *Exp. Gerontol.* **2015**, *69*, 103–110. [CrossRef]
19. Fried, L.P.; Tangen, C.M.; Walston, J.; Newman, A.B.; Hirsch, C.; Gottdiener, J.; Seeman, T.; Tracy, R.; Kop, W.J.; Burke, G.; et al. Frailty in older adults: Evidence for a phenotype. *J. Gerontol. Ser. A Biol. Sci. Med. Sci.* **2001**, *56*, M146–M157. [CrossRef]
20. Guigoz, Y.; Lauque, S.; Vellas, B.J. Identifying the elderly at risk for malnutrition. *Clin. Geriatr. Med.* **2002**, *18*, 737–757. [CrossRef]
21. Justice, J.N.; Ferrucci, L.; Newman, A.B.; Aroda, V.R.; Bahnson, J.L.; Divers, J.; Espeland, M.A.; Marcovina, S.; Pollak, M.N.; Kritchevsky, S.B.; et al. A framework for selection of blood-based biomarkers for geroscience-guided clinical trials: Report from the TAME Biomarkers Workgroup. *GeroScience* **2018**, *40*, 419–436. [CrossRef]
22. Adriaensen, W.; Mathei, C.; Vaes, B.; Van Pottelbergh, G.; Wallemacq, P.; Degryse, J.-M. Interleukin-6 predicts short-term global functional decline in the oldest old: Results from the BELFRAIL study. *AGE* **2014**, *36*, 1–14. [CrossRef]
23. Roberts, H.C.; Denison, H.J.; Martin, H.J.; Patel, H.P.; Syddall, H.; Cooper, C.; Sayer, A.A. A review of the measurement of grip strength in clinical and epidemiological studies: Towards a standardised approach. *Age Ageing* **2011**, *40*, 423–429. [CrossRef]
24. Guralnik, J.M.; Ferrucci, L.; Pieper, C.F.; Leveille, S.G.; Markides, K.S.; Ostir, G.V.; Studenski, S.; Berkman, L.F.; Wallace, R.B. Lower extremity function and subsequent disability: Consistency across studies, predictive models, and value of gait speed alone compared with the short physical performance battery. *J. Gerontol. Ser. A Boil. Sci. Med. Sci.* **2000**, *55*, M221–M231. [CrossRef]
25. Beaudart, C.; Rolland, Y.; Cruz-Jentoft, A.J.; Bauer, J.M.; Sieber, C.; Cooper, C.; Al-Daghri, N.; De Carvalho, I.A.; Bautmans, I.; Bernabei, R.; et al. Assessment of Muscle Function and Physical Performance in Daily Clinical Practice: A position paper endorsed by the European Society for Clinical and Economic Aspects of Osteoporosis, Osteoarthritis and Musculoskeletal Diseases (ESCEO). *Calcif. Tissue Int.* **2019**, *105*, 1–14. [CrossRef]
26. Tombaugh, T.N.; McIntyre, N.J. The Mini-Mental State Examination: A Comprehensive Review. *J. Am. Geriatr Soc.* **1992**, *40*, 922–935. [CrossRef]
27. Lawton, M.P.; Brody, E.M. Assessment of Older People: Self-Maintaining and Instrumental Activities of Daily Living. *Gerontology* **1969**, *9*, 179–186. [CrossRef]
28. Taylor, H.L.; Jacobs, D.R.; Schucker, B.; Knudsen, J.; Leon, A.S.; Debacker, G.; Jacobs, D.R., Jr. A questionnaire for the assessment of leisure time physical activities. *J. Chronic Dis.* **1978**, *31*, 741–755. [CrossRef]
29. Cruz-Jentoft, A.J.; Landi, F.; Schneider, S.M.; Zúñiga, C.; Arai, H.; Boirie, Y.; Chen, L.K.; Fielding, R.A.; Martin, F.C.; Michel, J.P.; et al. Prevalence of and interventions for sarcopenia in ageing adults: A systematic review. Report of the International Sarcopenia Initiative (EWGSOP and IWGS). *Age Ageing* **2014**, *43*, 748–759. [CrossRef]
30. Zadak, Z.; Hyspler, R.; Ticha, A.; Vlcek, J. Polypharmacy and malnutrition. *Curr. Opin. Clin. Nutr. Metab. Care* **2013**, *16*, 50–55. [CrossRef]
31. Sanders, C.; Behrens, S.; Schwartz, S.; Wengreen, H.; Corcoran, C.D.; Lyketsos, C.G.; Tschanz, J.T. Nutritional Status is Associated with Faster Cognitive Decline and Worse Functional Impairment in the Progression of Dementia: The Cache County Dementia Progression Study1. *J. Alzheimer's Dis.* **2016**, *52*, 33–42. [CrossRef]

32. Steffl, M.; Bohannon, R.W.; Sontakova, L.; Tufano, J.J.; Shiells, K.; Holmerova, I. Relationship between sarcopenia and physical activity in older people: A systematic review and meta-analysis. *Clin. Interv. Aging* **2017**, *12*, 835–845. [CrossRef]
33. Contreras-Bolívar, V.; Sánchez-Torralvo, F.J.; Ruiz-Vico, M.; González-Almendros, I.; Barrios, M.; Padín, S.; Alba, E.; Olveira, G. GLIM Criteria Using Hand Grip Strength Adequately Predict Six-Month Mortality in Cancer Inpatients. *Nutrients* **2019**, *11*, 2043. [CrossRef] [PubMed]
34. Yilmaz, M.; Atilla, F.D.; Sahin, F.; Saydam, G. The effect of malnutrition on mortality in hospitalized patients with hematologic malignancy. *Support. Care Cancer* **2019**, 1–8. [CrossRef] [PubMed]
35. Lindqvist, C.; Slinde, F.; Majeed, A.; Bottai, M.; Wahlin, S. Nutrition impact symptoms are related to malnutrition and quality of life-A cross-sectional study of patients with chronic liver disease. *Clin. Nutr.* **2019**. [CrossRef]
36. Karahalios, A.; English, D.R.; Simpson, J.A. Change in body size and mortality: A systematic review and meta-analysis. *Int. J. Epidemiol.* **2017**, *46*, 526–546. [CrossRef]
37. Vettoretti, S.; Caldiroli, L.; Armelloni, S.; Ferrari, C.; Cesari, M.; Messa, P. Sarcopenia is Associated with Malnutrition but Not with Systemic Inflammation in Older Persons with Advanced CKD. *Nutrition* **2019**, *11*, 1378. [CrossRef]
38. Marco, E.; Sánchez-Rodríguez, D.; Dávalos-Yerovi, V.N.; Duran, X.; Pascual, E.M.; Muniesa, J.M.; Rodríguez, D.A.; Aguilera-Zubizarreta, A.; Escalada, F.; Duarte, E. Malnutrition according to ESPEN consensus predicts hospitalizations and long-term mortality in rehabilitation patients with stable chronic obstructive pulmonary disease. *Clin. Nutr.* **2019**, *38*, 2180–2186. [CrossRef]
39. Sánchez-Rodríguez, D.; Marco, E.; Ronquillo-Moreno, N.; Miralles, R.; Vázquez-Ibar, O.; Escalada, F.; Muniesa, J.M. Prevalence of malnutrition and sarcopenia in a post-acute care geriatric unit: Applying the new ESPEN definition and EWGSOP criteria. *Clin. Nutr.* **2017**, *36*, 1339–1344. [CrossRef]
40. Martone, A.M.; Bianchi, L.; Abete, P.; Bellelli, G.; Bo, M.; Cherubini, A.; Corica, F.; Di Bari, M.; Maggio, M.; Manca, G.M.; et al. The incidence of sarcopenia among hospitalized older patients: Results from the Glisten study. *J. Cachex Sarcopenia Muscle* **2017**, *8*, 907–914. [CrossRef]
41. Mithal, A.; Bonjour, J.P.; Boonen, S.; Burckhardt, P.; Degens, H.; Fuleihan, G.A.E.; Josse, R.; Lips, P.; Torres, J.M.; Rizzoli, R.; et al. Impact of nutrition on muscle mass, strength, and performance in older adults. *Osteoporos. Int.* **2013**, *24*, 1555–1566. [CrossRef] [PubMed]
42. Beckwée, D.; Delaere, A.; Aelbrecht, S.; Baert, V.; Beaudart, C.; Bruyere, O.; de Saint-Hubert, M.; Bautmans, I. Exercise Interventions for the Prevention and Treatment of Sarcopenia. A Systematic Umbrella Review. *J. Nutr. Health Aging* **2019**, *23*, 494–502. [CrossRef] [PubMed]
43. Robinson, S.M.; Reginster, J.Y.; Rizzoli, R.; Shaw, S.C.; Kanis, J.A.; Bautmans, I.; Bischoff-Ferrariet, H.; Bruyère, O.; Cesari, M.; Dawson-Hughes, B.; et al. Does nutrition play a role in the prevention and management of sarcopenia? *Clin. Nutr.* **2018**, *37*, 1121–1132. [CrossRef] [PubMed]
44. Vellas, B.; Fielding, R.A.; Bens, C.; Bernabei, R.; Cawthon, P.M.; Cederholm, T.; Cruz-Jentoft, A.J.; Del Signore, S.; Donahue, S.; Morley, J.; et al. Implications of ICD-10 for Sarcopenia Clinical Practice and Clinical Trials: Report by the International Conference on Frailty and Sarcopenia Research Task Force. *J. Frailty Aging* **2018**, *7*, 2–9. [PubMed]
45. Dubard, C.A.; Jackson, C.T. Active Redesign of a Medicaid Care Management Strategy for Greater Return on Investment: Predicting Impactability. *Popul. Health Manag.* **2018**, *21*, 102–109. [CrossRef] [PubMed]
46. Juby, A.G.; Mager, D.R. A review of nutrition screening tools used to assess the malnutrition-sarcopenia syndrome (MSS) in the older adult. *Clin. Nutr. ESPEN* **2019**, *32*, 8–15. [CrossRef] [PubMed]

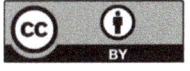

© 2019 by the authors. Licensee MDPI, Basel, Switzerland. This article is an open access article distributed under the terms and conditions of the Creative Commons Attribution (CC BY) license (http://creativecommons.org/licenses/by/4.0/).

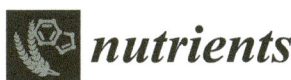

Article

Hochu-Ekki-To Improves Motor Function in an Amyotrophic Lateral Sclerosis Animal Model

Mudan Cai [1] and Eun Jin Yang [2],*

[1] Department of Herbal medicine Research, Korea Institute of Oriental Medicine, 1672 Yuseong-daero, Yuseong-gu, Daejeon 305-811, Korea; mudan126@kiom.re.kr
[2] Department of Clinical Research, Korea Institute of Oriental Medicine, 1672 Yuseong-daero, Yuseong-gu, Daejeon 305-811, Korea
* Correspondence: yej4823@gmail.com; Tel.: +82-42-863-9497; Fax: 82-42-868-9339

Received: 23 September 2019; Accepted: 31 October 2019; Published: 4 November 2019

Abstract: Hochu-ekki-to (Bojungikgi-Tang (BJIGT) in Korea; Bu-Zhong-Yi-Qi Tang in Chinese), a traditional herbal prescription, has been widely used in Asia. Hochu-ekki-to (HET) is used to enhance the immune system in respiratory disorders, improve the nutritional status associated with chronic diseases, enhance the mucosal immune system, and improve learning and memory. Amyotrophic lateral sclerosis (ALS) is pathologically characterized by motor neuron cell death and muscle paralysis, and is an adult-onset motor neuron disease. Several pathological mechanisms of ALS have been reported by clinical and *in vitro*/*in vivo* studies using ALS models. However, the underlying mechanisms remain elusive, and the critical pathological target needs to be identified before effective drugs can be developed for patients with ALS. Since ALS is a disease involving both motor neuron death and skeletal muscle paralysis, suitable therapy with optimal treatment effects would involve a motor neuron target combined with a skeletal muscle target. Herbal medicine is effective for complex diseases because it consists of multiple components for multiple targets. Therefore, we investigated the effect of the herbal medicine HET on motor function and survival in hSOD1^{G93A} transgenic mice. HET was orally administered once a day for 6 weeks from the age of 2 months (the pre-symptomatic stage) of hSOD1^{G93A} transgenic mice. We used the rota-rod test and foot printing test to examine motor activity, and Western blotting and H&E staining for evaluation of the effects of HET in the gastrocnemius muscle and lumbar (L4–5) spinal cord of mice. We found that HET treatment dramatically inhibited inflammation and oxidative stress both in the spinal cord and gastrocnemius of hSOD1^{G93A} transgenic mice. Furthermore, HET treatment improved motor function and extended the survival of hSOD1^{G93A} transgenic mice. Our findings suggest that HET treatment may modulate the immune reaction in muscles and neurons to delay disease progression in a model of ALS.

Keywords: amyotrophic lateral sclerosis; Hochu-ekki-to; herbal medicine; muscle dysfunction; motor neuronal cell death

1. Introduction

Amyotrophic lateral sclerosis (ALS), also known as Lou Gehrig's disease, is characterized by a loss of motor neurons, muscle weakness, and spasticity [1]. ALS can be divided into familiar ALS (fALS), which is caused by autosomal dominant mutations in genes such as superoxide dismutase (SOD)1, and sporadic ALS (sALS). However, some gene mutations have been found to be involved in both fALS and sALS, including mutations of TAR DNA-binding protein (TDP) 43, fused in sarcoma (FUS), valosin-containing protein (VCP), and TATA-binding protein-associated factor 15 (TAF15) [2].

Several pathological mechanisms underlying ALS have been reported, including proteasome and autophagy dysfunction, ER stress, oxidative stress, and mitochondrial disorders [3]. Most notably, a dysregulated immune response plays a critical role in disease progression, as revealed by both ALS animal model and clinical studies [4–6].

In the central nervous system (CNS), neuroinflammation that is mediated by microglia is involved in the pathogenesis of neurodegenerative diseases such as Alzheimer's Disease (AD), Parkinson's Disease (PD), and ALS. In ALS, specific gene mutations in the CNS have been found to contribute to immune dysfunction, including mutations of SOD1, TARDBP, and C9orf72 [7–9]. A mutant SOD1 overexpressed animal model was found to exhibit motor neuron dysfunction that was induced by an increase in activated microglia in the peripheral nervous system and CNS [10]. In addition, the expression of IL-6 has been reported to increase via activation of microglia and macrophages in both an animal model of and patients with ALS [11,12]. In the muscles, alternation of neuromuscular junction (NMJ) and muscle denervation that involves a loss of presynaptic terminals, Schwann cells, and axonal degeneration, has been found to lead to clinical weakness and an increased disease severity in patients with ALS [13]. Furthermore, activated macrophages reportedly surround NMJs in symptomatic and end-stage mouse models of ALS [14], and complement factors are upregulated to recruit macrophages in the denervated muscle of a SOD1^{G93A} mouse model [15]. Therefore, immune enhancers could be a candidate for attenuating disease progression and enhancing homeostasis of the body in patients with ALS.

Herbal medicine has been widely used in Asian countries for thousands of years because of antinociceptive, analgesic, and anti-inflammatory effects, both centrally and peripherally [16,17]. Simply put, herbal medicine can stimulate the immune system and maintain the internal balance of the body. In the case of AD, bioactive components from herbal medicines such as Radix Polygalae, *Panax ginseng*, and *Ginko biloba* have been shown to effectively improve AD symptoms by targeting autophagy [18]. In ALS, many experimental studies have demonstrated that Chinese prescriptions have anti-inflammatory and anti-oxidant effects. In patients with ALS, Chinese prescriptions, including Jiawei Sijunzi, and Dihuang Yinzi, have been found to improve phenotype symptoms and functional rating scales [19,20]. However, further evidence for the efficacy, mechanisms of action, and safety of herbal medicines in the treatment of ALS is required.

Hochu-ekki-to (HET) in Japanese herbal (Kampo) medicine is similar to Bojungikgi-Tang (BJIGT) in Korea and Bu-Zhong-Yi-Qi Tang in Chinese medicine. HET has ten component herbs, as follows: Astragali radix (16.7%, *A. membranaceus* Bunge), Atractylodes lancea Rhizome (16.7%, rhizomes of *A. lancea* DC.), Ginseng radix (16.7%, *P. ginseng* C.A. Meyer), Angelica Radix (12.5%, *Angelica acutiloba* Kitagawa), Bupleuri radix (8.3%, *Bupleurum falcatum* L.), Zizyphi fructus (8.3%, *Zizyphus jujuba* Miller var. inermis Rehder), Aurantii nobilis pericarpium (8.3%, *Citrus unshu* Markovich), Glycyrrhizae radix (6.3%, *Glycyrrhiza uralensis* Fisch et DC.), Cimicifugae Rhizoma (4.2%, *Cimicifuga simplex* Worms kjord), and Zingiberis Rhizoma (2%, *Zingiber officinale* Roscoe) and it was provided by Tsumura pharmaceutical company [21,22]. In addition, Dan et al., and Yae et al., had already reported chemical profile of HET by 3-dimensional HPLC.

HET has been used to enhance the immune system in respiratory disorders [23,24] and to improve the nutritional status associated with chronic diseases [25]. Thus, many studies have investigated the immunopharmacological activities of HET [26–28]. In addition, Kiyohara et al. reported that HET enhanced the mucosal immune system [29]. Shih et al. found that HET improved learning and memory, and had an anti-aging effects in a senescence-accelerated mouse model [29]. Furthermore, the authors suggested that HET can penetrate the blood–brain barrier by increasing dopamine and noradrenaline levels in the brain.

ALS causes both motor neuron death and skeletal muscle paralysis. A suitable therapy with optimal treatment effects for patients with ALS would involve a motor neuron target combined with a skeletal muscle target. In this sense, herbal medicine is effective for complex disease because herbal medicine consists of multiple components. Therefore, we investigated the effect of HET on neuroinflammation, motor function, and muscle weakness in a hSOD1^{G93A} animal model.

2. Materials and Methods

2.1. Animals

Male hemizygous hSOD1^{G93A} transgenic mice and female B6SJL mice were purchased from the Jackson Laboratory (Bar Harbor, ME, USA) and maintained as described previously [30]. hSOD1^{G93A} mice have a glycine-to-alanine base-pair mutation at the 93rd codon of the cytosolic Cu/Zn superoxide dismutase gene. Male hSOD1^{G93A} mice were housed at 3–4 per cage under specific pathogen-free conditions and had *ad libitum* access to food and water. The facilities were maintained under a constant temperature (21 ± 3 °C) and humidity (50 ± 10%) with a 12 hours light/dark cycle (lights on 07:00–19:00). All mice were treated in accordance with the animal care guidelines of the Korea Institute of Oriental Medicine (protocol number: 13–109).

2.2. Hochu-Ekki-To (HET) Treatment

Hochu-ekki-to (HET) was purchased from TSUMURA Co. Ltd (TSUMURA, Osaka, Japan) and diluted at 1 mg/g with autoclaved distilled water. The mice were randomly divided into three groups, as follows: a non-transgenic mice group (nTg, $n = 8$), a hSOD1^{G93A} transgenic mice group (Tg, $n = 11$), and a HET treated hSOD1^{G93A} transgenic mice group (Tg-HET, $n = 11$) (Figure 1). HET (1 mg/g) was orally administered with a disposable oral gavage syringe (FUCHIGAMI, Kurume, Japan) once a day for 6 weeks from the age of 2 months (the pre-symptomatic stage). The dose was translated from human to animal based on a previous study [31].

2.3. Rota-Rod Test

The rota-rod test is used to assess motor activity and balance in rodents. Mice were trained every other day for 2 weeks to adapt to the apparatus (Rotarod, B.S Technolab Inc., Korea). During training, the rota-rod was maintained at a constant speed of 10 rpm for 180 seconds. After the last administration of HET, mice performed the test, and we recorded the time mice remained on the rod before falling. Each mouse performed three trials and the average time spent on the rod was determined for each group.

2.4. Foot Print Test

The day before mice were sacrificed, the footprint test was used to measure gait. To record stride length, mice hind paws were stained with nontoxic water-soluble black ink, and the alley floor (70 cm length, 6 cm width, and 16 cm height) was covered with white paper to absorb the ink. Each mouse performed three trials and the average of stride length was determined for each group.

2.5. Survival Test

To measure lifespan, male transgenic mice were randomly divided into the following treatment groups: distilled water-treated ALS mice ($n = 8$) and ALS mice treated with HET for 6 weeks ($n = 8$/group). Death was defined according to our previous paper [32].

2.6. Tissue Preparation

Body weight of mice was measured and mice were anesthetized using pentobarbital sodium (Entobar, Hanlim Pharm, Co., Ltd., Seoul, Korea) and perfused with phosphate-buffered saline (PBS). The gastrocnemius muscle and spinal cord of the mice were dissected and stored at −80 °C until use. The gastrocnemius muscle weight was recorded and the average value for each group recorded. For hematoxylin and eosin (H&E) staining, the gastrocnemius muscle of the mice was fixed in 4% paraformaldehyde at 4 °C before embedding in paraffin. The tissues were cut into transverse sections (5 μm thick) using a microtome (Leica biosystems, IL, USA) and mounted on glass slides.

2.7. Western Blotting

For Western blotting, the gastrocnemius muscle and lumbar (L4–5) spinal cord of mice were homogenized in radioimmunoprecipitation assay buffer (50 mM, Tris-HCl (pH 7.4); 1% Nonidet P–40; 0.1% sodium dodecyl sulfate; 150 mM NaCl) containing protease and a phosphatase inhibitor cocktail (Thermo, Waltham, MA, USA). Homogenized tissues were centrifuged at 20,800 × g for 15 minutes at 4 °C. The protein concentration was determined using the Bicinchoninic Acid Assay Kit (Pierce, IL, USA). The samples (20 μg of protein) were denatured with sodium dodecyl sulfate sampling buffer, separated using SDS-PAGE electrophoresis, and transferred to a Polyvinylidene difluoride membrane (Bio-Rad, Hercules, CA, USA). Membranes were incubated in a blocking solution (5% skim milk in TBS) for 1 hour at room temperature then incubated in the various primary antibodies (anti-iba-1, anti-GFAP, anti-TLR4, anti-BAX, anti-HO1, anti-transferrin, anti-CD11b, anti-Ferritin, anti-tubulin, and anti-actin) overnight at 4 °C. The next day, blots were washed and incubated with horseradish peroxidase-conjugated secondary antibodies, and then visualized using the SuperSignal West Femto Substrate Maximum Sensitivity Substrate (Thermo Fisher Scientific, Waltham, MA, USA). For detection of the other antibodies, membranes were stripped in a stripping buffer (Thermo Fisher Scientific, Waltham, MA, USA). The blots were analyzed using the ChemiDoc imaging system (Bio-Rad, Hercules, CA, USA), which were then quantified using the NIH ImageJ program (National Institutes of Health, Bethesda, MD, USA).

2.8. H&E Staining and Immunohistohcemistry

For H&E staining, the paraffin sections were de-paraffinized in xylene and rehydrated in a graded alcohol series (100%, 95%, 80% ethanol), followed by deionized H_2O. Slices were incubated in hematoxylin (Sigma-Aldrich Corp., St. Louis, MO, USA) for 6 minutes and washed under flowing distilled water for 5 minutes, then incubated in eosin for 45 seconds, dehydrated (95%, 100%, xylene), and mounted using a Histomount medium (Sigma-Aldrich Corp.). Immunohistochemistry was performed with previous paper described [32]. In brief, de-paraffinized slides were incubated with 3% hydrogen peroxide (H_2O_2) and 5% bovine serum albumin (BSA) in 0.01% PBS-Triton X–100 (Sigma-Aldrich, Oakville, ON, Canada). The sections were incubated with anti-IL-1β (Abcam, Cambridge, UK) and then secondary antibody. For observation, the ABC kit and 3,3'-diaminobenzidine (DAB)/H_2O_2 substrate were used with a hematoxylin counterstain. Immunostained tissues were observed with a light microscope (Olympus, Tokyo, Japan). The central nuclei (as a marker of abnormal nuclei) were counted and expressed as a percentage: the number of myocytes with central nuclei divided by the total number of myocytes in each captured image. For the quantification of myocyte cross-sectional area (CSA), the average area of individual myocytes was measured using the NIH ImageJ program.

2.9. Statistical Analysis

All values are expressed as the mean ± SEM. The results were analyzed using a one-way analysis of variance (ANOVA) followed by the Newman-Keuls's *post hoc* test for multiple comparisons. For survival test, the data were analyzed by Kaplan–Meier survival curves. Data were analyzed using GraphPad Prism 5.0 (GraphPad Software, San Diego, CA, USA). Statistical significance was set at $p < 0.05$.

3. Results

3.1. Hochu-Ekki-(HET) Extended Survival and Improved Motor Function

To examine the effects of HET on physical function, we measured the body and muscle weight of symptomatic HET-treated hSOD1^{G93A} mice (Tg-HET). As shown in Figure 1A, body weight of hSOD1^{G93A} mice (Tg) was lower than that of age-matched non-Tg (nTg); however, there was no significant difference in body weight between the Tg and Tg-HET groups. HET treatment resulted in a 1.6-fold significant increase in the weight of the gastrocnemius muscle compared to that of Tg mice

(Figure 1B). Furthermore, we found that HET treatment resulted in a 2.8-fold improvement in motor function in symptomatic hSOD1^{G93A} mice, as revealed in the rota-rod test (Figure 1C). Motor activity was assessed by measuring stride length through the foot print test. The stride length of Tg-HET mice was 1.5-fold greater than age-matched Tg mice (Figure 1D). Furthermore, HET treatment extended the survival rate compared to that of Tg mice (Figure 1E). These findings suggest that HET treatment can prevent motor neuron death and skeletal muscle paralysis in hSOD1^{G93A} mice.

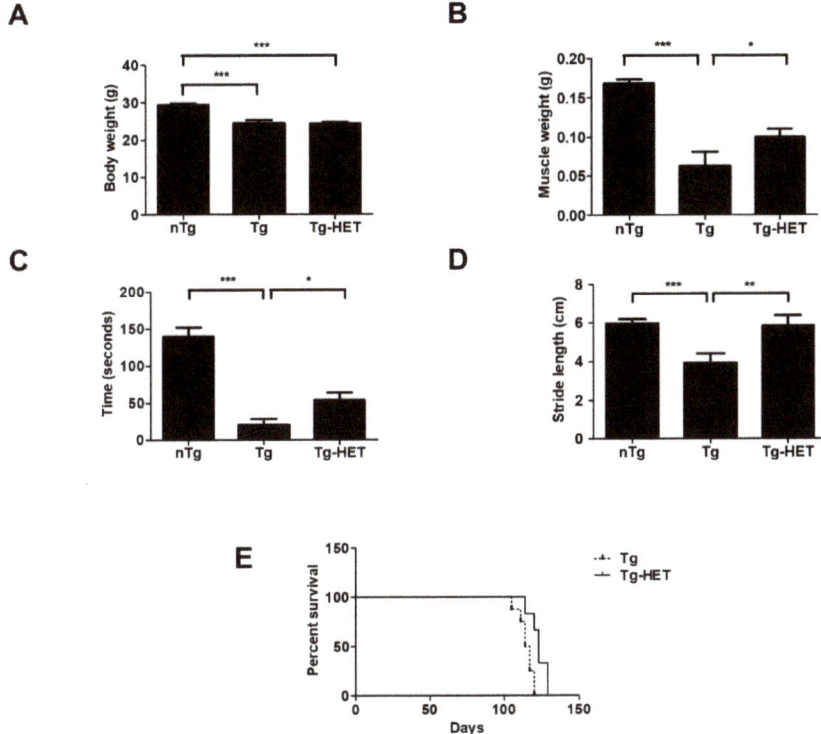

Figure 1. Hochu-ekki-to (HET) treatment ameliorates motor activity and prolongs the life span of a mouse model of amyotrophic lateral sclerosis (ALS). HET (1 mg/g) was orally administered once a day for 6 weeks from the age of 2 months. (**A**) Comparison of body weight between the nTg, Tg, and HET-treated Tg groups. (**B**) Comparison of gastrocnemius weight between the nTg, Tg, and HET-treated Tg groups. (**C**) Motor function was measured by the rota-rod test in all groups. (**D**) The representative average of stride length (n = 7/group) of each group, measured using the foot print test. (**E**) Survival rate was calculated by Kaplan-Meyer analysis in Tg and HET-treated Tg (n = 8/group). Data are shown as the mean ± SEM. * p < 0.05, ** p < 0.01, *** p < 0.001. nTg: non-transgenic mice, Tg: hSOD1^{G93A}, Tg-HET:HET-treated hSOD1^{G93A}.

3.2. Hochu-Ekki-To (HET) Reduces Neuroinflammation and Oxidative Stress in the Spinal Cord of hSOD1^{G93A} Mice

In our previous study, we found that hSOD1^{G93A} transgenic mice had increased neuroinflammation, indicated by an increase in CD11b, GFAP, Iba-1, and TLR4 (inflammatory proteins in spinal cord) [33,34]. To investigate the effect of HET on neuroinflammation of the spinal cord in hSOD1^{G93A} mice, we investigated the expression of neuroinflammation-related proteins (Iba-1, GFAP, and TLR4) using immunoblotting. As shown in Figure 2A,B, the expression levels of Iba-1, GFAP, and TLR4 in the spinal cord were significantly greater by 18-, 2.1-, and 2.8-fold in symptomatic Tg mice compared to those of nTg mice. However, HET treatment dramatically reduced the levels of Iba-1, GFAP, and TLR4 proteins by 2.3-, 2.7-, and 1.7-fold compared to that of Tg mice. In addition, proinflammatory cytokine, IL-1β immunoreactivity was increased in anterior horn of spinal cord of symptomatic Tg mice, but it was reduced by treatment with HET (Figure 2C). Furthermore, we found evidence for anti-neuroinflammatory effects of HET, and observed a reduction of oxidative stress in the spinal cord of Tg mice. Oxidative stress-related proteins HO1, transferrin, and BAX were significantly lower by 7-, 2.6-, and 1.6-fold in the spinal cord of Tg-HET mice compared to that of age-matched Tg mice (Figure 2D,E). Taken together, HET treatment seems to enhance neuroimmune systems to maintain motor neuron survival and consequently improve motor function in the ALS animal model.

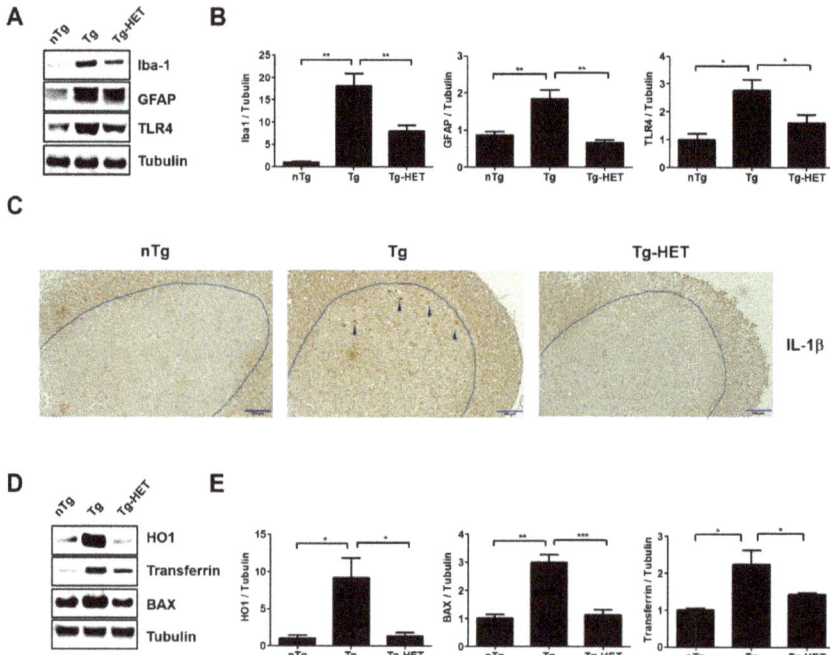

Figure 2. Hochu-ekki-to (HET) increases anti-inflammation and anti-oxidative stress effects in the spinal cord of an ALS mouse model. (**A**) Representative Western blots on inflammatory protein levels of Iba-1 (a marker of microglia), GFAP (a marker of astrocytes), and TLR4 in the spinal cord of each group (nTg, Tg, and Tg- HET). Tubulin was used as a loading control. (**B**) Quantification of the expression level of Iba-1/Tubulin, GFAP/Tubulin, and TLR4/Tubulin in each immunoblot. (**C**) Representative images of IL-1β immunoreatcivity in the anterior horn of the spinal cord in each group. Scale bars = 100 μm (**D**) Representative images of oxidative stress-related proteins (BAX, HO1, and Transferrin) in the spinal cord of each group mice. (**E**) Quantification of the expression levels of BAX/Tubulin, HO1/Tubulin, and transferrin/Tubulin. Data are presented as the mean ± SEM ($n = 3$/group). * $p < 0.05$, ** $p < 0.01$, *** $p < 0.001$. nTg: non-transgenic mice, Tg: hSOD1^{G93A}, Tg-HET:HET-treated hSOD1^{G93A}.

3.3. Hochu-Ekki-To (HET) Attenuates Muscle Dysfunction

In our previous study, we found that HO1, Transferrin, BAX, and Ferritin (as oxidative stress-related proteins) were increased in the spinal cord of hSOD1^{G93A} mice [35,36]. To examine the effect of HET on the weakness of skeletal muscle during ALS progression, we investigated the expression level of inflammatory and oxidative stress-related proteins in the gastrocnemius muscle of symptomatic hSOD1^{G93A} mice. The smaller myocytes with abnormal nuclei that had moved to the center of the cells in the gastrocnemius of hSOD1^{G93A} mice. As shown in Figure 3A,B, we found that the percentage of central nuclei was increased by 7.8-fold in the gastrocnemius muscle of symptomatic hSOD1^{G93A} mice compared to nTg mice (Figure 3B). In addition, the average CSA of myocytes was reduced by 2.2-fold in symptomatic hSOD1^{G93A} mice compared to nTg mice (Figure 3B). However, HET treatment led to decrease 4.8-fold in the percentage of central nuclei and increase 2.4-fold the average CSA of myocytes in the gastrocnemius of hSOD1^{G93A} mice.

In addition, myocyte was small in the gastrocnemius muscle of symptomatic hSOD1^{G93A} mice. However, HET treatment inhibited the muscle atrophy seen in the gastrocnemius by H&E staining (Figure 3). This suggests that HET treatment can reduce muscle damage and inflammation in the gastrocnemius of symptomatic hSOD1^{G93A} mice. To address this hypothesis, we investigated the expression level of inflammatory proteins including CD11b and GFAP and oxidative stress-related proteins such as Ferritin, HO1, and BAX in gastrocnemius of symptomatic hSOD1^{G93A} mice. As expected, HET treatment significantly reduced the expression levels of GFAP and CD11b by 1.7- and 2.5-fold, respectively, in the gastrocnemius of hSOD1^{G93A} mice (Figure 4A,B). In addition, proinflammatory cytokine, IL-1β immunoreactivity was increased in the gastrocnemius of symptomatic Tg mice, but it was reduced by treatment with HET (Figure 4C). Furthermore, HET treatment significantly reduced the levels of Ferritin, HO1, and BAX by 1.9-, 1.6-, and 2.2-fold, respectively, in the gastrocnemius of hSOD1^{G93A} mice (Figure 4D,E). These findings suggest that HET treatment may boost the immune system to protect from muscle loss and damage in this model of ALS.

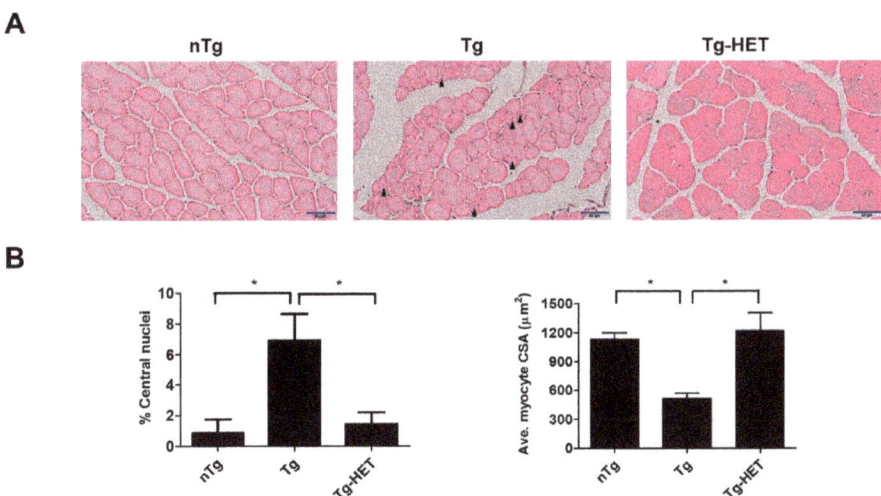

Figure 3. Hochu-ekki-to (HET) treatment has a protective effect against muscle atrophy in the gastrocnemius of an ALS mouse model. (**A**) Representative images of H&E staining showing the muscle atrophy condition, such as smaller myocytes and abnormal nuclei in gastrocnemius of hSOD1^{G93A} mice. Arrowheads indicate abnormal nuclei (central nucleation) in myocytes. (**B**) Abnormal nuclei were expressed as a percentage of abnormal nuclei (left panel). Quantified average myocyte cross-sectional area (CSA) (right panel). Scale bar = 50 μm Data are presented as the mean ± SEM (n = 3/group). * p < 0.05. nTg: non-transgenic mice, Tg: hSOD1^{G93A}, Tg-HET:HET-treated hSOD1^{G93A}.

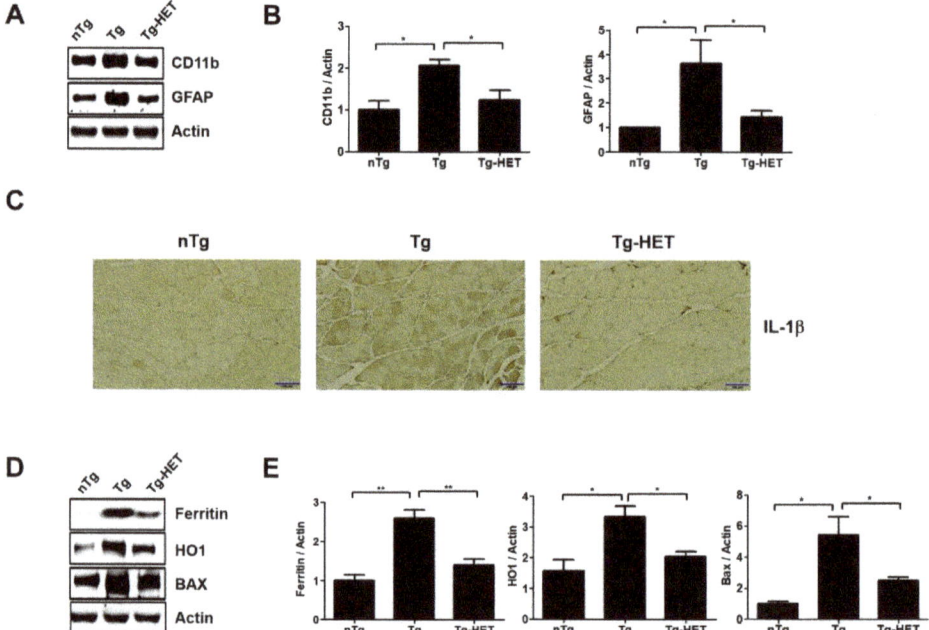

Figure 4. Hochu-ekki-to (HET) treatment enhances anti-inflammation, anti-oxidative stress effects, and regulates autophagy in the gastrocnemius of an ALS mouse model. (**A**) Representative Western blots of inflammatory related proteins, CD11b and GFAP, in the gastrocnemius of each group. Actin was used as a loading control. (**B**) Quantification of the expression levels of CD11b/Actin and GFAP/Actin. (**C**) Representative images of IL-1β immunostaining in the gastrocnemius of each group. Scale bars = 100 μm (**D**) Representative images of oxidative stress-related proteins (Ferratin, HO1, and BAX) in the gastrocnemius of each group. (**E**) Quantification of the expression levels of Ferritin/Actin, HO1/Actin, and BAX/Actin. Data are presented as the mean ± SEM (n = 3/group). * $p < 0.05$, ** $p < 0.01$. nTg: non-transgenic mice, Tg: hSOD1^{G93A}, Tg-HET:HET-treated hSOD1^{G93A}.

4. Discussion

ALS is a disease with complex pathological mechanisms and no effective drug treatment. Herbal medicine is composed of multiple components and is used for multi-targets. In addition, herbal medicine focuses on boosting the immune system and maintaining an internal balance of the body. To investigate the possibility of using herbal medicine as treatment for ALS, we investigated the effect of HET treatment on the spinal cord and skeletal muscle in an animal model of ALS.

Neuroinflammation in the brain occurred via microglial proliferation and astrocytic hypertrophy. Microglia are immune cells in the CNS that play a role in clearing pathogens through phagocytosis and play a critical role in homeostasis [37]. Microglial cell activation increases the expression of inflammatory cytokines such as IL-6 and IL1β and leads to oxidative stress and neuroinflammation, which results in augmented microglial NADPH-derived ROS accumulation [38,39]. In ALS, microglial activation is correlated with neuroinflammation and disease progression [40]. Correspondingly, minocycline treatment has been found to reduce neuroinflammation and microglial activation in clinical trials with patients with ALS [41]. However, it is not effective in patients with ALS who have other neurological disorders. Hence, herbal medicine may be a good, more effective candidate for protecting neurons and skeletal muscle from degeneration, primarily because herbal medicine contains multiple compounds and targets. In this study, HET treatment reduced the expression levels of CD11b and GFAP in the spinal cord and gastrocnemius of symptomatic hSOD1^{G93A} mice. This suggests that HET treatment can enhance the body's immune system and extend the survival rate of these mice. As expected, we found that HET treatment increases gastrocnemius weight and survival rate of hSOD1^{G93A} mice.

Oxidative stress and inflammation are significant factors in ALS pathogenesis, and lead to motor neuron death and severe muscle degeneration. While motor neurons control muscle function, retrograde signals can pass from the muscle back to motor neurons via the NMJ [42]. In addition, previous work has found that oxidative stress leading to muscle atrophy was increased in the pre-symptomatic stages in hSOD1^{G86R} mice [43]. In our study, we found that oxidative stress-related proteins such as Ferritin, HO1, Transferrin, and BAX were dramatically increased in the gastrocnemius and the spinal cord of symptomatic hSOD1^{G93A} mice. Furthermore, HET treatment significantly attenuated the expression level of oxidative stress-related proteins in the muscle and spinal cord of hSOD1^{G93A} mice. Patients with ALS have defective energy homeostasis, and skeletal muscle degeneration is a critical factor in the pathogenesis of ALS and its symptoms. Some studies have provided consistent evidence by demonstrating that atrophy occurred before motor neuron loss and neurodegeneration [44,45]. Furthermore, studies with patients with ALS (fALS and sALS) and animal models of ALS (hSOD1^{G93A} and ^{G86R} models) have reported increased energy expenditure and a defective energy balance due to increased oxidative stress, mitochondrial dysfunction, and inflammation [46–48].

5. Conclusions

In this study, HET treatment improved muscle function and the survival rate via a reduction of inflammation-related events in both the spinal cord and gastrocnemius of symptomatic hSOD1^{G93A} mice. This suggests that HET treatment can be used to boost immune responses and homeostasis in not only ALS, but also other neurodegenerative diseases. Since ALS is a heterogeneous disease, our findings of a protective effect of HET against muscle atrophy should be verified using other genetic mutation models involving ALS mice of both sexes. Furthermore, patients with ALS have a diverse range of pathologies compared to hSOD1^{G93A} mice. Therefore, future work could examine tissue or cells from patients with ALS treated with HET. Another future challenge would be to identify the bioactive compound of HET, which is composed of ten herbs, to pinpoint the specific molecular mechanisms underlying the positive effects of this herbal medicine.

Author Contributions: M.C. performed with experimental works and wrote a part of the manuscript. Data were analyzed by M.C. and E.J.Y. E.J.Y. designed research and wrote final proof. All authors have read and approved the final manuscript.

Funding: This study was supported by the Korea Institute of Oriental Medicine (KIOM) under Grant C18040 and KSN1621051.

Acknowledgments: We thank Sun Hwa Lee for helping animal care.

Conflicts of Interest: The authors declare that they have no competing interests.

References

1. Orsini, M.; Oliveira, A.B.; Nascimento, O.J.; Reis, C.H.; Leite, M.A.; de Souza, J.A.; Pupe, C.; de Souza, O.G.; Bastos, V.H.; de Freitas, M.R.; et al. Amyotrophic Lateral Sclerosis: New Perpectives and Update. *Neurol. Int.* **2015**, *7*, 5885. [CrossRef] [PubMed]
2. Robberecht, W.; Philips, T. The changing scene of amyotrophic lateral sclerosis. *Nat. Rev. Neurosci.* **2013**, *14*, 248–264. [CrossRef] [PubMed]
3. Mesika, R.; Reichmann, D. When safeguarding goes wrong: Impact of oxidative stress on protein homeostasis in health and neurodegenerative disorders. *Adv. Protein Chem. Struct. Biol.* **2019**, *114*, 221–264. [CrossRef] [PubMed]
4. Rusconi, M.; Gerardi, F.; Santus, W.; Lizio, A.; Sansone, V.A.; Lunetta, C.; Zanoni, I.; Granucci, F. Inflammatory role of dendritic cells in Amyotrophic Lateral Sclerosis revealed by an analysis of patients' peripheral blood. *Sci. Rep.* **2017**, *7*, 7853. [CrossRef] [PubMed]

5. McCauley, M.E.; Baloh, R.H. Inflammation in ALS/FTD pathogenesis. *Acta. Neuropathol.* **2019**, *137*, 715–730. [CrossRef] [PubMed]
6. Lyon, M.S.; Wosiski-Kuhn, M.; Gillespie, R.; Caress, J.; Milligan, C. Inflammation, Immunity, and amyotrophic lateral sclerosis: I. Etiology and pathology. *Muscle Nerve* **2019**, *59*, 10–22. [CrossRef]
7. Rosen, D.R.; Siddique, T.; Patterson, D.; Figlewicz, D.A.; Sapp, P.; Hentati, A.; Donaldson, D.; Goto, J.; O'Regan, J.P.; Deng, H.X.; et al. Mutations in Cu/Zn superoxide dismutase gene are associated with familial amyotrophic lateral sclerosis. *Nature* **1993**, *362*, 59–62. [CrossRef]
8. Neumann, M.; Sampathu, D.M.; Kwong, L.K.; Truax, A.C.; Micsenyi, M.C.; Chou, T.T.; Bruce, J.; Schuck, T.; Grossman, M.; Clark, C.M.; et al. Ubiquitinated TDP-43 in frontotemporal lobar degeneration and amyotrophic lateral sclerosis. *Science* **2006**, *314*, 130–133. [CrossRef]
9. DeJesus-Hernandez, M.; Mackenzie, I.R.; Boeve, B.F.; Boxer, A.L.; Baker, M.; Rutherford, N.J.; Nicholson, A.M.; Finch, N.A.; Flynn, H.; Adamson, J.; et al. Expanded GGGGCC hexanucleotide repeat in noncoding region of C9ORF72 causes chromosome 9p-linked FTD and ALS. *Neuron* **2011**, *72*, 245–256. [CrossRef]
10. Boillee, S.; Yamanaka, K.; Lobsiger, C.S.; Copeland, N.G.; Jenkins, N.A.; Kassiotis, G.; Kollias, G.; Cleveland, D.W. Onset and progression in inherited ALS determined by motor neurons and microglia. *Science* **2006**, *312*, 1389–1392. [CrossRef]
11. Zhao, W.; Beers, D.R.; Hooten, K.G.; Sieglaff, D.H.; Zhang, A.; Kalyana-Sundaram, S.; Traini, C.M.; Halsey, W.S.; Hughes, A.M.; Sathe, G.M.; et al. Characterization of Gene Expression Phenotype in Amyotrophic Lateral Sclerosis Monocytes. *JAMA Neurol.* **2017**, *74*, 677–685. [CrossRef] [PubMed]
12. Patin, F.; Baranek, T.; Vourc'h, P.; Nadal-Desbarats, L.; Goossens, J.F.; Marouillat, S.; Dessein, A.F.; Descat, A.; Hounoum, B.M.; Bruno, C.; et al. Combined Metabolomics and Transcriptomics Approaches to Assess the IL-6 Blockade as a Therapeutic of ALS: Deleterious Alteration of Lipid Metabolism. *Neurotherapeutics* **2016**, *13*, 905–917. [CrossRef] [PubMed]
13. Arbour, D.; Vande Velde, C.; Robitaille, R. New perspectives on amyotrophic lateral sclerosis: The role of glial cells at the neuromuscular junction. *J. Physiol.* **2017**, *595*, 647–661. [CrossRef] [PubMed]
14. Nardo, G.; Trolese, M.C.; de Vito, G.; Cecchi, R.; Riva, N.; Dina, G.; Heath, P.R.; Quattrini, A.; Shaw, P.J.; Piazza, V.; et al. Immune response in peripheral axons delays disease progression in SOD1(G93A) mice. *J. Neuroinflammation* **2016**, *13*, 261. [CrossRef] [PubMed]
15. Heurich, B.; El Idrissi, N.B.; Donev, R.M.; Petri, S.; Claus, P.; Neal, J.; Morgan, B.P.; Ramaglia, V. Complement upregulation and activation on motor neurons and neuromuscular junction in the SOD1 G93A mouse model of familial amyotrophic lateral sclerosis. *J. Neuroimmunol.* **2011**, *235*, 104–109. [CrossRef] [PubMed]
16. Almeida, R.N.; Navarro, D.S.; Barbosa-Filho, J.M. Plants with central analgesic activity. *Phytomedicine* **2001**, *8*, 310–322. [CrossRef]
17. Bahmani, M.; Shirzad, H.; Majlesi, M.; Shahinfard, N.; Rafieian-Kopaei, M. A review study on analgesic applications of Iranian medicinal plants. *Asian Pac. J. Trop. Med.* **2014**, *7S1*, S43–S53. [CrossRef]
18. Zeng, Q.; Siu, W.; Li, L.; Jin, Y.; Liang, S.; Cao, M.; Ma, M.; Wu, Z. Autophagy in Alzheimer's disease and promising modulatory effects of herbal medicine. *Exp. Gerontol.* **2019**, *119*, 100–110. [CrossRef]
19. Qiu, H.; Li, J.H.; Yin, S.B.; Ke, J.Q.; Qiu, C.L.; Zheng, G.Q. Dihuang Yinzi, a Classical Chinese Herbal Prescription, for Amyotrophic Lateral Sclerosis: A 12-Year Follow-up Case Report. *Medicine (Baltimore)* **2016**, *95*, e3324. [CrossRef]
20. Pan, W.; Su, X.; Bao, J.; Wang, J.; Zhu, J.; Cai, D.; Yu, L.; Zhou, H. Open Randomized Clinical Trial on JWSJZ Decoction for the Treatment of ALS Patients. *Evid. Based Complement Alternat. Med.* **2013**, *2013*, 347525. [CrossRef]
21. Yae, S.; Takahashi, F.; Yae, T.; Yamaguchi, T.; Tsukada, R.; Koike, K.; Minakata, K.; Murakami, A.; Nurwidya, F.; Kato, M.; et al. Hochuekkito (TJ-41), a Kampo Formula, Ameliorates Cachexia Induced by Colon 26 Adenocarcinoma in Mice. *Evid. Based Complement Alternat. Med.* **2012**, *2012*, 976926. [CrossRef] [PubMed]
22. Dan, K.; Akiyoshi, H.; Munakata, K.; Hasegawa, H.; Watanabe, K. A Kampo (traditional Japanese herbal) medicine, Hochuekkito, pretreatment in mice prevented influenza virus replication accompanied with GM-CSF expression and increase in several defensin mRNA levels. *Pharmacology* **2013**, *91*, 314–321. [CrossRef] [PubMed]
23. Yang, S.H.; Kao, T.I.; Chiang, B.L.; Chen, H.Y.; Chen, K.H.; Chen, J.L. Immune-modulatory effects of bu-zhong-yi-qi-tang in ovalbumin-induced murine model of allergic asthma. *PLoS ONE* **2015**, *10*, e0127636. [CrossRef] [PubMed]

24. Liu, L.; Hu, L.; Yao, Z.; Qin, Z.; Idehara, M.; Dai, Y.; Kiyohara, H.; Yamada, H.; Yao, X. Mucosal immunomodulatory evaluation and chemical profile elucidation of a classical traditional Chinese formula, Bu-Zhong-Yi-Qi-Tang. *J. Ethnopharmacol.* **2019**, *228*, 188–199. [CrossRef] [PubMed]
25. Tatsumi, K.; Shinozuka, N.; Nakayama, K.; Sekiya, N.; Kuriyama, T.; Fukuchi, Y. Hochuekkito improves systemic inflammation and nutritional status in elderly patients with chronic obstructive pulmonary disease. *J. Am. Geriatr. Soc.* **2009**, *57*, 169–170. [CrossRef] [PubMed]
26. Utsuyama, M.; Seidlar, H.; Kitagawa, M.; Hirokawa, K. Immunological restoration and anti-tumor effect by Japanese herbal medicine in aged mice. *Mech. Ageing Dev.* **2001**, *122*, 341–352. [CrossRef]
27. Suzuki, T.; Takano, I.; Nagai, F.; Fujitani, T.; Ushiyama, K.; Okubo, T.; Seto, T.; Ikeda, S.; Kano, I. Suppressive effects of Hochu-ekki-to, a traditional Chinese medicine, on IgE production and histamine release in mice immunized with ovalbumin. *Biol. Pharm. Bull.* **1999**, *22*, 1180–1184. [CrossRef] [PubMed]
28. Kaneko, M.; Kawakita, T.; Yamaoka, Y.; Nomoto, K. Development of the susceptibility to oral tolerance induction in infant mice administered a herbal drug, Hochu-ekki-to (Bu-Zhong-Yi-Qi-Tang). *Int. Immunopharmacol.* **2001**, *1*, 219–227. [CrossRef]
29. Kiyohara, H.; Nagai, T.; Munakata, K.; Nonaka, K.; Hanawa, T.; Kim, S.J.; Yamada, H. Stimulating effect of Japanese herbal (kampo) medicine, hochuekkito on upper respiratory mucosal immune system. *Evid. Based Complement Alternat. Med.* **2006**, *3*, 459–467. [CrossRef]
30. Jiang, J.H.; Yang, E.J.; Baek, M.G.; Kim, S.H.; Lee, S.M.; Choi, S.M. Anti-inflammatory effects of electroacupuncture in the respiratory system of a symptomatic amyotrophic lateral sclerosis animal model. *Neurodegener. Dis.* **2011**, *8*, 504–514. [CrossRef]
31. Reagan-Shaw, S.; Nihal, M.; Ahmad, N. Dose translation from animal to human studies revisited. *FASEB J.* **2008**, *22*, 659–661. [CrossRef] [PubMed]
32. Cai, M.; Lee, S.H.; Yang, E.J. Bojungikgi-tang Improves Muscle and Spinal Cord Function in an Amyotrophic Lateral Sclerosis Model. *Mol. Neurobiol.* **2019**, *56*, 2394–2407. [CrossRef] [PubMed]
33. Yang, E.J.; Jiang, J.H.; Lee, S.M.; Yang, S.C.; Hwang, H.S.; Lee, M.S.; Choi, S.M. Bee venom attenuates neuroinflammatory events and extends survival in amyotrophic lateral sclerosis models. *J. Neuroinflammation* **2010**, *7*, 69. [CrossRef] [PubMed]
34. Cai, M.; Choi, S.M.; Yang, E.J. The effects of bee venom acupuncture on the central nervous system and muscle in an animal hSOD1G93A mutant. *Toxins (Basel)* **2015**, *7*, 846–858. [CrossRef]
35. Lee, S.H.; Yang, E.J. Anti-Neuroinflammatory Effect of Jaeumganghwa-Tang in an Animal Model of Amyotrophic Lateral Sclerosis. *Evid. Based Complement Alternat. Med.* **2019**, *2019*, 1893526. [CrossRef]
36. Cai, M.; Yang, E.J. Gamisoyo-San Ameliorates Neuroinflammation in the Spinal Cord of hSOD1(G93A) Transgenic Mice. *Mediators Inflamm.* **2018**, *2018*, 5897817. [CrossRef]
37. Schafer, D.P.; Stevens, B. Microglia Function in Central Nervous System Development and Plasticity. *Cold Spring Harb. Perspect. Biol.* **2015**, *7*, a020545. [CrossRef]
38. Weiss, A.; Attisano, L. The TGFbeta superfamily signaling pathway. *Wiley Interdiscip. Rev. Dev. Biol.* **2013**, *2*, 47–63. [CrossRef]
39. Zuroff, L.; Daley, D.; Black, K.L.; Koronyo-Hamaoui, M. Clearance of cerebral Abeta in Alzheimer's disease: Reassessing the role of microglia and monocytes. *Cell Mol. Life Sci.* **2017**, *74*, 2167–2201. [CrossRef]
40. Henkel, J.S.; Beers, D.R.; Zhao, W.; Appel, S.H. Microglia in ALS: The good, the bad, and the resting. *J. Neuroimmune Pharmacol.* **2009**, *4*, 389–398. [CrossRef]
41. Gordon, P.H.; Moore, D.H.; Miller, R.G.; Florence, J.M.; Verheijde, J.L.; Doorish, C.; Hilton, J.F.; Spitalny, G.M.; MacArthur, R.B.; Mitsumoto, H.; et al. Efficacy of minocycline in patients with amyotrophic lateral sclerosis: A phase III randomised trial. *Lancet Neurol.* **2007**, *6*, 1045–1053. [CrossRef]
42. Nguyen, Q.T.; Son, Y.J.; Sanes, J.R.; Lichtman, J.W. Nerve terminals form but fail to mature when postsynaptic differentiation is blocked: In vivo analysis using mammalian nerve-muscle chimeras. *J. Neurosci.* **2000**, *20*, 6077–6086. [CrossRef] [PubMed]
43. Halter, B.; Gonzalez de Aguilar, J.L.; Rene, F.; Petri, S.; Fricker, B.; Echaniz-Laguna, A.; Dupuis, L.; Larmet, Y.; Loeffler, J.P. Oxidative stress in skeletal muscle stimulates early expression of Rad in a mouse model of amyotrophic lateral sclerosis. *Free Radic. Biol. Med.* **2010**, *48*, 915–923. [CrossRef] [PubMed]
44. Dadon-Nachum, M.; Melamed, E.; Offen, D. The "dying-back" phenomenon of motor neurons in ALS. *J. Mol. Neurosci.* **2011**, *43*, 470–477. [CrossRef] [PubMed]

45. Marcuzzo, S.; Zucca, I.; Mastropietro, A.; de Rosbo, N.K.; Cavalcante, P.; Tartari, S.; Bonanno, S.; Preite, L.; Mantegazza, R.; Bernasconi, P. Hind limb muscle atrophy precedes cerebral neuronal degeneration in G93A-SOD1 mouse model of amyotrophic lateral sclerosis: A longitudinal MRI study. *Exp. Neurol.* **2011**, *231*, 30–37. [CrossRef]
46. Dupuis, L.; Pradat, P.F.; Ludolph, A.C.; Loeffler, J.P. Energy metabolism in amyotrophic lateral sclerosis. *Lancet Neurol.* **2011**, *10*, 75–82. [CrossRef]
47. Pi-Sunyer, F.X. Overnutrition and undernutrition as modifiers of metabolic processes in disease states. *Am. J. Clin. Nutr.* **2000**, *72*, 533S–537S. [CrossRef]
48. Dupuis, L.; Oudart, H.; Rene, F.; Gonzalez de Aguilar, J.L.; Loeffler, J.P. Evidence for defective energy homeostasis in amyotrophic lateral sclerosis: Benefit of a high-energy diet in a transgenic mouse model. *Proc. Natl. Acad. Sci. USA* **2004**, *101*, 11159–11164. [CrossRef]

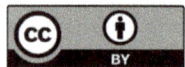

© 2019 by the authors. Licensee MDPI, Basel, Switzerland. This article is an open access article distributed under the terms and conditions of the Creative Commons Attribution (CC BY) license (http://creativecommons.org/licenses/by/4.0/).

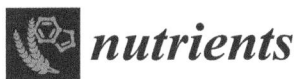

Article

Influence of Diets with Varying Essential/Nonessential Amino Acid Ratios on Mouse Lifespan

Claudia Romano [1,†], Giovanni Corsetti [1,*,†], Vincenzo Flati [2,†], Evasio Pasini [3], Anna Picca [4,5], Riccardo Calvani [4,5], Emanuele Marzetti [4] and Francesco Saverio Dioguardi [6,*]

1. Division of Human Anatomy and Physiopathology, Department of Clinical and Experimental Sciences, University of Brescia, 25124 Brescia, Italy; cla300482@gmail.com
2. Department of Biotechnological and Applied Clinical Sciences, University of L'Aquila, 67100 L'Aquila, Italy; vincenzo.flati@univaq.it
3. Istituti Clinici Scientifici Maugeri - IRCCS Lumezzane - Cardiac Rehabilitation Division, 25065 Lumezzane (Brescia), Italy; evpasini@gmail.com
4. Fondazione Policlinico Universitario "Agostino Gemelli" IRCCS, 00168 Rome, Italy; anna.picca1@gmail.com (A.P.); riccardo.calvani@gmail.com (R.C.); emarzetti@live.com (E.M.)
5. Institute of Internal Medicine and Geriatrics, Università Cattolica del Sacro Cuore, 00168 Rome, Italy
6. Department of Internal Medicine, University of Cagliari, 09042 Monserrato (Cagliari), Italy
* Correspondence: giovanni.corsetti@unibs.it (G.C.); fsdioguardi@gmail.com (F.S.D.); Tel.: +39-030-3717484 (G.C.); +39-02-58318096 (F.S.D.); Fax: +39-030-371-7486 (G.C.)
† These authors contributed equally to this work.

Received: 27 March 2019; Accepted: 13 June 2019; Published: 18 June 2019

Abstract: An adequate intake of essential (EAA) and non-essential amino acids (NEAA) is crucial to preserve cell integrity and whole-body metabolism. EAA introduced with diet may be insufficient to meet the organismal needs, especially under increased physiological requirements or in pathological conditions, and may condition lifespan. We therefore examined the effects of iso-caloric and providing the same nitrogenous content diets, any diet containing different stoichiometric blends of EAA/NEAA, on mouse lifespan. Three groups of just-weaned male Balb/C mice were fed exclusively with special diets with varying EAA/NEAA ratios, ranging from 100%/0% to 0%/100%. Three additional groups of mice were fed with different diets, two based on casein as alimentary proteins, one providing the said protein, one reproducing the amino acidic composition of casein, and the third one, the control group, was fed by a standard laboratory diet. Mouse lifespan was inversely correlated with the percentage of NEAA introduced with each diet. Either limiting EAA, or exceeding NEAA, induced rapid and permanent structural modifications on muscle and adipose tissue, independently of caloric intake. These changes significantly affected food and water intake, body weight, and lifespan. Dietary intake of varying EAA/NEAA ratios induced changes in several organs and profoundly influenced murine lifespan. The balanced content of EAA provided by dietary proteins should be considered as the preferable means for "optimal" nutrition and the elevated or unbalanced intake of NEAA provided by food proteins may negatively affect the health and lifespan of mice.

Keywords: amino acids intake; essential amino acids; diet; extended lifespan; mice

1. Introduction

Proteins are macromolecules serving a vast array of functions within the cell, and a balanced protein synthesis and degradation is crucial for preserving cell homeostasis. Hence, increased proteolysis and reduced protein synthesis have been associated with the severe depletion of body protein reserves, eventually resulting in malnutrition. This may impact the progression of several disease-associated conditions [1]. For example, muscle wasting in people aged over 65 years old, hospitalized for a variety of chronic disease conditions, has been related with the disarrangement of protein balance [2].

Therefore, an adequate nutritional supply of protein may represent a relevant means for the management of patients who are malnourished as a consequence of reduced food intake or increased metabolic demand (i.e., chronic and acute diseases).

Dietary proteins with their various compositions of amino acids (AAs) are nitrogen (N) sources for almost all organisms. From a nutritional point of view, AAs can be classified as non-essential (NEAA) or essential (EAA), depending on their potential to be synthesized endogenously or not [3,4], although the original definitions of the two terms focused on their efficiency in promoting protein deposition [5,6].

Adequate dietary provision of AAs is essential for the growth, development, health, and survival of animals and humans [7]. It is also established that the administration of an adequate EAA+NEAA mix favors an increase in rat body weight, which is considered an appropriate parameter to evaluate the success of the animal in terms of growth and wellness [3,7–9]. However, this concept should be profoundly reconsidered if associated to lifespan. Indeed, caloric restriction and short-term caloric deficit improve the efficiency of mitochondria in humans just as in rodents, which might have the potential to increase their longevity [10].

Previous work by our group showed that the supplementation of a laboratory standard diet, containing special EAA formulations, increased rodents' lifespan in older mice [11]. At the molecular level, such a dietary regimen was able to promote mitochondrial biogenesis and to induce organelle ultrastructural changes in the heart, skeletal muscle and adipose tissue [12–14]. In addition, an EAA-rich diet prevented liver damage induced by chronic ethanol consumption [15,16], boosted the effects of rosuvastatin on the kidneys [17] and accelerated wound healing in late middle-aged rats, by promoting collagen integrity [18]. Furthermore, in vitro data showed that variations in the EAA/NEAA ratio might be crucial for the fate of cancer cells via the induction of apoptosis [19]. Taken as a whole, these findings indicate that varying dietary EAA/NEAA ratios may affect cell metabolism.

While dietary proteins are the major source of AAs, the exact amounts of EAA contained in animal and vegetable proteins, introduced daily with diet, are difficult to establish. Indeed, the EAA content varies considerably depending on the source. However, any dietary protein has an EAA/NEAA ratio ≤0.9 at best. In other words, we introduce a very large amount of NEAA to meet the need for EAA and the excess of NEAA must be eliminated through complex metabolic pathways [20].

Many individual AAs have been tested by dietary exclusion studies in rodents, in order to demonstrate their influence on metabolism and health. For example, the restriction of methionine increases the expression of FGF21 with fall-out effects on insulin-dependent glucose uptake [21]. Other studies have been carried out in rodents with the restriction of branched-chain-AAs [22] or leucine alone [23], assessing their effects on various metabolic aspects (e.g., improving glucose tolerance or white and brown adipose tissue remodeling, respectively). The effects of caloric, protein and carbohydrate restriction on animal survival and welfare have also been studied [24–26]. While the restriction of individual AAs and groups of AAs has been looked at extensively in terms of metabolism and ageing, no studies have been performed specifically about EAA/NEAA ratio in the context of longevity.

Recent data from our studies on late middle-aged animals, fed for one month with iso-caloric and iso-nitrogenous diets containing different EAA/NEAA ratios, showed significant changes in body mass and blood parameters [27]. We therefore investigated the lifelong effects on male mice of iso-caloric and iso-nitrogenous special diets containing five specific EAA/NEAA ratios, compared to a standard laboratory rodent diet.

2. Materials and methods

2.1. Animals

Three-week old outbred male Balb/C mice (Envigo, Holland) were housed in plastic cages with white wood chips for bedding, in a quiet room under controlled lighting (12 h day/night cycle) and temperature (22 ± 1°C) conditions. Animals were regularly examined by veterinary doctors for their health, the maintenance of normal daily and nocturnal behavioral activities, and for criteria of increased disease burden, according to ethics standards for animal studies. The experimental protocol was conducted in accordance with the directives of the Italian Ministry of Health and complied with 'The National Animal Protection Guidelines'. The Ethics Committee for animal experiments of IZSLER (Brescia, Italy) (the "National Reference Centre for Animal Welfare" (http://www.izsler.it)), and the Italian Ministry of Health approved all of the procedures.

2.2. Diet Composition

We used three specific diets with different EAA/NEAA ratios ranging from 100%/0% to 0%/100%, as previously described [27]. A summary of diet composition and EAA/NEAA ratios is shown in Table 1.

(1) EAA-100% diet contained exclusively EAA as the source of nitrogen [11,17,18,28].
(2) EAA-30% diet (EAA-poor diet) and thus NEAA-rich diet (70% of NEAA).
(3) NEAA-100% diet contained exclusively NEAA as the source of nitrogen (thus 0% of EAA).
(4) Casein-Prot diet contained only whole casein protein of highest quality.
(5) Casein-AA (casein-like) diet contained free AAs equivalent to the composition of casein (EAA/NEAA = 49/51).
(6) A commercial standard rodent laboratory diet (StD) (Mucedola srl, Milan, Italy) was also used.

The Casein-Prot and Casein-AA diets were used as special test diets, since no composition of AAs in StD proteins was available even for the producer, and we needed to test the safety of life-long nutrition by free AAs.

All special diets provided quantitatively equal amounts of lipids, carbohydrate and micronutrients. All diets were thus iso-caloric and provided the same amounts of nitrogen, although nitrogen content was provided by different formulations of AAs or proteins, according to those presented in Table 1. All special diets were prepared for Nutriresearch s.r.l. (Milan, Italy) by Dottori Piccioni (Milan, Italy) in accordance with AIN76-A/NIH-7 rules [29].

Animals were randomly assigned to one of the six groups. Each group was fed exclusively with a specific diet [i.e., EAA-100% diet ($n = 30$), Casein-AA diet ($n = 30$), Casein-Prot ($n = 30$), StD ($n = 40$), EAA-30% diet ($n = 30$), or NEAA-100% diet ($n = 30$)]. All animals had free access to food and water.

Table 1. Diet composition.

Nutrients	EAA-100%	Casein-AA	Casein-Prot	StD	EAA-30%	NEAA-100%
KCal/Kg	3995	3995	3995	3952	3995	3995
Carbohydrates %	61.76	61.76	61.76	54.61	61.76	61.76
Lipids %	6.12	6.12	6.12	7.5	6.12	6.12
Nitrogen %	20 *	20 *	20 ^	21.8 °	20 *	20 *
Proteins: % of total nitrogen content	0	0	100	95.93	0	0
Free AAs: % of total nitrogen content	100	100	0	4.07	100	100
EAA/NEAA (% in grams)	100/0	49/51	-	-	30/70	0/100
Free AAs composition (%)						
L-Leucine (bcaa)	31.25	9.5	–	–	9.4	–
L-Isoleucine (bcaa)	15.62	6	–	–	4.7	–
L-Valine (bcaa)	15.62	6.5	–	–	4.7	–
L-Lysine	16.25	7	–	0.97	6.24	–
L-Threonine	8.75	4	–	–	2.7	–
L-Hystidine	3.75	2.8	–	–	1.1	–
L-Phenylalanine	2.5	5	–	–	0.8	–
L-Cysteine	–	0.8	–	–	–	–
L-Cystine	3.75	–	–	0.39	1.1	–
L-Methionine	1.25	2.5	–	0.45	0.4	–
L-Tyrosine	0.75	5	–	–	2.6	1.0
L-Triptophan	0.5	1.3	–	0.28	0.01	–
L-Alanine	–	3.2	–	–	24.0	35.0
L-Glycine	–	2.4	–	0.88	10.39	15.0
L-Arginine	–	3.4	–	1.1	13.5	14.0
L-Proline	–	9.5	–	–	8.2	12.0
L-Glutamine	–	9.5	–	–	3.0	12.0
L-Serine	–	5.1	–	–	4.1	6.0
L-Glutamic Acid	–	9.5	–	–	2.5	2.0
L-Asparagine	–	3.5	–	–	0.79	2.0
L-Aspartic Acid	–	3.5	–	–	1.1	1.0

* Nitrogen (%) from free amino acids (AAs) only. ° Nitrogen (%) from vegetable and animal proteins and added AAs. ^ whole casein protein. EAA-100% = free essential amino acid-exclusive diet; Casein-AA = Casein-like free AAs diet; Casein-Prot = Casein whole protein diet; StD = Standard diet; EAA-30% = free essential amino acid-poor diet; NEAA-100% = non-essential free amino acid-exclusive diet. The black line represents the limit between EAA (above) and NEAA (below). bcaa = branched-chain amino acids.

2.3. Data and Sample Collections

Body weight (BW), mean food and water consumption (g/days and mL/day, respectively) were calculated weekly in all groups. Mortality was monitored daily.

Animals from the two groups fed with NEAA-100% and EAA-30% had a mortality > 70% at the 7th week, and all those still surviving were euthanized for ethical reasons linked to a drop in weight, as discussed in results. Five animals from each of the other groups were euthanized after 12 and 18 months to check their morphometric and clinical parameters. Specifically, BW and nose–tail length (body length, BL) were measured. Blood samples from the hearts and urine from the bladders were immediately collected for further analysis. Glycaemia was also measured by a glucometer in venous blood samples collected from tail veins. Subsequently, the heart, kidneys, liver, spleen, *triceps surae*, retroperitoneal white adipose tissue (rpWAT) pad and brown adipose tissue (BAT) were quickly removed and weighed [30].

2.4. Blood and Urine Analysis

Blood samples were collected either in tubes containing the K3-EDTA anti-coagulant for cell count analysis, or in tubes without anti-coagulants for serum separation. The blood cell count was performed with a Cell-Dyn 3700 laser-impedance cell counter (Abbott Diagnostics Division, Abbott Laboratories, IL, USA). Serum and urine levels of albumin and creatinine were assessed with an ILab Aries (Instrumentation Laboratory, Lexington, MA, USA) automatic analyzer. Serum levels of haptoglobin (Hpg) [31] and the neutrophils to lymphocytes ratio (NLR) [32,33] were also assessed as inflammatory markers. These analyses were carried out by personnel of the "Division of Laboratory Animals" of IZSLER (Brescia, Italy).

2.5. Statistical Analysis

Differences between experimental groups were evaluated by one-way analysis of variance (ANOVA) followed by a Bonferroni test or Student t-test when appropriate. All analyses were performed using the Primer of Biostatistics software, with statistical significance set at $p < 0.05$.

Spearman (r) regression values were calculated and reported where appropriate. A Mantel–Cox test (z) was used to test survival differences between diets [34].

3. Results

The average survival time was markedly reduced in animals fed with the two diets where EAA were absent or deficient. Indeed, NEAA-100% diet allowed a lifespan of 44.56 ± 3.85 days, while the lifespan of EAA-30%-fed animals was slightly prolonged at 53 ± 1.97 days, on average <20%. Animals fed with Casein-Prot and Casein-AA diets survived for maximum 14 and 16 months, respectively. StD-fed animals survived for maximum 22 months. The longest survival time (25 months) was observed for the EAA-100%-fed animals (Figure 1). The percentage of EAA in the diet is correlated with survival ($r = 0.901$, $p < 0.001$).

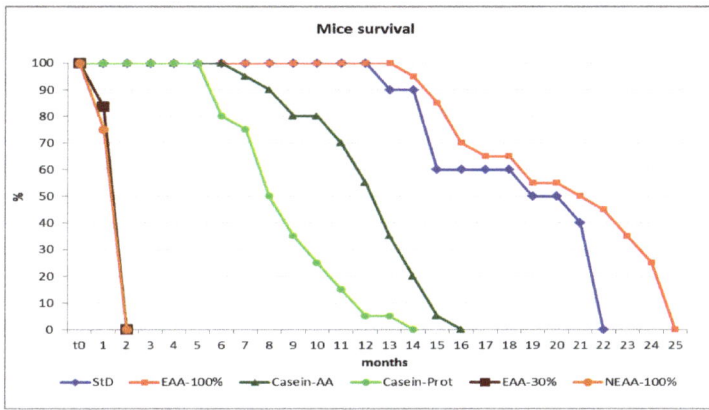

Figure 1. Percentage of mice's survival according to diet. Animals fed with NEAA-100% and EAA-30% diets (orange and brown lines) had shorter lifespans when compared to StD (blue line). It is interesting to observe the different survival curves between the animals fed with the diet containing casein whole protein (light-green line) and those fed with free AAs of casein (dark-green line). In addition, note the longest survival of the mice fed with EAA-100% diet (red line). Mantel–Cox test: Casein-AA vs. Casein-Prot, $z = 3.95$, $p < 0.001$; Casein-AA vs. StD, $z = 5.17$, $p < 0.001$; EAA-100% vs. StD, $z = 2.28$, $p = 0.0226$; EAA-30% vs. NEAA-100%, $z = 0.21$, $p = 0.83$.

3.1. Parameters Evaluation after 2 Months

3.1.1. Body Weight (BW) and Length (BL)

BW and BL are determined by the quality of nitrogen intake. For the diets poorest in EAA, NEAA-100% and EAA-30% diets, there is a rapid mortality correlating with BW loss ($r = 0.92$, $p < 0.000$)

and also BL (r = 0.99, $p < 0.000$) when compared to all diets. A relatively modest increase in EAA provided by Casein-AA or Casein-Prot diet (which each contain about 19% more EAA than EAA-30% diet), drives a BL increase comparable to those observed in EAA-100% diet and StD. On the contrary, BW is most increased by StD and either Casein-Prot or Casein-AA diet. Instead, EAA-100% diet allows a growth in BL comparable to StD, Casein-Prot and Casein-AA.

EAA-100% diet induced the smallest BW increase among animals fed all diets compatible with prolonged lifespan. That is, the BW of EAA-100%-fed animals, while increasing if compared with the diets poorest in EAA (NEAA-100% and EAA-30%), is significantly less increased ($p < 0.001$) when compared to both StD and either Casein-Prot or Casein-AA diets.

The BW and BL of mice fed with Casein-Prot and Casein-AA diets were comparable to those of animals fed StD (see Table 2).

Table 2. Body weight (BW), body length (BL) and organ weight after 2, 12 and 18 months (mean ± sd).

	NEAA-100%	EAA-30%	EAA-100%	StD	Casein-Prot	Casein-AA	F	p
2 months								
Body W. (g)	7.09 ± 0.41 *^	7.31 ± 0.52 *^	14.93 ± 0.62 *	22.35 ± 1.9	22.02 ± 1.2	21.84 ± 0.9	238.26	0.000
Body L. (cm)	6.61 ± 0.1 *^	6.63 ± 0.12 *^	9.15 ± 0.13 *	9.66 ± 0.1	9.62 ± 0.2	9.47 ± 0.17	1024.88	0.000
Heart (g)	0.08 ± 0.015 *	0.08 ± 0.01 *	0.08 ± 0.03 *	0.13 ± 0.006	-	-	9.75	0.000
Kidneys (g)	0.12 ± 0.008 *^	0.12 ± 0.009 *^	0.24 ± 0.028 *	0.40 ± 0.05	-	-	105.71	0.000
Liver (g)	0.32 ± 0.049 *^	0.34 ± 0.61 *^	0.75 ± 0.066 *	1.10 ± 0.17	-	-	70.95	0.000
Spleen (g)	0.02 ± 0.004 *	0.02 ± 0.003 *	0.05 ± 0.008 *	0.11 ± 0.032	-	-	32.35	0.000
rpWAT (g)	0 *	0 *	0.02 ± 0.002 *	0.11 ± 0.02	-	-	123.97	0.000
BAT (g)	0.02 ± 0.01 *	0.02 ± 0.009 *^	0.09 ± 0.01 *	0.13 ± 0.015	-	-	112.59	0.000
Triceps (g)	0.07 ± 0.01 *^	0.06 ± 0.002 *^	0.10 ± 0.011 *	0.19 ± 0.01	-	-	215.38	0.000
12 months							F	p
Body W. (g)	-	-	24.51 ± 1.9 *	31.78 ± 1.69	30.39 ± 2.79 ^	29.56 ± 1.0 ^	12.95	0.000
Body L. (cm)	-	-	9.82 ± 0.12	10.0 ± 0.13	10.01 ± 0.14	9.87 ± 0.13	2.65	0.085
Heart (g)	-	-	0.15 ± 0.02 *°	0.23 ± 0.03	0.18 ± 0.02	0.22 ± 0.05	6.51	0.000
Kidneys (g)	-	-	0.46 ± 0.06 *°§	0.8 ± 0.1	0.7 ± 0.05	0.69 ± 0.06	21.0	0.000
Liver (g)	-	-	1.36 ± 0.13 *°	1.79 ± 0.2	1.56 ± 0.2	1.7 ± 0.2	5.13	0.011
Spleen (g)	-	-	0.12 ± 0.03	0.15 ± 0.06	0.18 ± 0.02	0.15 ± 0.04	1.85	0.179
rpWAT (g)	-	-	0.07 ± 0.02 *§	0.17 ± 0.01	0.16 ± 0.08	0.09 ± 0.03 *	6.39	0.005
BAT (g)	-	-	0.13 ± 0.02 §	0.2 ± 0.04	0.23 ± 0.06	0.17 ± 0.03	5.62	0.008
Triceps (g)	-	-	0.18 ± 0.01 *°§	0.26 ± 0.02	0.31 ± 0.02 *	0.34 ± 0.03 *	54.35	0.000
18 months							t	p
Body W. (g)	-	-	23.67 ± 1.15 *	28.31 ± 1.04	-	-	6.692	0.000
Body L. (cm)	-	-	9.79 ± 0.11	9.95 ± 0.13	-	-	2.101	0.069
Heart (g)	-	-	0.15 ± 0.01 *	0.2 ± 0.01	-	-	7.906	0.000
Kidneys (g)	-	-	0.47 ± 0.04 *	0.68 ± 0.07	-	-	5.824	0.000
Liver (g)	-	-	1.18 ± 0.09 *	1.6 ± 0.15	-	-	5.369	0.000
Spleen (g)	-	-	0.08 ± 0.03 *	0.13 ± 0.04	-	-	2.236	0.038
rpWAT (g)	-	-	0.07 ± 0.03 *	0.11 ± 0.02	-	-	2.481	0.038
BAT (g)	-	-	0.12 ± 0.01 *	0.17 ± 0.01	-	-	7.906	0.000
Triceps (g)	-	-	0.15 ± 0.01 *	0.21 ± 0.01	-	-	9.487	0.000
22 months							t	p
Body W. (g)	-	-	22.2 ± 1.56 *	25.01 ± 1.2	-	-	4.515	0.000
Body L. (cm)	-	-	9.75 ± 0.12	9.81 ± 0.14	-	-	0.794	0.444

Note the similar changes in organ weight in EAA-30% and NEAA-100%-fed animals compared to StD after 2 months. Furthermore, it should be noted that the EAA-100% diet causes a slowdown in the BW and OW at all times compared to StD. ANOVA and Bonferroni t-test: * $p < 0.05$ vs. StD, ^ $p < 0.05$ vs. EAA-100%, ° $p < 0.05$ vs. Casein-AA, § $p < 0.05$ vs. Casein-Prot. WAT, white adipose tissue. BAT, brown adipose tissue.

3.1.2. Food and Water Consumption

The amounts of food and water consumed daily were influenced markedly by different diets. NEAA-100%-fed groups rapidly stopped growing in BL and showed a dramatically rapid BW loss similar to that of EAA-30% (Figure 2A), although the food consumption and therefore caloric intake of NEAA-100% during the first two weeks was significantly higher than any other diet except StD. With the proceeding of BW loss, and particularly in the 80% animals surviving after the sixth week, food consumption also declined, and all animals died in the following two weeks (Figure 2A,B). In NEAA-100%-fed animals, a striking difference between the grams of daily food intake, and thus calories, and BW was evident. Indeed, NEAA-100% and EAA-30%-fed animals progressively decreased in BW although their caloric intake was similar to that of EAA-100%-fed animals. Indeed, the correlation (r) between NEAA-100% or EAA-30% food intake and BW was –0.3 or –0.5, respectively. On the contrary, there was a higher correlation between EAA-100% food intake and BW ($r = 0.9$, $p < 0.001$) (Figure 2A,B). Only in the case of the NEAA-100% group, water consumption increased significantly from the first week of treatment ($p < 0.001$, about six-fold), and then decreased progressively to around the average water intake in StD-fed animals, before dying (Figure 2C).

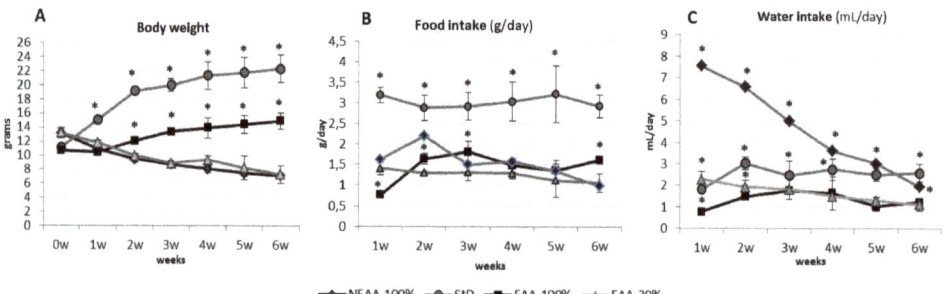

Figure 2. Comparison between BW (**A**), food (g/day) (**B**), and water (mL/day) consumption (**C**) (mean ± sd) of animals fed with NEAA-100% and EAA-30% diets, StD and EAA-100% diet after 6 weeks. NEAA-100% and EAA-30% diets drive rapid BW decrease, whereas EAA-100% diet slowly increases BW compared to StD (**A**). Note that EAA-100% diet was consumed in the same amount as NEAA-100% and EAA-30% diets (**B**). NEAA-100%-fed animals showed a higher water intake compared to StD, whereas EAA-30% and EAA-100%-fed animals had a lower water consumption than StD (**C**). Black square, EAA-100%; gray rhombus, NEAA-100%; gray triangle, EAA-30%; gray circle, StD. ANOVA and Bonferroni t-test, * $p < 0.05$ vs. all diets.

3.1.3. Organ Weights

The weights of specific organs (organ weight, OW) in animals fed with NEAA-100%, EAA-30% and EAA-100% diets were significantly lower than those in animals fed with StD. The weights of the kidneys, livers, BAT and *triceps surae* of the animals fed with NEAA-100% and EAA-30% diets were significantly less than those of the EAA-100%-fed animals. The OW of animals was similar in both NEAA-100% and EAA-30% diets but, interestingly, the rpWAT was near absent in those groups (Table 2).

3.1.4. Blood and Urinary Parameters

The two groups fed with NEAA-100% and EAA-30% diets had altered blood and urine parameters when compared to StD and EAA-100%-fed mice. This is especially evident in the reduction in blood concentration of hemoglobin and albumin, in the increase in neutrophils to lymphocytes ratio (NLR), and in the reduction of albumin and increase of creatinine in the urine. Blood and urine parameters from the EAA-100%-fed group did not differ from those of the StD-fed group, except for the Hpg value which was found to be lower (Table 3).

Table 3. Blood and urine data (mean ± sd) after 2, 12 and 18 months of treatment. See text for description.

	NEAA-100%	EAA-30%	EAA-100%	StD	Casein-Prot	Casein-AA	F	p
Blood 2 months								
Glucose (mg/dL)	108.3 ± 6.7 *^	111.7 ± 7.9 *	122.04 ± 8.1	127.3 ± 9.6	-	-	8.47	0.000
Erythrocytes (M/μL)	7.75 ± 1.93	8.01 ± 1.32	9.04 ± 0.58	9.13 ± 0.29	-	-	1.69	0.210
Hemoglobin (g/dL)	10.23 ± 2.37 *^	11.46 ± 2.15 *^	14.18 ± 1.16	14.8 ± 0.46	-	-	8.04	0.002
NLR	1.88 ± 1.02 *^	1.64 ± 0.93 *^	0.68 ± 0.26	0.67 ± 0.25	-	-	3.95	0.028
Albumin (g/L)	22.58 ± 1.68 *	24.75 ± 1.56 *	26.8 ± 1.83	28.66 ± 2.57	-	-	9.03	0.000
Creatinine (μmol/L)	25.92 ± 4.54	24.95 ± 3.9	22.8 ± 1.75	23.82 ± 1.89	-	-	0.86	0.480
Haptoglobin (mg/mL)	0.02 ± 0.01 *^	0.04 ± 0.01 *^	0.13 ± 0.02 *	0.18 ± 0.02	-	-	113.83	0.000
Urine 3 months								
Albumin (g/L)	0.9 ± 0.4 *^	0.8 ± 0.6 *^	2.2 ± 0.4	1.8 ± 0.3	-	-	12.19	0.000
Creatinine (μmol/L)	5502 ± 443 *^	5653 ± 520 *^	3956 ± 824	4066 ± 1027	-	-	7.49	0.002
Blood 12 months							F	p
Glucose (mg/dL)	-	-	119.3 ± 11.4	124.3 ± 19.4	127.25 ± 14	113.25 ± 4.3	1.04	0.40
Erythrocytes (M/μL)	-	-	9.65 ± 0.62	9.93 ± 0.37	9.28 ± 0.33	9.8 ± 0.28	2.23	0.124
Hemoglobin (g/dL)	-	-	13.35 ± 1.02	14.4 ± 1.5	14.32 ± 0.3	14.4 ± 0.2	1.54	0.243
NLR	-	-	0.71 ± 0.1	0.72 ± 0.12	0.65 ± 0.07	0.67 ± 0.14	0.45	0.723
Albumin (g/L)	-	-	29.7 ± 1.7	30.88 ± 2.1	46.2 ± 8.03 *^	31.6 ± 6.6 ^	11.09	0.000
Creatinine (μmol/L)	-	-	46.9 ± 2.3	42.9 ± 5.7	72.33 ± 12.7 *^	57.0 ± 12.4	9.75	0.000
Haptoglobin (mg/mL)	-	-	0.10 ± 0.04 *	0.15 ± 0.07	4.53 ± 0.15 *^	4.97 ± 0.06 *^	3968	0.000
Urine 12 months								
Albumin (g/L)	-	-	2.13 ± 0.23	1.94 ± 0.21	1.3 ± 0.19 *^	1.02 ± 0.35 *^	21.46	0.000
Creatinine (μmol/L)	-	-	3581 ± 526	3832 ± 364	2934 ± 355 *^	2595 ± 222.7 *^	11.13	0.000
Blood 18 months							t	p
Glucose (mg/dL)	-	-	127.2 ± 8.3	133.4 ± 12.6	-	-	0.919	0.385
Erythrocytes (M/μL)	-	-	9.73 ± 0.25	9.97 ± 1.06	-	-	0.493	0.635
Hemoglobin (g/dL)	-	-	14.23 ± 0.15	14.87 ± 1.4	-	-	1.016	0.339
NLR	-	-	0.95 ± 0.2 *	1.44 ± 0.08	-	-	5.087	0.000
Albumin (g/L)	-	-	29.1 ± 0.7 *	27.4 ± 0.78	-	-	2.332	0.04
Creatinine (μmol/L)	-	-	38.3 ± 2.69	37.8 ± 1.45	-	-	0.366	0.724
Haptoglobin (mg/mL)	-	-	0.33 ± 0.15 *	0.56 ± 0.16	-	-	2.268	0.05
Urine 18 months								
Albumin (g/L)	-	-	1.58 ± 0.99 *	3.49 ± 0.87	-	-	3.241	0.01
Creatinine (μmol/L)	-	-	2954.9 ± 927	3421.7 ± 670	-	-	0.913	0.388

NLR = Neutrophils lymphocytes ratio. ANOVA and Bonferroni t-test. * $p < 0.05$ vs. StD, ^ $p < 0.05$ vs. EAA-100%.

3.2. Parameter Evaluation after 12 Months.

3.2.1. Body Weight and Length

After one year of follow-up, BW and length were still determined by the quality of nitrogen intake. The growth of mice on Casein-Prot-based diets did not differ from that of StD-fed mice. On the contrary, the EAA-100%-fed animals showed a more modest increase in BW, which remained significantly lower than the BW of the StD, Casein-Prot and EAA-100%-fed groups (Figure 3A, Table 2).

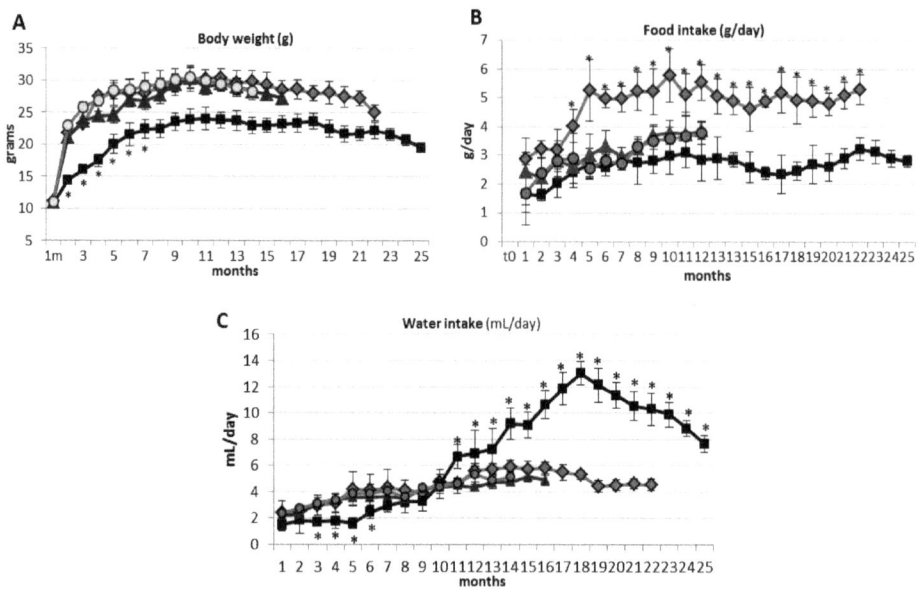

Figure 3. BW (**A**), food (**B**) and water (**C**) consumption (mean ± sd) according to StD, EAA-100%, Casein-Prot and Casein-AA diets during the whole survival period of mice. After about eight months, EAA-100%-fed mice significantly increase their water consumption (**C**), although food consumption (**B**) and BW (**A**) remain unchanged. See text for description. Black square, EAA-100%; gray rhombus, StD; gray triangle, Casein-AA; gray circle, Casein-Prot. ANOVA and Bonferroni t-test: * $p < 0.05$ vs. all diets.

3.2.2. Food and Water Consumption

The Casein-AA, Casein-Prot and EAA-100%-fed animals showed a substantially comparable daily food intake (g/day). All those groups registered a daily food consumption that was significantly reduced compared to that of the StD-fed animals, from the 4th month onwards. Water consumption (ml/day) was similar among StD, Casein-AA and Casein-Prot, whereas EAA-100%-fed mice showed a significantly increased water consumption starting from the eighth month and continuing all along the remaining follow-up (Figure 3C).

3.2.3. Organ Weights

Comparable to BW, mice from the EAA-100% group showed the lowest OW except for spleen. In particular, kidney and *triceps surae* weights were significantly lower than those recorded in all other groups. The heart weights of the EAA-100%-fed animals were significantly lower than in the StD and Casein-AA groups, whereas the rpWAT weights were lower in EAA-100% than in both StD and Casein-Prot groups. Liver weight was significantly higher in the StD and Casein-Prot and Casein-AA groups than in EAA-100%. BAT weight in EAA-100% was significantly lower than the Casein-Prot group, while animals fed with Casein-AA and Casein-Prot diets had a significantly increased *triceps surae* weight, when compared to the StD group. Interestingly, the Casein-AA diet induced a significant weight decrease for rpWAT, similar to that observed in EAA-100%-fed animals. On the other hand, rpWAT weights of mice fed Casein-Prot did not differ from those of mice fed with StD (Table 1).

3.2.4. Blood and Urinary Parameters

Serum concentrations of Hpg were markedly increased (about fifty times, $p < 0.001$) in animals fed with the Casein-AA and Casein-Prot diets as compared to StD-fed animals. In addition, mice fed with the Casein-AA and Casein-Prot diets had increased levels of serum and lowered levels of urinary albumin and creatinine. On the other hand, EAA-100%-fed animals had normal blood parameters and urinary concentrations of albumin and creatinine, and also showed a significantly lower Hpg level even compared to the StD-fed mice (Table 3).

3.3. Parameter Evaluation after 18 Months.

3.3.1. Body Weight and Length.

After 18 months, only animals fed with the StD and EAA-100% diets survived (Figure 1). EAA-100%-fed animals had lower BW than the StD-fed animals, whereas BL did not vary (Table 2). The fur appearance and spontaneous motor activity of EAA-100%-fed animals seemed to be preserved far better than in StD-fed ones. In fact, the animals fed with EAA-100% showed greater vitality than the others and often clung to the cage, keeping themselves suspended without difficulty.

3.3.2. Food and Water Consumption

The food consumption of EAA-fed animals was consistently lower than in StD-fed ones (Figure 3B). On the contrary, EAA-100%-fed animals showed a progressively and significantly increased water consumption (Figure 3C).

3.3.3. Organ Weights.

All OW of EAA-100%-fed animals were significantly smaller than StD-fed animals (Table 2).

3.3.4. Blood and Urinary Parameters

EAA-100%-fed mice had lower NLR, lower Hpg and higher serum albumin levels in comparison to StD-fed mice. Noticeably, urinary albumin losses were also the lowest in EAA-100%-fed animals (Table 3).

3.4. Parameter Evaluation after 22 Months

After 22 months, we were able to measure only BW and BL of the few surviving animals, i.e., four animals fed with StD and nine animals fed with the EAA-100% diet (Table 2). The four StD-fed mice died a few days after these last measurements. The EAA-100% fed mice, albeit showing lower BW, appeared vital, with thick and shiny furs (Figure 1). The last mouse died at the age of 25 months and belonged to the EAA-100% group.

4. Discussion

The main result of our study was the observation that the lifespan of mice was affected by the quality of the AAs content in the diets. Here, we have shown that the EAA-100%-fed animals lived the longest, although they had the lowest total energy (calories) intake, and the lowest BW compared to animals fed with the other diets, while growth in BL was unaffected. These observations confirm and extend previous studies in mice whose diets were supplemented with particular EAA blends, where a prolonged lifespan paralleled improved mitochondrial biogenesis and other parameters connected with healthy aging [11–13].

Furthermore, we also showed that the EAA-30% diet induced a progressive BW decrease by rapid loss of muscle mass and stopped growth in BL. This was followed by precocious death.

The diet without EAA (alias NEAA-100% diet) quickly arrested development and induced a rapid decay of animals' health, as the availability of EAA is, for instance, the main promoter of muscle protein anabolism [35]. However, the effects of NEAA-100% and EAA-30% diets were similar, suggesting that diets providing even a relatively modestly unbalanced lowering of the EAA/NEAA ratio, in our case a diet only about <20% poorer in EAA than the Casein-Prot and Casein-AA diets (common food proteins), may trigger a severe catabolic imbalance leading to body consumption and premature death. Since the animals fed with NEAA-100% and EAA-30% diets ate less than those fed with StD, at least in the last weeks of their short lives, this could lead to the obvious conclusion that the effects were due to quantitative (and thus caloric) malnutrition. However, the daily consumption of the NEAA-100% and EAA-30% diets was comparable to the consumption of the EAA-100% diet, but in this latter case, the animals survived the longest and even longer than the StD-fed animals, albeit with reduced growth in weight (BW), but not length (BL). On this basis, we suggest that the EAA/NEAA ratio played a more prominent role than calories in ensuring animal well-being and survival.

Special NEAA-100% and EAA-30% (thus NEAA-70%) diets strongly reduced the mass of organs and determined a complete loss of rpWAT with a proportional decrease of BAT. This was unexpected, especially for the EAA-30% diet, suggesting again that a minor reduction in the EAA/NEAA ratio (EAA were <20% lower than in the Casein diets) can lead to extremely serious consequences for the whole body. In addition, we observed that malnutrition induced by NEAA-100% and EAA-30% diets led to a decrease in serum hemoglobin and albumin values. This was probably due to reduced protein synthesis and higher turnover, dependent on a poor EAA availability. However, direct and inhibitory effects exerted by elevated plasma NEAA on albumin synthesis cannot be excluded. In fact, this would be in agreement with previous observations in adult animals [27] and in undernourished patients [36,37].

Significant changes, induced by NEAA-100% and EAA-30% diets, were also observed for serum Hpg levels. Hpg is a hemoglobin-binding protein synthesized in the liver and released into the circulation, where it acts as an acute phase reactant protein. In fact, it increases during acute conditions such as infection, injury, tissue destruction, some cancers, burns, surgery or trauma, in response to inflammation. On the contrary, it decreases under other pathological conditions such as chronic liver disease, hematoma and hemolytic anemia. Because Hpg levels become depleted in the presence of large amounts of free hemoglobin, a decreased Hpg is considered a good marker of hemolysis [38,39]. In our experimental setup, the NEAA-100% and EAA-30% diets induced a sharp decrease in the serum Hpg level, but also induced higher NLR, with a concomitant decrease in hemoglobin concentration, red blood cell number and spleen mass. So, we believe that the very low level of Hpg observed in NEAA and EAA-30% diets was due not only to hemolytic events, but also to an impairment of Hpg synthesis by the liver. We also observed that the EAA-100% diet reduced Hpg level, but not NLR ratio, more than StD. This confirms that EAA have anti-inflammatory activity as observed previously [11,40].

All special diets were consumed in significantly lower quantities than StD, thus leading to a decreasing proportion of caloric intake. It is possible that StD has a more pleasing taste than other diets. However, in our recent work, we have observed that when mice can choose between special diets and StD, the StD is not the first choice [27]. Instead, previous studies have indicated an association between increased plasma AA concentration and decreased appetite [41]. So, the quick and free AAs availability provided by special diets can trigger satiety signals, thereby decreasing food intake. Interestingly, in the case of the diets containing casein, low intake did not influence BW and OW in comparison to StD. This suggests that caloric intake is not the only parameter that influenced BW. This agree with previous works showing that EAA/NEAAA ratio plays a pivotal role in changes in body composition [3,9,27]. In addition, according to previous authors, a difference in BW and OW between

EAA-100% diet and StD was observed, and we believe that this depends on the slowdown in growth caused by the EAA-100% diet.

Curiously, NEAA-100%-fed mice had an early and sharp increase in water intake without an increase in water retention. This finding agrees with previous observations in adult mice [27]. We believe that this may be related to enhanced muscle proteolysis and hyperosmolarity due to the increased release of different N-related products (such as creatinine) into the bloodstream. Indeed, all NEAA-100% and EAA-30%-fed mice had higher urinary creatinine levels compatible with muscular wasting induced by EAA deficiency. On this basis, we propose that animals fed with these diets could be used as an experimental model for muscle loss, since such a model would be inexpensive, easy to reproduce, and can be efficiently reversed by re-nutrition.

Besides StD, in line with previous studies [29,42], as a comparison we used two diets containing, respectively, casein in the form of the whole protein (Casein-Prot) or in the form of free AAs (Casein-AA) equivalent to the composition of casein, establishing a composition of reference (see Table 1). This was suitable for the purpose of comparing a whole protein needing digestion to its free AAs composition, which was more rapidly and completely available for absorption. Casein is a widely used protein in rodent pellets, but it has been shown not to provide sufficient amounts of sulphur-containing AAs, and therefore should be integrated with other proteins from animal sources in order to match the animals' needs for sulphur-providing AAs [29].

We compared two casein diets (-Prot and -AA) to evaluate possible biological differences between feeding proteins, which must be digested prior to absorption, and free AAs. Our choice was dictated by the fact that, unfortunately, an AAs composition of the commercially available StD was not available, since it contains 15% of unspecified "fish-based proteins" whose AAs composition is unknown to producers. On the contrary, casein-based diets were fully controlled in terms of AAs composition. Furthermore, an earlier study showed that the minimum concentration of casein which supports adequate growth, reproduction and lactation in mice was 13.6%, supplying 5.9 mg of total nitrogen/Cal [43]. Our Casein-Prot diet provided a 20% concentration of protein, thus ensuring adequate amounts of nitrogen to support growth, albeit with the cited and well known deficiencies in methionine and cisteine that identify this protein as not fully adequate to maintain a maximally prolonged life [29]. This is why we found that animals fed with Casein-Prot and Casein-AA diets had a drastically reduced survival in comparison to StD. Furthermore, Casein-Prot-fed animals lived shorter than Casein-AA-fed animals. These results might be interpreted on the basis of two main points: First, protein digestion was incomplete, since efficiency of protein digestion is <80% [44], indigested proteins contribute to fecal composition, and may thus have influenced both intestinal microbiota and promoted syntheses of some toxic metabolites [35,45]; second, the more efficient absorption of free AAs, coupled with the reduced metabolic costs of producing digestive enzymes [46] may have been responsible for survival differences. Thus, in line with previous clinical studies [47], we have shown here that the ingestion of EAA in a free form is a more efficient anabolic stimulus than the ingestion of a similar amount of AAs in the form of proteins, and that this kind of superior N intake can significantly affect life expectancy.

Animals fed with casein diets had no evident modifications of BW and BL, but lifespan was shorter compared to those on StD. However, although the animals ate significantly less calories and macronutrients than those on StD, their muscle mass increased significantly. This is in line with a previous work which has shown that casein protein intake could stimulate muscle protein synthesis without influencing lipid metabolism [48]. This observation opens some questions about the possible puzzling roles of methionine and cysteine in controlling protein syntheses and healthy life in humans and rodents. It is interesting to notice also that, by a different protocol, methionine restriction has been linked to improved lifespan in rodents, but administration of cisteine in a ratio suitable to match total sulphur containing amino acids needs, and also reducing methionine-linked toxicity, was not contemplated [20,49].

In any case, after 12 months, animals fed with casein diets had higher serum albumin (particularly in those fed with the Casein-Prot diet). High serum albumin, concomitantly with decreased urine albumin, suggests an improvement in both globular blood proteins synthesis and nephron function [50]. However, both casein diets also resulted in very high values of Hpg, suggesting that these diets provided some deficit-inducing high levels of chronic inflammation and potentially leading animals to their premature death when compared with StD or EAA-100% diet.

Indeed, after 12 months, the urinary creatinine excretion in the Casein-Prot-fed mice was lower, whereas the blood creatinine was higher than in the StD-fed animals. This finding would suggest an impairment of kidney function [51], although urinary albumin losses were unaffected. On the contrary, in Casein-AA-fed mice, although their urinary creatinine level reached lower values than in StD-fed mice, blood creatinine did not differ from that of StD-fed mice. This would suggest a more beneficial effect on the kidneys by the free AAs intake and absorption, when compared to feeding the whole proteins. Perhaps this unidentified mechanism also provides some effects connected to a potential advantage responsible for the longer lifespan observed in Casein-AA-fed animals when compared to the Casein-Prot-fed animals.

Animals fed with the EAA-100% diet survived longer than all other groups. This is in agreement with a previous study showing that this particular EAA-blend supplementation improves mitochondrial biogenesis, thus increasing lifespan [11]. However, we also observed that these mice had slower body growth and were always (at all times) smaller than those fed with control diets. However, since no significant difference in food consumption was observed between EAA-100% and other special diets, the weight difference was not attributable to the amount of calories introduced, but was very likely due to the quality of nitrogen (thus of AAs) present in the diet. This is in agreement with a recent work where animals fed with a special blend of EAA-100% diet for one month showed similar outcomes [27]. Furthermore, other studies have demonstrated that a prolonged life is correlated with a smaller body size, both in mice [52] and in humans [53], an effect also provided by caloric restriction, which also supports our thesis.

Unexpectedly, in animals fed with EAA-100% diet, we also observed a progressive increase in water intake after eight months on this diet, although hematologic and urinary parameters did not differ from StD-fed mice. Unfortunately, to our knowledge, there is no literature that can help us to explain this behavior which, however, had no adverse effect upon or even promoted animal health.

We also observed that the EAA-100% diet reduced inflammation, as suggested by the lower Hpg level found in animals on this diet, even when compared to StD. This is in agreement with the anti-inflammatory activity of EAA observed in previous experimental [11,40] and clinical settings [1,54,55]. Those effects on inflammation modulation could represent one of the mechanisms underpinning the longer lifespan reached by these animals.

The EAA-100% and Casein-AA diets induced a partial loss of rpWAT. rpWAT is a very plastic tissue capable of storing and releasing lipids in response to metabolic needs. A WAT decrease suggests a change in the balance of substrates used for energy production and/or an increased energy expenditure. However, it has been shown that mice fed with an L-leucine-deficient diet quickly reduced in their fat mass and lipogenic activity [56]. Our Casein-AA diet contained an adequate amount of L-leucine, whereas the EAA-Ex diet contained an even higher amount of L-leucine. Therefore, other factors besides leucine concentration are probably involved in fat loss. The reason why free AAs decreased rpWAT, and through which mechanisms, remains unclear, and further studies are necessary to have a clear picture of the mechanisms involved. In our opinion, it is the nitrogen quality in food, and not the amount of caloric intake, that determines the balance of deposited/consumed rpWAT in our study.

4.1. Clinical Implications

Our data suggest that it may be useful to reconsider some aspects of metabolic roles of dietary nitrogen supply in animals, as well as in humans. NEAA should be considered hidden enemies introduced through proteins, which, when introduced in excess, shorten lifespan and probably directly modulate, inhibit or blunt the synthetic activities promoted by EAA. We believe that integrating the nitrogen supply provided by diets through the supplementation of EAA, in order to increase the EAA/NEAA ratio to at least >1, should be the pivotal intervention that may most efficiently improve the life expectancy of malnourished people of any age.

The usual paradigm of clinical nutrition assumes that whatever is lacking should be provided. However, this does not seem to be true for NEAA. A better alternative would be the provision of sufficient amounts of balanced formulations of EAA, because these would better promote and maintain those metabolic pathways responsible for the synthesis of the NEAA as needed, and also of their precursors and derivatives. Indeed, balanced formulations of EAA and the unbalancing of EAA/NEAA ratios >1, promote the gene expression and activity of mTOR, PGC-1-alpha, SIRT-1, eNOS and also promote mitochondriogenesis [11]. These factors are known to be involved with optimal metabolic performances in any physiological or pathological condition and at any age, and also are effective in vitro in inducing apoptosis in cancer cells [19]. An unresolved question is now if NEAA, on the contrary, inhibit some of the pathways epigenetically activated by EAA.

4.2. Study limitations

Our study has some limitations that need to be discussed. We used an EAA-100% formulation tailored to human needs, and thus presently used as a nutritional supplement for humans. Furthermore, the impossibility, in our experimental settings, to conduct precise bromatological analyses of the AAs content provided by the StD, so to control the possible variations that may exist among batches even when provided by the same producer, is of some concern and causes possible unexpected bias.

We also did not separately evaluate the contributions of individual AAs with respect to body changes. However, these probably had a mild influence on the overall results of the study. Therefore, investigating the effects of individual, or of a few, AAs, although interesting from a doctrinal point of view, would not reflect the complexity of nutritional needs and survival requirements linked to optimal animal nutrition and metabolism. This complexity is also demonstrated by testing with a known deficiency diet, such as that based only on casein protein and the peculiar amino acids ratios provided by casein.

5. Conclusions

We investigated the effects of different diets providing the same amount of carbohydrates, lipids, micronutrients and nitrogen, but containing various proteins or free EAA/NEAA ratios, on lifespan in mice. To our knowledge, this is the first report showing that diets providing nitrogen as free EAA are compatible with a prolonged lifespan in mice. The most relevant finding of our study was the inverse relationship between NEAA dietary content and lifespan. On the contrary, the diet with the highest amount of EAA increased lifespan and maintained low BW, while reducing systemic inflammation and preserving a balanced protein metabolism. On the contrary, the diet with a reduction of just less than 20% in EAA content compared to that usually provided by food proteins (about 45/49%) triggered the rapid catabolic processes characterized by rapid muscle mass loss, and led to precocious death of animals. We confirmed that casein, although among the reference proteins for rodents, is a protein that does not allow a lifespan comparable to that allowed by standard laboratory diets and providing adequate amounts of sulphur-containing AAs, which are insufficiently present in casein. However, in casein diets we could observe that a formulation of free AAs reproducing casein AAs content promoted the longest survival, in our opinion probably consequent to a more elevated absorption of methionine and cisteine.

It is commonly claimed that lifespan is affected by the amount of calories consumed [57]. Our data suggest that this is an oversimplified assumption. On the contrary, lifespan is conditioned by EAA and NEAA dietary content, since this ratio modulates phenotypic modifications in different organs, especially adipose and muscle tissues, and induces profound biological modifications. If we evaluate a diet in terms of the extension of lifespan, the total AAs content provided by any dietary protein should not be considered the optimal parameter. Indeed, our study suggests that an elevated intake of NEAA, provided by normal nutritional and food proteins, negatively affects health and correlates with lifespan, at least in mice. So, the concept of "optimal nutrition", being very hard to define anyway because it depends on so many variables (the aims of diet, sex, age, health, environment, species etc.), should be deeply revised on the basis of the present data. We think that the ratio among EAA and NEAA is the most likely factor responsible for the health-promoting effects of proteins in any diet, and eventually for prolonged or reduced survival, at least in rodents.

These data also led us to the question of why some AAs are provided exclusively with diet, whereas others can be synthesized by the organism itself. The origin and evolutionary significance of the relationships between EAA and NEAA is not known. We suggest as an hypothesis worth to be further explored, that the excessive introduction of NEAA may trigger certain natural selection mechanisms connected with the shortening of lifespan.

Author Contributions: Conceptualization, F.S.D., G.C. and C.R.; Methodology, G.C. and C.R.; Software, C.R. and G.C.; Formal Analysis, V.F., E.P., G.C.; Investigation, G.C. and C.R.; Data Curation, G.C., C.R. V.F.; Writing—Original Draft Preparation, G.C., C.R., V.F. and E.P.; Writing—Review, E.M., A.P., R.C. and F.S.D.; Writing—Editing. C.R., G.C., V.F.; Supervision, F.S.D.; Project Administration, F.S.D.; Funding Acquisition, F.S.D. and G.C.

Funding: This work was supported by grants from Nutriresearch s.r.l. (Milan, Italy) (G.C.). It was also partially supported by a grant provided by Dolomite-Franchi S.p.a. (Marone, Brescia, Italy) to G.C.

Conflicts of Interest: All authors have no competing financial interests to declare.

Compliance with Ethical Standards: All animal procedures followed the European Communities Council Directive of November 24, 1986 (86/609/EEC), and complied with the Italian Ministry of Health and The National Animal Protection Guidelines.

Abbreviations

AAs, amino acids; BAT, brown adipose tissue; BW, body weight; BL, body length; EAA, essential amino acids; Hpg, haptoglobin; NEAA, non-essential amino acids; N, nitrogen; NLR, neutrophils-lymphocytes ratio; OW, organ weight; rpWAT, retroperitoneal white adipose tissue; StD, standard diet.

References

1. Pasini, E.; Corsetti, G.; Aquilani, R.; Romano, C.; Picca, A.; Calvani, R.; Dioguardi, F.S. Protein-amino acid metabolism disarrangements: The hidden enemy of chronic age-related conditions. *Nutrients* **2018**, *10*, 391. [CrossRef] [PubMed]
2. Guigoz, Y. The mini nutritional assessment review of the literature: What does it tell us? *J. Nutr. Health Aging* **2006**, *10*, 466–485. [PubMed]
3. Wu, G. Amino acids: Metabolism, functions, and nutrition. *Amino Acids* **2009**, *37*, 1–17. [CrossRef] [PubMed]
4. Hou, Y.; Yin, Y.; Wu, G. Dietary essentiality of "nutritionally non-essential amino acids" for animals and humans. *Exp. Biol. Med. (Maywood)* **2015**, *240*, 997–1007. [CrossRef] [PubMed]
5. Borman, A.; Wood, T.R.; Balck, H.C.; Anderson, E.G.; Oesterling, M.J.; Womack, M.; Rose, W.C. The role of arginine in growth with some observations on the effects of argininic acid. *J. Biol. Chem.* **1946**, *166*, 585–594. [PubMed]
6. Reeds, P.J. Dispensable and indispensable amino acids for humans. *J. Nutr.* **2000**, *130*, 1835S–1840S. [CrossRef] [PubMed]
7. Ren, W.; Yin, Y.; Liu, G.; Yu, X.; Li, Y.; Yang, G.; Li, T.; Wu, G. Effect of dietary arginine supplementation on reproductive performance of mice with porcine circovirus type 2 infection. *Amino Acids* **2012**, *42*, 2089–2094. [CrossRef]
8. Rose, W.C.; Oesterling, M.J.; Womack, M.J. Comparative growth on diets containing ten and 19 amino acids, with further observations upon the role of glutamic and aspartic acids. *Biol. Chem.* **1948**, *176*, 753–762.
9. Wu, G.; Wu, Z.; Dai, Z.; Yang, Y.; Wang, W.; Liu, C.; Wang, B.; Wang, J.; Yin, Y. Dietary requirements of "nutritionally non-essential amino acids" by animals and humans. *Amino Acids* **2013**, *44*, 1107–1113. [CrossRef]

10. Civitarese, A.E.; Carling, S.; Heilbronn, L.K.; Hulver, M.H.; Ukropcova, B.; Deutsch, W.A.; Smith, S.R.; Ravussin, E.; CALERIE Pennington Team. Calorie restriction increases muscle mitochondrial biogenesis in healthy humans. *PLoS Med.* **2007**, *4*, e76. [CrossRef]
11. D'Antona, G.; Ragni, M.; Cardile, A.; Tedesco, L.; Dossena, M.; Bruttini, F.; Caliaro, F.; Corsetti, G.; Bottinelli, R.; Carruba, M.O.; et al. Branched-chain amino acid supplementation promotes survival and supports cardiac and skeletal muscle mitochondrial biogenesis in middle-aged mice. *Cell Metab.* **2010**, *12*, 362–372. [CrossRef] [PubMed]
12. Corsetti, G.; Pasini, E.; D'Antona, G.; Nisoli, E.; Flati, V.; Assanelli, D.; Dioguardi, F.S.; Bianchi, R. Morphometric changes induced by amino acid supplementation in skeletal and cardiac muscles of old mice. *Am. J. Cardiol.* **2008**, *101*, S26–S34. [CrossRef] [PubMed]
13. Flati, V.; Pasini, E.; D'Antona, G.; Speca, S.; Toniato, E.; Martinotti, S. Intracellular mechanisms of metabolism regulation: The role of signaling via the mammalian target of rapamycin pathway and other routes. *Am. J. Cardiol.* **2008**, *101*, 16E–21E. [CrossRef] [PubMed]
14. Stacchiotti, A.; Corsetti, G.; Lavazza, A.; Rezzani, R. Microscopic features of mitochondria rejuvenation by amino acids. In *Current Microscopy Contributions to Advances in Science and Technology*; Méndez-Vilas, A., Ed.; Formatex Research Center: Badajoz, Spain, 2012; pp. 286–294.
15. Corsetti, G.; Stacchiotti, A.; Tedesco, L.; D'Antona, G.; Pasini, E.; Dioguardi, F.S.; Nisoli, E.; Rezzani, R. Essential amino acid supplementation decreases liver damage induced by chronic ethanol consumption in rats. *Int. J. Immunopathol. Pharmacol.* **2011**, *24*, 611–619. [CrossRef] [PubMed]
16. Tedesco, L.; Corsetti, G.; Ruocco, C.; Ragni, M.; Rossi, F.; Carruba, M.O.; Valerio, A.; Nisoli, E. A specific amino acid formula prevents alcoholic liver disease in rodents. *Am. J. Physiol. Gastrointest. Liver Physiol.* **2018**, *314*, G566–G582. [CrossRef] [PubMed]
17. Corsetti, G.; D'Antona, G.; Ruocco, C.; Stacchiotti, A.; Romano, C.; Tedesco, L.; Dioguardi, F.S.; Rezzani, R.; Nisoli, E. Dietary supplementation with essential amino acids boots the beneficial effects of rosuvastatin on mouse kidney. *Amino Acids* **2014**, *6*, 2189–2203. [CrossRef]
18. Corsetti, G.; Romano, C.; Pasini, E.; Marzetti, E.; Calvani, R.; Picca, A.; Flati, V.; Dioguardi, F.S. Diet enrichment with a specific essential free amino acid mixture improves healing of undressed wounds in aged rats. *Exp. Geront.* **2017**, *96*, 138–145. [CrossRef] [PubMed]
19. Bonfili, L.; Cecarini, V.; Cuccioloni, M.; Angeletti, M.; Flati, V.; Corsetti, G.; Pasini, E.; Dioguardi, F.S.; Eleuteri, A.M. Essential amino acid mixtures drive cancer cells to apoptosis through proteasome inhibition and autophagy activation. *FEBS J.* **2017**, *284*, 1726–1737. [CrossRef]
20. Dioguardi, F.S. Clinical use of amino acids as dietary supplement: Pros and cons. *J. Cachexia Sarcopenia Muscle* **2011**, *2*, 75–80. [CrossRef]
21. Wanders, D.; Forney, L.A.; Stone, K.P.; Burk, D.H.; Pierse, A.; Gettys, T.W. FGF21 mediates the thermogenic and insulin-sensitizing effects of dietary methionine restriction but not its effects on hepatic lipid metabolism. *Diabetes* **2017**, *66*, 858–867. [CrossRef]
22. Cummings, N.E.M.; Williams, E.M.; Kasza, I. Restoration of metabolic health by decreased consumption of branched-chain amino acids. *J. Physiol.* **2018**, *596*, 623–645. [CrossRef] [PubMed]
23. Wanders, D.; Stone, K.P.; Dille, K.; Simon, J.; Pierse, A.; Gettys, T.W. Metabolic responses to dietary leucine restriction involve remodeling of adipose tissue and enhanced hepatic insulin signaling. *Biofactors* **2015**, *41*, 391–402. [CrossRef] [PubMed]
24. Simpson, S.J.; Le Couteur, D.G.; Raubenheimer, D.; Solon-Biet, S.M.; Cooney, G.J.; Cogger, V.C.; Fontana, L. Dietary protein, aging and nutritional geometry. *Ageing Res. Rev.* **2017**, *39*, 78–86. [CrossRef] [PubMed]
25. Le Couteur, D.G.; Solon-Biet, S.; Wahl, D.; Cogger, V.C.; Willcox, B.J.; Willcox, D.C.; Raubenheimer, D.; Simpson, S.J. New Horizons: Dietary protein, ageing and the Okinawan ratio. *Age Ageing* **2016**, *45*, 443–447. [CrossRef] [PubMed]
26. Le Couteur, D.G.; Solon-Biet, S.; Cogger, V.C.; Mitchell, S.J.; Senior, A.; de Cabo, R.; Raubenheimer, D.; Simpson, S.J. The impact of low-protein high-carbohydrate diets on aging and lifespan. *Cell Mol. Life Sci.* **2016**, *73*, 1237–1252. [CrossRef]
27. Corsetti, G.; Pasini, E.; Romano, C.; Calvani, R.; Picca, A.; Marzetti, E.; Flati, V.; Dioguardi, F.S. Body weight loss and tissue wasting in late middle-aged mice on slightly imbalanced essential/non-essential amino acids diet. *Front. Med. (Lausanne)* **2018**, *17*, 136. [CrossRef] [PubMed]

28. Pasini, E.; Aquilani, R.; Dioguardi, F.S.; D'Antona, G.; Gheorghiade, M.; Taegtmeyer, H. Hypercatabolic syndrome: Molecular basis and effects of nutritional supplements with amino acids. *Am. J. Cardiol.* **2008**, *101*, 11E–15E. [CrossRef]
29. Reeves, P.G.; Forrest, H.; Nielsen, F.H.; Fahey, G.C., Jr. AIN-93 Purified diets for laboratory rodents: Final report of the american institute of nutrition ad hoc writing committee on the reformulation of the AIN-76A rodent diet. *J. Nutr.* **1993**, *123*, 1939–1951. [CrossRef] [PubMed]
30. Blouet, C.; Mariotti, F.; Azzout-Marniche, D.; Bos, C.; Mathé, V.; Tomé, D.; Huneau, J.F. The reduced energy intake of rats fed a high-protein low-carbohydrate diet explains the lower fat deposition, but macronutrient substitution accounts for the improved glycemic control. *J. Nutr.* **2006**, *136*, 1849–1854. [CrossRef] [PubMed]
31. French, T. Acute phase proteins. In *The Clinical Chemistry of Laboratory Animals*; Loeb, W.F., Quimby, F.W., Eds.; Pergamon Press: Oxford, UK, 1989; Volume 1, pp. 201–235.
32. Ouellet, G.; Malhotra, R.; Penne, E.L.; Usvya, L.; Levin, N.W.; Kotanko, P. Neutrophil-lymphocyte ratio as a novel predictor of survival in chronic hemodialysis patients. *Clin. Nephrol.* **2016**, *85*, 191–198. [CrossRef]
33. Prats-Puig, A.; Gispert-Saüch, M.; Díaz-Roldán, F.; Carreras-Badosa, G.; Osiniri, I.; Planella-Colomer, M.; Mayol, L.; de Zegher, F.; Ibáñez, L.; Bassols, J.; et al. Neutrophil-to-lymphocyte ratio: An inflammation marker related to cardiovascular risk in children. *Thromb. Haemost.* **2015**, *114*. [CrossRef]
34. Evan's Awesome A/B Tools. Available online: http://www.evanmiller.org/ab-testing/survival-curves.html (accessed on 8 May 2019).
35. Volpi, E.; Kobayashi, H.; Sheffield-Moore, M.; Mittendorfer, B.; Wolfe, R.R. Essential amino acids are primarily responsible for the amino acid stimulation of muscle protein anabolism in healthy elderly adults. *Am. J. Clin. Nutr.* **2003**, *78*, 250–258. [CrossRef] [PubMed]
36. Mitrache, C.; Passweg, J.R.; Libura, J.; Petrikkos, L.; Seiler, W.O.; Gratwohl, A.; Stähelin, H.B.; Tichelli, A. Anemia: An indicator for malnutrition in the elderly. *Ann. Hematol.* **2001**, *80*, 295–298. [CrossRef] [PubMed]
37. Ou, S.M.; Chen, Y.T.; Hung, S.C.; Shih, C.J.; Lin, C.H.; Chiang, C.K.; Tarng, D.C. Taiwan Geriatric Kidney Disease (TGKD) Research Group: Association of estimated glomerular filtration rate with all-cause and cardiovascular mortality: The role of malnutrition-inflammation-cachexia syndrome. *J. Cachexia Sarcopenia Muscle* **2016**, *7*, 144–151. [CrossRef] [PubMed]
38. Shih, A.W.; McFarlane, A.; Verhovsek, M. Haptoglobin testing in hemolysis: Measurement and interpretation. *Am. J. Hematol.* **2014**, *89*, 443–447. [CrossRef] [PubMed]
39. Irwin, D.C.; Hyen Baek, J.; Hassell, K.; Nuss, R.; Eigenberger, P.; Lisk, C.; Loomis, Z.; Maltzahn, J.; Stenmark, K.R.; Nozik-Grayck, E.; et al. Hemoglobin-induced lung vascular oxidation, inflammation, and remodeling contribute to the progression of hypoxic pulmonary hypertension and is attenuated in rats with repeated-dose haptoglobin administration. *Free Radic. Biol. Med.* **2015**, *82*, 50–62. [CrossRef] [PubMed]
40. Romano, C.; Corsetti, G.; Pasini, E.; Flati, V.; Dioguardi, F.S. Dietary modifications of nitrogen intake decreases inflammation and promotes rejuvenation of spleen in aged mice. *J. Food Nutr. Res.* **2018**, *6*, 419–432. [CrossRef]
41. Potier, M.; Darcela, N.; Tome, D. Protein, amino acids and the control of food intake. *Curr. Opin. Clin. Nutr. Metab. Care* **2009**, *12*, 54–58. [CrossRef]
42. Dubos, R.; Schaedler, R.W.; Costello, R. Lasting biological effects of early environmental influences. 1. Conditioning of adult size by prenatal and postnatal nutrition. *J. Exp. Med.* **1968**, *127*, 783–799. [CrossRef]
43. Goettsch, M. Comparative protein requirement of the rat and mouse for growth, reproduction and lactation using casein diets. *J. Nutr.* **1960**, *70*, 307–312. [CrossRef]
44. Miner-Williams, W.; Deglaire, A.; Benamouzig, R.; Fuller, M.F.; Tomé, D.; Moughan, P.J. Endogenous proteins in terminal ileal digesta of adult subjects fed a casein-based diet. *Am. J. Clin. Nutr.* **2012**, *96*, 508–515. [CrossRef] [PubMed]
45. Jin, U.-H.; Lee, S.-O.; Sridharan, G.; Lee, K.; Davidson, L.A.; Jayaraman, A.; Chapkin, R.S.; Alaniz, R.; Safe, S. Microbiome-derived tryptophan metabolites and their aryl hydrocarbon receptor-dependent agonist and antagonist activities. *Mol. Pharmacol.* **2014**, *85*, 777–788. [CrossRef] [PubMed]
46. He, L.; Wu, L.; Xu, Z.; Li, T.; Yao, K.; Cui, Z.; Yin, Y.; Wu, G. Low-protein diets affect ileal amino acid digestibility and gene expression of digestive enzymes in growing and finishing pigs. *Amino Acids* **2015**, *48*, 21–30. [CrossRef] [PubMed]

47. Rondanelli, M.; Aquilani, R.; Verri, M.; Boschi, F.; Pasini, E.; Perna, S.; Faliva, A.; Condino, A.M. Plasma kinetics of essential amino acids following their ingestion as free formula or as dietary protein components. *Aging Clin. Exp. Res.* **2017**, *29*, 801–805. [CrossRef] [PubMed]
48. Jäger, R.; Kerksick, C.M.; Campbell, B.I.; Cribb, P.J.; Wells, S.D.; Skwiat, T.M.; Purpura, M.; Ziegenfuss, T.N.; Ferrando, A.A.; Arent, S.M.; et al. International Society of Sports Nutrition Position Stand: Protein and exercise. *J. Int. Soc. Sports Nutr.* **2017**, *14*, 20. [CrossRef] [PubMed]
49. Ables, G.P.; Johnson, J.E. Pleiotropic responses to methionine restriction. *Exp. Gerontol.* **2017**, *94*, 83–88. [CrossRef] [PubMed]
50. Levitt, D.G.; Levitt, M.D. Human serum albumin homeostasis: A new look at the roles of synthesis, catabolism, renal and gastrointestinal excretion, and the clinical value of serum albumin measurements. *Int. J. Gen. Med.* **2016**, *9*, 229–255. [CrossRef] [PubMed]
51. Gowda, S.; Desai, P.B.; Kulkarni, S.S.; Hull, V.V.; Math, A.A.; Vernekar, S.N. Markers of renal function tests. *N. Am. J. Med. Sci.* **2010**, *2*, 170–173.
52. Miller, R.A.; Chrisp, C.; Atchley, W. Differential longevity in mouse stocks selected for early life growth trajectory. *J. Gerontol. A Biol. Sci. Med. Sci.* **2000**, *55*, B455–B461. [CrossRef]
53. He, Q.; Morris, B.J.; Grove, J.S.; Petrovitch, H.; Ross, W.; Masaki, K.H.; Rodriguez, B.; Chen, R.; Donlon, T.A.; Willcox, D.C.; et al. Shorter men live longer: Association of height with longevity and FOXO3 genotype in american men of japanese ancestry. *PLoS ONE* **2014**, *9*, e94385. [CrossRef] [PubMed]
54. Aquilani, R.; Zuccarelli, G.C.; Condino, A.M.; Catani, M.; Rutili, C.; Del Vecchio, C.; Pisano, P.; Verri, M.; Iadarola, P.; Viglio, S.; et al. Despite inflammation, supplemented essential amino acids may improve circulating levels of albumin and hemoglobin in patients after hip fractures. *Nutrients* **2017**, *9*, 637. [CrossRef] [PubMed]
55. Boselli, M.; Aquilani, R.; Maestri, R.; Achilli, M.P.; Arrigoni, N.; Pasini, E.; Condino, A.M.; Boschi, F.; Dossena, M.; Buonocore, D.; et al. Inflammation and rehabilitation outcomes in patients with nontraumatic intracranial hemorrhage. *NeuroRehabilitation* **2018**, *42*, 449–456. [CrossRef] [PubMed]
56. Cheng, Y.; Meng, Q.; Wang, C.; Li, H.; Huang, Z.; Chen, S.; Xiao, F.; Guo, F. Leucine deprivation decreases fat mass by stimulation of lipolysis in white adipose tissue and upregulation of uncoupling protein 1 (UCP1) in brown adipose tissue. *Diabetes* **2010**, *59*, 17–25. [CrossRef] [PubMed]
57. Fontana, L.; Partridge, L.; Longo, V.D. Extending healthy life span–from yeast to humans. *Science* **2010**, *328*, 321–326. [CrossRef]

© 2019 by the authors. Licensee MDPI, Basel, Switzerland. This article is an open access article distributed under the terms and conditions of the Creative Commons Attribution (CC BY) license (http://creativecommons.org/licenses/by/4.0/).

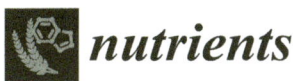

Article

Lactate Stimulates a Potential for Hypertrophy and Regeneration of Mouse Skeletal Muscle

Yoshitaka Ohno [1], Koki Ando [1], Takafumi Ito [1], Yohei Suda [1], Yuki Matsui [1], Akiko Oyama [1], Hikari Kaneko [1], Shingo Yokoyama [1], Tatsuro Egawa [2] and Katsumasa Goto [1,3,*]

1. Laboratory of Physiology, School of Health Sciences, Toyohashi SOZO University, Toyohashi 440-8511, Japan; yohno@sozo.ac.jp (Y.O.); r1482701@sc.sozo.ac.jp (K.A.); r1482703@sc.sozo.ac.jp (T.I.); r1482716@sc.sozo.ac.jp (Y.S.); r1482724@sc.sozo.ac.jp (Y.M.); r1382605@sc.sozo.ac.jp (A.O.); r1382606@sc.sozo.ac.jp (H.K.); s-yokoyama@sozo.ac.jp (S.Y.)
2. Laboratory of Sports and Exercise Medicine, Graduate School of Human and Environmental Studies, Kyoto University, Kyoto 606-8501, Japan; egawa.tatsuro.4u@kyoto-u.ac.jp
3. Department of Physiology, Graduate School of Health Sciences, Toyohashi SOZO University, Toyohashi 440-8511, Japan
* Correspondence: gotok@sepia.ocn.ne.jp; Tel.: +81-50-2017-2272

Received: 16 March 2019; Accepted: 15 April 2019; Published: 17 April 2019

Abstract: The effects of lactate on muscle mass and regeneration were investigated using mouse skeletal muscle tissue and cultured C2C12 cells. Male C57BL/6J mice were randomly divided into (1) control, (2) lactate (1 mol/L in distilled water, 8.9 mL/g body weight)-administered, (3) cardio toxin (CTX)-injected (CX), and (4) lactate-administered after CTX-injection (LX) groups. CTX was injected into right tibialis anterior (TA) muscle before the oral administration of sodium lactate (five days/week for two weeks) to the mice. Oral lactate administration increased the muscle weight and fiber cross-sectional area, and the population of Pax7-positive nuclei in mouse TA skeletal muscle. Oral administration of lactate also facilitated the recovery process of CTX-associated injured mouse TA muscle mass accompanied with a transient increase in the population of Pax7-positive nuclei. Mouse myoblast-derived C2C12 cells were differentiated for five days to form myotubes with or without lactate administration. C2C12 myotube formation with an increase in protein content, fiber diameter, length, and myo-nuclei was stimulated by lactate. These observations suggest that lactate may be a potential molecule to stimulate muscle hypertrophy and regeneration of mouse skeletal muscle via the activation of muscle satellite cells.

Keywords: lactate; skeletal muscle; hypertrophy; regeneration; muscle satellite cell

1. Introduction

Muscle satellite cells are known as skeletal muscle-specific stem cells that reside between the basal lamina and sarcolemma of mature myo-fibers [1]. Muscle satellite cells, which express the paired box transcription factor 7 (Pax7), are normally quiescent but become activated in response to exercise or injury [2–4]. Activated muscle satellite cells proliferate and undergo differentiation into myoblasts. Then the myoblasts differentiate and fuse into preexisting myofibers or fuse to form new myofibers, which result in skeletal muscle hypertrophy or regeneration [5–7].

Muscle satellite cells are considered to play a crucial role in exercise-associated muscle hypertrophy in human skeletal muscles [6,8] even though the studies using rodent models indicated that satellite cells may not contribute to exercise-associated hypertrophy of skeletal muscle [9,10]. Furthermore, exercise-associated stimuli, such as mechanical and heat stresses, are proposed to be potential stimuli to activate the regenerative process of injured skeletal muscle [11–13]. However, the mechanism of exercise-induced hypertrophy and regeneration of skeletal muscle is not fully elucidated.

Recent studies demonstrate that the number of biologically active molecules, so-called myokines, are released from resting as well as contracting skeletal muscle cells [14]. It is generally accepted that intensive exercise induces the release of lactate from contracting skeletal muscle. Extracellular lactate is re-uptaken by skeletal muscle to utilize it for an energy source [15,16]. On the other hand, the previous study using C2C12 skeletal muscle cells showed that a high level of extracellular lactate changed the expression of follistatin and myostatin [17], which regulate the proliferation of muscle satellite cells [18]. Furthermore, we recently demonstrated extracellular lactate-associated C2C12 myotube hypertrophy by activating the anabolic intracellular signals, such as p42/44 extracellular signal-regulated kinase-1/2 (ERK1/2) pathway [19], which stimulates muscle cell proliferation and differentiation [20–22]. Judging from published results, we hypothesize that increasing extracellular lactate level, which is generally induced by intensive exercise, may induce muscle hypertrophy as well as regeneration of injured skeletal muscle by activating muscle satellite cells.

In the present study, we investigated the effects of oral lactate administration on hypertrophy and regeneration in mouse skeletal muscle. Since previous studies have reported that an increase of satellite cells, which is caused by extracellular stimuli including electrical and heat stimulation [11,23], facilitated muscle regeneration, we evaluated the population of satellite cells following lactate administration. The effects of lactate on the formation of myotubes were also investigated by using cultured C2C12 cells.

2. Materials and Methods

2.1. Animal Experiments

All animal experimental procedures were conducted in accordance with the Guide for the Care and Use of Laboratory Animals, as adopted and promulgated by the National Institutes of Health (Bethesda, MD, USA). The Animal Use Committee of Toyohashi SOZO University (A2016003, A2017002) approved the procedures of animal experiments in this study. Male C57BL/6J mice aged 8-week old were used. To investigate the effects of lactate on skeletal muscle hypertrophy or regeneration, mice were randomly divided into control (C) and lactate-administered (L) groups ($n = 24$), or cardio-toxin (CTX)-injected (CX) and lactate-administered after CTX injection (LX) groups ($n = 28$). All mice were housed in a clean room controlled at approximately 23 °C with a 12/12 h light-dark cycle. Solid diet and water were provided ad libitum.

Muscle injury-regeneration cycle was induced by injecting 0.1 mL cardiotoxin (CTX, 10 µmol/L in physiological saline, Sigma-Aldrich, St. Louis, MO, USA) of Naja naja atra venom into right tibialis anterior (TA) muscles in the CX and LX groups. After epilation of right hind limb with a commercial hair remover for human, injection of CTX into right TA muscle was performed using a 27-gauge needle. During this procedure, all mice were under anesthesia with intraperitoneal injection of sodium pentobarbital (50 mg/kg) [23].

In the L and LX group, sodium lactate (1 mol/L in distilled water, 8.9 mL/g body weight, Otsuka Pharmaceutical Factory, Inc., Naruto, Tokushima, Japan) was administered to the mice by using an oral sonde 5 days a week for 2 weeks after CTX injection. The dose (or amount) of lactate was selected considering the previous rat study [18]. The same volume of ultrapure water was administered to the C and CX groups. In a pilot study, the changes of blood lactate concentration, which was collected from the tail vein of mice after oral lactate administration, were evaluated using the Lactate Pro2 blood lactate test meter (ARKRAY, Inc., Kyoto, Japan). Before the administration of lactate, the blood lactate concentration of mice ($n = 7$) was 2.9 ± 0.2 mmol/L (Table 1). Two hours after the lactate administration, blood lactate level significantly increased up to 4.1 ± 0.3 mmol/L. Similar to this observation, the oral administration of lactic acid to rats led to a rise in the blood level [24].

Table 1. Blood lactate concentration of mice following orally administered sodium lactate.

	Pre	2 h	6 h	24 h
Concentration, mmol/L	2.9 ± 0.2	4.1 ± 0.3 [†]	2.9 ± 0.3 [§]	3.0 ± 0.4

Pre: before oral lactate administration (base line); 2 h, 6 h, and 24 h: 2, 6, and 24 h after the lactate administration. Values are means ± SEM. $n = 7$. [†] and [§]: $p < 0.05$ vs. Pre and 2 h, respectively.

Mice were sacrificed by cervical dislocation under anesthesia with intraperitoneal injection of sodium pentobarbital (50 mg/kg) 1 and 2 weeks after CTX injection. Immediately after the sacrification, right TA muscle was excised. Dissected TA muscles were rapidly weighed and frozen in isopentane cooled in liquid nitrogen. All samples were then stored at −80 °C until analyses.

Serial transverse cryo-sections (8-μm thick) of the samples were cut at −20 °C and immediately mounted onto glass slides. Sections were stained to analyze the cross-sectional area (fiber CSA) of muscle fibers by hematoxylin and eosin (H&E), and the profiles of Pax7-positive nuclei by a standard immuno-histochemical technique [23]. Monoclonal anti-Pax7 antibody (Developmental Studies Hybridoma Bank, Iowa, IA, USA) was used for the detection of muscle satellite cells [3]. The sections were fixed in 4% paraformaldehyde, and were then post-fixed in ice-cooled methanol. After blocking by using 1% Roche blocking reagent (Roche Diagnostic, Penzberg, Germany), sections were incubated with the primary antibodies for Pax7 and rabbit polyclonal anti-laminin (Z0097, DakoCytomation, Glostrup, Denmark). Following an incubation period at 4 °C, sections were incubated with secondary antibodies for Cy3-conjugated anti-mouse IgG (Jackson Immuno Research, West Grove, PA, USA) and with fluorescein isothiocyanate-conjugated anti-rabbit IgG (Sigma-Aldrich) at room temperature. Nuclear counterstaining was performed in a solution of 4′,6-diamidino-2-phenylindole dihydrochloride (DAPI, Sigma-Aldrich). The number of Pax7-positive nuclei located within the laminin-positive basal membrane per muscle fiber (approximately 250 fibers) from each muscle was calculated. Using H&E stained sections, mean fiber CSA was measured from approximately 250 fibers of each muscle using the National Institutes of Health Image J 1.38X (NIH, Bethesda, MD, USA) software for Windows.

2.2. Cell Culture Experiments

Mouse myoblast-derived C2C12 cells (6×10^4 cells/well) were cultured on 6-well culture plates, coated with type I collagen (Biocoat, Corning, NY, USA). Cells were maintained in 2 mL of growth medium that consisted of Dulbecco's modified Eagle's medium (DMEM, Thermo Fisher Scientific, Yokohama, Japan) supplemented with 10% heat-inactivated fetal bovine serum containing high glucose (4.5 g/L glucose, 4.0 mM L-glutamine, without sodium pyruvate) for proliferation. During the third day of the proliferation phase (at ~80% confluence), the culture medium was then changed to the same amount of differentiation medium, which consisted of DMEM supplemented with 2% heat-inactivated horse serum containing low glucose (1.0 g/L glucose, 4.0 mM L-glutamine, and 110 mg/L sodium pyruvate) for differentiation, as was described previously [19]. Every 2 days, cells were replenished with fresh differentiation medium and cultures were maintained for 5 days. All cells were maintained at 37 °C, under a humidified atmosphere with 5% CO_2 and 95% air.

Sodium lactate was administered into the conditioned medium throughout the differentiation phase. The concentration of lactate was set at 20 mM in the conditioned culture medium, which took into account previous studies using skeletal muscle cells [19,25]. Ultrapure water alone was added to the conditioning medium for the control group ($n = 6$ well in each group).

The images of myotubes at the 5th day of the differentiation phase were visualized at x40 magnification using a calibrated color imaging camera (DP12, Olympus, Tokyo, Japan) set up to a phase contrast light microscope (CK40, Olympus). In order to measure the myotube diameter, we used a modified method of a previous study [26]. We first randomly selected fields of view from 6 wells of each condition. Using Image J, the diameters of at least 100 myotubes in each well were measured at three randomly selected portions taken along the length of the myotube. Then, the average diameter of a myotube was calculated as the mean of three measurements. The myotubes were also used for the evaluation of myotube length and the myo-nuclei number as described below. Cells were fixed with 4% paraformaldehyde. After blocking, cells were incubated with the primary antibodies for skeletal myosin (M4276, Sigma-Aldrich). Cells were then incubated with the secondary antibodies for Cy3-conjugated anti-mouse IgG. Then nuclei were counterstained with DAPI. Since a muscle cell containing 3 or more nuclei was considered to be a myotube [27], the myotube length and myonuclei number in differentiated myotubes (>2 myonuclei) were measured using Image J.

In addition, the myotubes at the 5th day of differentiation were used to analyze muscular protein content as described below. In order to extract protein from C2C12 cells, the cells were lysed in a cell lysis reagent (CelLytic^{TM}-M, Sigma-Aldrich), in accordance with the previously reported method [19]. The cells in each well were rinsed twice in 1 mL of ice-cooled phosphate-buffered saline. The cells of each well were then scraped into 0.3 mL of cell lysis reagent on ice. The cell lysate was sonicated and centrifuged at 20,000 g at 4 °C for 10 min. The supernatant was collected for the analysis of protein content. Protein content in the supernatant was determined using the Bradford technique (protein Assay kit, Bio-Rad, Hercules, CA, USA) and bovine serum albumin (Sigma-Aldrich) as the standard.

2.3. Animal Experiments

All values were expressed as means ± SEM. In animal experiments, the statistically significant level of blood lactate concentration was analyzed using one-way analysis of variance (ANOVA) followed by the Tukey-Kramer test. Other significant levels were tested using a two-way (lactate administration and time) ANOVA for multiple comparisons followed by the Tukey-Kramer test. When a significant interaction between main factors was observed, one-way ANOVA followed by the Tukey-Kramer test was performed. Statistically significant levels in cell experiments were evaluated using unpaired Student's *t*-test following F-test. The significance level was accepted at $p < 0.05$.

3. Results

3.1. Effect of Lactate on Skeletal Muscle Hypertrophy

The body weight, TA muscle weight, and fiber CSA in response to oral lactate administration were shown in Figure 1. There was no significant difference in body weight between groups. A significant increase in the absolute TA muscle weight and the muscle weight relative to body weight was observed in the lactate-administered L group (Figure 1A, $p < 0.05$). Similarly, the fiber CSA in the L group was significantly larger than that in the C group (Figure 1B, $p < 0.05$).

There was no significant change in the population number of Pax7-positive nuclei a fiber of TA muscle in the C group during the experimental period. In the L group, the population of Pax7-positive nuclei was significantly increased (200% and 138% at 1 and 2 weeks after lactate administration, respectively), compared with that in the C group (Figure 1C, $p < 0.05$).

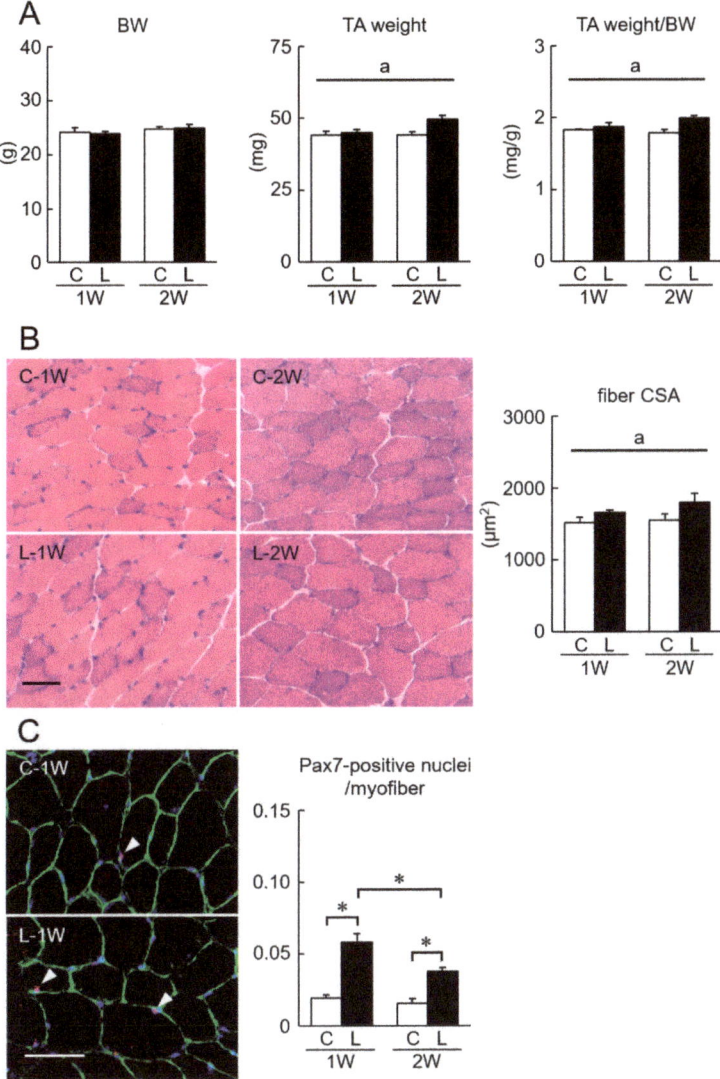

Figure 1. (**A**) Effects of oral lactate administration on body weight (BW) and tibialis anterior (TA) weight in mice. Effect of oral lactate administration on the TA muscle fiber cross-sectional area (CSA) (**B**) and the number of Pax7-positive nuclei per muscle fiber (**C**). Representative images of histochemical and immuno-histochemical staining in TA muscle are shown. Arrowheads indicate the Pax7-positive nuclei. Scale bar = 50 μm. TA weight/BW: relative TA weight to BW. C: control group. L: lactate-administered group. 1W and 2W: 1 and 2 weeks of lactate administration, respectively. Values are means ± SEM. $n = 6$ per group. a: Significant main effect of lactate, $p < 0.05$. *: $p < 0.05$.

3.2. Effect of Lactate on Skeletal Muscle Regeneration

Many regenerating fibers with centrally located nuclei in CTX-injected TA muscle were observed 1 and 2 weeks after the injection (Figure 2B). There was no significant change in body weight of not only CX but also LX groups during the experimental period (Figure 2A). Both TA muscle weight (24% and 29% of absolute and relative levels, respectively) and fiber CSA (44%) 2 weeks after CTX injection increased, compared with those 1 week after the injection. Two weeks after CTX injection, lactate administration-associated increase in the absolute TA muscle weight was observed ($p < 0.05$). A significant main effect of lactate administration was observed in the relative muscle weight as well as fiber CSA ($p < 0.05$).

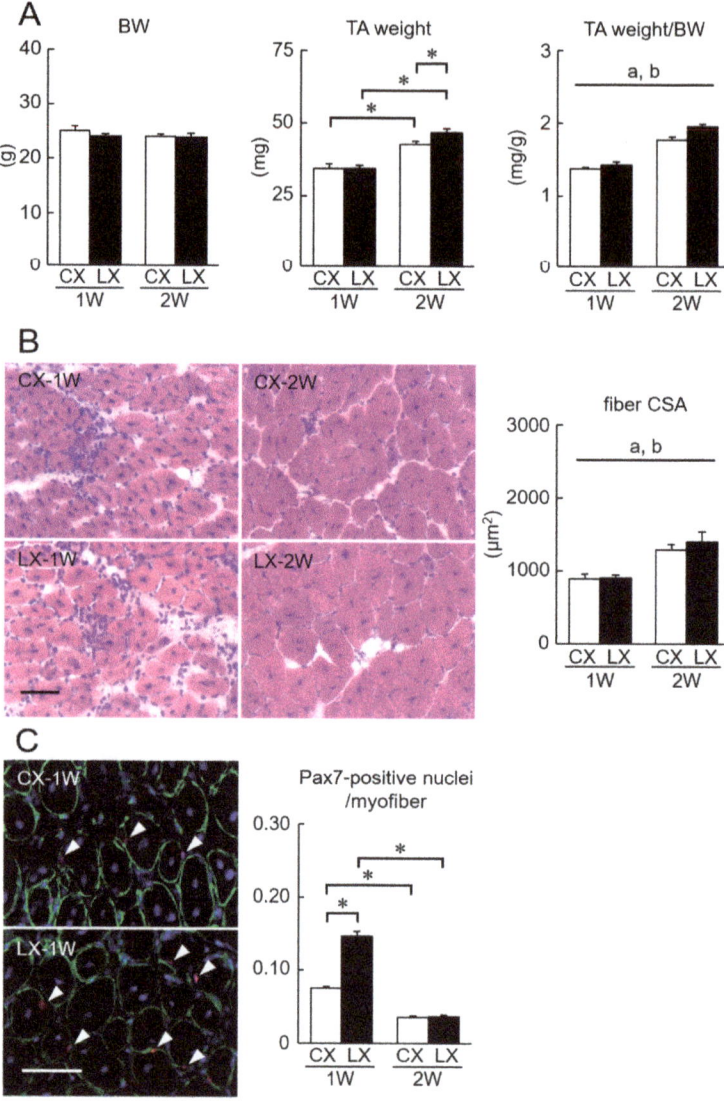

Figure 2. (**A**) Effects of oral lactate administration on BW and TA weight in cardio-toxin (CTX)-injected mice. Effect of oral lactate administration on CTX-injected TA muscle fiber CSA (**B**) and the number of Pax7-positive nuclei per muscle fiber (**C**). Representative images of histochemical and immuno-histochemical staining in CTX-injected TA muscle are shown. Arrowheads indicate the Pax7-positive nuclei. Scale bar = 50 µm. CX: CTX-injected group. LX: lactate-administered after the CTX-injection group. 1W and 2W: 1 and 2 weeks after CTX injection, respectively. See Figure 1 for other abbreviations. Values are means ± SEM. $n = 7$ per group. a and b: Significant main effect of lactate and time, respectively. $p < 0.05$. *: $p < 0.05$.

One week after CTX injection, the population of Pax7-positive nuclei was increased (0.08/myofiber), compared with that in the C group (0.02/myofiber). Furthermore, the additional increase in the population of Pax7-positive nuclei was observed in the lactate-administered LX group, when compared with the CX group, 1 week after CTX injection ($p < 0.05$).

3.3. Effects of Lactate on Myotube Formation

We examined the effects of lactate on myotube formation of C2C12 cells. The typical images of myotubes, on the 5th day of differentiation, with or without lactate in the medium were shown in Figure 3. In the lactate-administered cells, myotubes have a wider diameter, longer length, and more myonuclei compared with the control. A significant increase in the myotube diameter and muscular protein content was induced by lactate (Figure 3A,B, $p < 0.05$). Lactate administration also increased myotube length as well as myo-nuclei number (Figure 3C, $p < 0.05$).

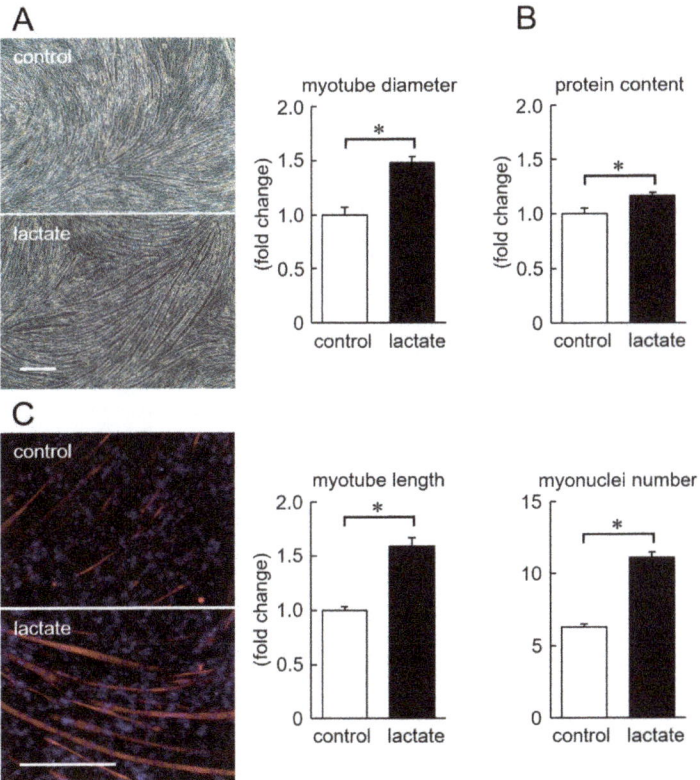

Figure 3. Myo-tube diameter (**A**), muscular protein content (**B**), myo-tube length, and myonuclei number (**C**) of C2C12 cells in response to lactate. Scale bar = 300 μm. Values are means ± SEM. $n = 6$ wells per group. *: $p < 0.05$.

4. Discussion

The present study demonstrated that oral lactate administration induced muscle hypertrophy accompanied with an increase of Pax7-positive nuclei in mouse TA muscle. In injured TA muscle, the increase of muscle mass and Pax7-positive nuclei population was stimulated by lactate administration. Furthermore, lactate-induced myotube formation including higher protein content, wider diameter, longer length, and more myo-nuclei were observed in C2C12 cells.

4.1. Muscle Hypertrophy

In the present study, oral lactate administration increased TA muscle weight and fiber CSA in mice. This is the first report showing the effect of lactate on skeletal muscle mass in animals. Furthermore, the population of Pax7-positive nuclei in TA muscle was increased by lactate administration. Since the previous study using C2C12 skeletal muscle cells reported that extracellular lactate increased follistatin and decreased myostatin expressions involved in the proliferation of satellite cells [17,18], oral lactate administration-associated increase of blood lactate concentration may enhance the proliferation of muscle satellite cells. Recently, we demonstrated an extracellular lactate-associated increase in the diameter of C2C12 myo-tubes [19]. These observations suggest that lactate administration, which could increase blood lactate levels, stimulated the hypertrophy of skeletal muscle with the activation of muscle satellite cells. Training with a blood flow restriction, which is exercise with vascular occlusion, is known to increase muscle size [28,29] and the blood lactate level [29,30] in humans. Therefore, there is a possibility that the blood lactate level may contribute to muscle size following occlusion training.

4.2. Muscle Regeneration

In the present study, increase in muscle weight and fiber CSA in CTX-injected TA muscle was observed during a 2-week experimental period. In addition, the population of Pax7-positive nuclei was increased by CTX injection. These phenomena are consistent with the previously reported data in mice [23]. Larger muscle mass and Pax7-positive nuclei population were also observed in lactate-administered mouse, which suggests that lactate stimulates the regenerative potential of injured skeletal muscle by activating muscle satellite cells.

4.3. Myotube Formation

In the present study, lactate increased the myotube diameter and protein content in C2C12 cells. These results are supported by the previous report that lactate caused the activation of anabolic signals for hypertrophy and myogenesis in skeletal muscle cells [18]. Our previous data also showed that extracellular lactate increased the diameter of C2C12 myotubes in a dose-dependent manner [19]. In addition, the present study demonstrated that extracellular lactate caused the extension of the myotube length and the increase of the myonuclei number. Therefore, it was suggested that lactate may stimulate the fusion of myoblasts, which results in myotube formation. This contributes to muscle hypertrophy and regeneration [5–7].

It has been a debatable argument that various metabolites, including lactate, may be involved in exercise-associated skeletal muscle hypertrophy [31]. In the present study, cell culture experiments demonstrated lactate induces an increase in muscle mass even though no myotube contraction is observed. On the other hand, lactate may also stimulate the hypertrophic effects of physical activity on skeletal muscle, since mice moved freely immediately after the administration of lactate in the present study. Additional results are needed to elucidate the difference and interaction between lactate and muscle contraction in skeletal muscle hypertrophy.

5. Conclusions

The present study demonstrated oral lactate administration-associated hypertrophy and regeneration of mouse skeletal muscle. Extracellular lactate might contribute to the regulation of skeletal muscle plasticity.

Author Contributions: Conceptualization, Y.O., T.E., and K.G. Investigation, Y.O., K.A., T.I., Y.S., Y.M., A.O., H.K., and S.Y. Formal analysis, Y.O., K.A., T.I., Y.S., Y.M., A.O., and H.K. Writing—original draft preparation, Y.O., T.E., and K.G. Funding acquisition, Y.O and K.G.

Funding: MEXT/JSPS KAKENHI Grant Number (16K12942, Y.O.; 16K13022, K.G.; 17K01762, K.G.; 18K10796; Y.O.; 18H03160, K.G.), the Uehara Memorial Foundation (Y.O.; K.G.), the Meiji Yasuda Life Foundation of Health and Welfare (Y.O.), the Naito Foundation (K.G.), the Descente Sports Foundation (K.G.), the All Japan Coffee Association (K.G.), the Science Research Promotion Fund from the Promotion and Mutual Aid Corporation for

Private Schools of Japan (K.G.), and Graduate School of Health Sciences, Toyohashi SOZO University (K.G.) supported this study.

Conflicts of Interest: The authors declare no conflict of interest. The funders had no role in the design of the study, in the collection, analyses, or interpretation of data, in the writing of the manuscript, or in the decision to publish the results.

References

1. Mauro, A. Satellite cell of skeletal muscle fibers. *J. Biophys. Biochem. Cytol.* **1961**, *9*, 493–495. [CrossRef] [PubMed]
2. Bazgir, B.; Fathi, R.; Rezazadeh Valojerdi, M.; Mozdziak, P.; Asgari, A. Satellite cells contribution to exercise mediated muscle hypertrophy and repair. *Cell J.* **2017**, *18*, 473–484. [PubMed]
3. Seale, P.; Sabourin, L.A.; Girgis-Gabardo, A.; Mansouri, A.; Gruss, P.; Rudnicki, M.A. Pax7 is required for the specification of myogenic satellite cells. *Cell* **2000**, *102*, 777–786. [CrossRef]
4. Tidball, J.G. Inflammatory processes in muscle injury and repair. *Am. J. Physiol. Regul. Integr. Comp. Physiol.* **2005**, *288*, R345–R353. [CrossRef] [PubMed]
5. Bischoff, R. Analysis of muscle regeneration using single myofibers in culture. *Med. Sci. Sports Exerc.* **1989**, *21*, S164–S172. [CrossRef] [PubMed]
6. Petrella, J.K.; Kim, J.S.; Mayhew, D.L.; Cross, J.M.; Bamman, M.M. Potent myofiber hypertrophy during resistance training in humans is associated with satellite cell-mediated myonuclear addition: A cluster analysis. *J. Appl. Physiol.* **2008**, *104*, 1736–1742. [CrossRef]
7. Relaix, F.; Zammit, P.S. Satellite cells are essential for skeletal muscle regeneration: The cell on the edge returns centre stage. *Development* **2012**, *139*, 2845–2856. [CrossRef]
8. Bellamy, L.M.; Joanisse, S.; Grubb, A.; Mitchell, C.J.; McKay, B.R.; Phillips, S.M.; Baker, S.; Parise, G. The acute satellite cell response and skeletal muscle hypertrophy following resistance training. *PLoS ONE* **2014**, *9*, e109739. [CrossRef] [PubMed]
9. Jackson, J.R.; Mula, J.; Kirby, T.J.; Fry, C.S.; Lee, J.D.; Ubele, M.F.; Campbell, K.S.; McCarthy, J.J.; Peterson, C.A.; Dupont-Versteegden, E.E. Satellite cell depletion does not inhibit adult skeletal muscle regrowth following unloading-induced atrophy. *Am. J. Physiol. Cell Physiol.* **2012**, *303*, C854–C861. [CrossRef]
10. McCarthy, J.J.; Mula, J.; Miyazaki, M.; Erfani, R.; Garrison, K.; Farooqui, A.B.; Srikuea, R.; Lawson, B.A.; Grimes, B.; Keller, C.; et al. Effective fiber hypertrophy in satellite cell-depleted skeletal muscle. *Development* **2011**, *138*, 3657–3666. [CrossRef] [PubMed]
11. Kojima, A.; Goto, K.; Morioka, S.; Naito, T.; Akema, T.; Fujiya, H.; Sugiura, T.; Ohira, Y.; Beppu, M.; Aoki, H.; et al. Heat stress facilitates the regeneration of injured skeletal muscle in rats. *J. Orthop. Sci.* **2007**, *12*, 74–82. [CrossRef]
12. Matsuba, Y.; Goto, K.; Morioka, S.; Naito, T.; Akema, T.; Hashimoto, N.; Sugiura, T.; Ohira, Y.; Beppu, M.; Yoshioka, T. Gravitational unloading inhibits the regenerative potential of atrophied soleus muscle in mice. *Acta Physiol.* **2009**, *196*, 329–339. [CrossRef] [PubMed]
13. Morioka, S.; Goto, K.; Kojima, A.; Naito, T.; Matsuba, Y.; Akema, T.; Fujiya, H.; Sugiura, T.; Ohira, Y.; Beppu, M.; et al. Functional overloading facilitates the regeneration of injured soleus muscles in mice. *J. Physiol. Sci.* **2008**, *58*, 397–404. [CrossRef] [PubMed]
14. So, B.; Kim, H.J.; Kim, J.; Song, W. Exercise-induced myokines in health and metabolic diseases. *Integr. Med. Res.* **2014**, *3*, 172–179. [CrossRef]
15. Brooks, G.A. Cell-cell and intracellular lactate shuttles. *J. Physiol.* **2009**, *587*, 5591–5600. [CrossRef] [PubMed]
16. Gladden, L.B. Lactate metabolism: A new paradigm for the third millennium. *J. Physiol.* **2004**, *558*, 5–30. [CrossRef]
17. Gilson, H.; Schakman, O.; Kalista, S.; Lause, P.; Tsuchida, K.; Thissen, J.P. Follistatin induces muscle hypertrophy through satellite cell proliferation and inhibition of both myostatin and activing. *Am. J. Physiol. Endocrinol. Metab.* **2009**, *297*, E157–E164. [CrossRef] [PubMed]
18. Oishi, Y.; Tsukamoto, H.; Yokokawa, T.; Hirotsu, K.; Shimazu, M.; Uchida, K.; Tomi, H.; Higashida, K.; Iwanaka, N.; Hashimoto, T. Mixed lactate and caffeine compound increases satellite cell activity and anabolic signals for muscle hypertrophy. *J. Appl. Physiol.* **2015**, *118*, 742–749. [CrossRef] [PubMed]

19. Ohno, Y.; Oyama, A.; Kaneko, H.; Egawa, T.; Yokoyama, S.; Sugiura, T.; Ohira, Y.; Yoshioka, T.; Goto, K. Lactate is a potential hypertrophic stimulus for myotubes via activation of MEK/ERK pathway. *Acta Physiol.* **2018**, *223*, e13042. [CrossRef]
20. Coolican, S.A.; Samuel, D.S.; Ewton, D.Z.; McWade, F.J.; Florini, J.R. The mitogenic and myogenic actions of insulin-like growth factors utilize distinct signaling pathways. *J. Biol. Chem.* **1997**, *272*, 6653–6662. [CrossRef]
21. Li, J.; Johnson, S.E. ERK2 is required for efficient terminal differentiation of skeletal myoblasts. *Biochem. Biophys. Res. Commun.* **2006**, *345*, 1425–1433. [CrossRef]
22. Wu, Z.; Woodring, P.J.; Bhakta, K.S.; Tamura, K.; Wen, F.; Feramisco, J.R.; Karin, M.; Wang, J.Y.; Puri, P.L. p38 and extracellular signal-regulated kinases regulate the myogenic program at multiple steps. *Mol. Cell. Biol.* **2000**, *20*, 3951–3964. [CrossRef]
23. Fujiya, H.; Ogura, Y.; Ohno, Y.; Goto, A.; Nakamura, A.; Ohashi, K.; Uematsu, D.; Aoki, H.; Musha, H.; Goto, K. Microcurrent electrical neuromuscular stimulation facilitates regeneration of injured skeletal muscle in mice. *J. Sports Sci. Med.* **2015**, *14*, 297–303.
24. Morotomi, M.; Sakai, K.; Yazawa, K.; Suegara, N.; Kawai, Y.; Mutai, M. Effect and fate of orally administered lactic acid in rats. *J. Nutr. Sci. Vitaminol.* **1981**, *27*, 117–128. [CrossRef]
25. Hashimoto, T.; Hussien, R.; Oommen, S.; Gohil, K.; Brooks, G.A. Lactate sensitive transcription factor network in L6 cells: Activation of MCT1 and mitochondrial biogenesis. *FASEB J.* **2007**, *21*, 2602–2612. [CrossRef]
26. Williamson, D.L.; Butler, D.C.; Always, S.E. AMPK inhibits myoblast differentiation through a PGC-1alpha-dependent mechanism. *Am. J. Physiol. Endocrinol. Metab.* **2009**, *297*, E304–E314. [CrossRef]
27. Ge, X.; Zhang, Y.; Park, S.; Cong, X.; Gerrard, D.E.; Jiang, H. Stac3 inhibits myoblast differentiation into myotubes. *PLoS ONE* **2014**, *9*, e95876. [CrossRef]
28. Abe, T.; Kearns, C.F.; Sato, Y. Muscle size and strength are increased following walk training with restricted venous blood flow from the leg muscle, Kaatsu-walk training. *J. Appl. Physiol.* **2006**, *100*, 1460–1466. [CrossRef]
29. Takarada, Y.; Takazawa, H.; Sato, Y.; Takebayashi, S.; Tanaka, Y.; Ishii, N. Effects of resistance exercise combined with moderate vascular occlusion on muscular function in humans. *J. Appl. Physiol.* **2000**, *88*, 2097–2106. [CrossRef]
30. Takarada, Y.; Nakamura, Y.; Aruga, S.; Onda, T.; Miyazaki, S.; Ishii, N. Rapid increase in plasma growth hormone after low-intensity resistance exercise with vascular occlusion. *J. Appl. Physiol.* **2000**, *88*, 61–65. [CrossRef]
31. Dankel, S.J.; Mattocks, K.T.; Jessee, M.B.; Buckner, S.L.; Mouser, J.G.; Loenneke, J.P. Do metabolites that are produced during resistance exercise enhance muscle hypertrophy? *Eur. J. Appl. Physiol.* **2017**, *117*, 2125–2135. [CrossRef]

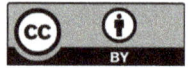

© 2019 by the authors. Licensee MDPI, Basel, Switzerland. This article is an open access article distributed under the terms and conditions of the Creative Commons Attribution (CC BY) license (http://creativecommons.org/licenses/by/4.0/).

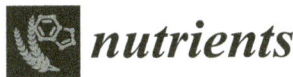

Review

Poor Oral Health as a Determinant of Malnutrition and Sarcopenia

Domenico Azzolino [1,2,*,†], Pier Carmine Passarelli [3,†], Paolo De Angelis [3], Giovan Battista Piccirillo [3], Antonio D'Addona [3] and Matteo Cesari [1,2]

1. Geriatric Unit, Fondazione IRCCS Ca' Granda Ospedale Maggiore Policlinico, 20122 Milan, Italy; matteo.cesari@unimi.it
2. Department of Clinical Sciences and Community Health, University of Milan, 20122 Milan, Italy
3. Department of Head and Neck, Oral Surgery and Implantology Unit, Institute of Clinical Dentistry, Catholic University of Sacred Hearth, Fondazione Policlinico Universitario Gemelli, 00168 Rome, Italy; piercarminepassarelli@hotmail.it (P.C.P.); dr.paolodeangelis@gmail.com (P.D.A.); giovanbpiccirillo@gmail.com (G.B.P.); antonio.daddona@unicatt.it (A.D.)

* Correspondence: domenico.azzolino@policlinico.mi.it
† These authors contributed equally to this work.

Received: 7 November 2019; Accepted: 27 November 2019; Published: 29 November 2019

Abstract: Aging is accompanied by profound changes in many physiological functions, leading to a decreased ability to cope with stressors. Many changes are subtle, but can negatively affect nutrient intake, leading to overt malnutrition. Poor oral health may affect food selection and nutrient intake, leading to malnutrition and, consequently, to frailty and sarcopenia. On the other hand, it has been highlighted that sarcopenia is a whole-body process also affecting muscles dedicated to chewing and swallowing. Hence, muscle decline of these muscle groups may also have a negative impact on nutrient intake, increasing the risk for malnutrition. The interplay between oral diseases and malnutrition with frailty and sarcopenia may be explained through biological and environmental factors that are linked to the common burden of inflammation and oxidative stress. The presence of oral problems, alone or in combination with sarcopenia, may thus represent the biological substratum of the disabling cascade experienced by many frail individuals. A multimodal and multidisciplinary approach, including personalized dietary counselling and oral health care, may thus be helpful to better manage the complexity of older people. Furthermore, preventive strategies applied throughout the lifetime could help to preserve both oral and muscle function later in life. Here, we provide an overview on the relevance of poor oral health as a determinant of malnutrition and sarcopenia.

Keywords: sarcopenia; nutrition; oral health; older people; malnutrition; swallowing; life course approach

1. Introduction

Advancing age is characterized by a progressive decline in multiple physiological functions, leading to an increased vulnerability to stressors and augmented risk of adverse outcomes [1–3]. During the aging process, several factors may affect body shape from both clinical and functional perspectives. Reduction in smell and taste senses, poor appetite (the so-called "anorexia of aging"), and decreased energy expenditure may all contribute to poor nutrition. Moreover, illnesses, medications, as well as poor oral health (for example, due to teeth loss and poorly fitting dentures) can exacerbate anorexia [4–6]. Nutritional status among older people may be also influenced by living or eating alone, poor financial status, dismobility, and decreased ability to shop or prepare meals [7,8]. Psychosocial factors including loneliness, sleep disorders, dementia, and depression are also recognized to have a negative impact on the dietary intake of older subjects [9].

Furthermore, with aging, there is a progressive loss in muscle mass and strength, whereas fat mass and fat infiltration of muscle increase [10,11]. Sarcopenia is the term, introduced for the first time in 1988 by Irwin Rosenberg, to indicate the pathologic reduction in muscle mass and strength leading to a poor function [12,13]. Interestingly, in recent years, it has been highlighted that sarcopenia is not limited to lower limbs, but is a whole-body process [14–16], also affecting the muscles devoted to chewing and swallowing [10,17], with a negative impact on food intake. In fact, atrophy of muscles critical for the respiratory and swallowing functions has been reported [14,18–22].

The variety of dental problems experienced by older people can result in chewing difficulties determining changes in food selection, thus leading to malnutrition and consequently to frailty [23] and sarcopenia [10,23]. Poor oral status may also predispose one to a chronic low-grade systemic inflammation through periodontal disease [24,25], which has an increased prevalence in those who are not able to perform the daily oral hygiene procedures [26], and it is a well-known risk factor in the pathogenesis of frailty [27] and sarcopenia [28]. Furthermore, periodontal disease has been associated with faster decline in handgrip strength [29], and recent studies showed an association between chewing difficulties and frailty [24].

Therefore, a hypothetical triangle oral status–nutrition–sarcopenia, exposing the older person to the frailty disabling cascade, may be suggested, as seen in Figure 1.

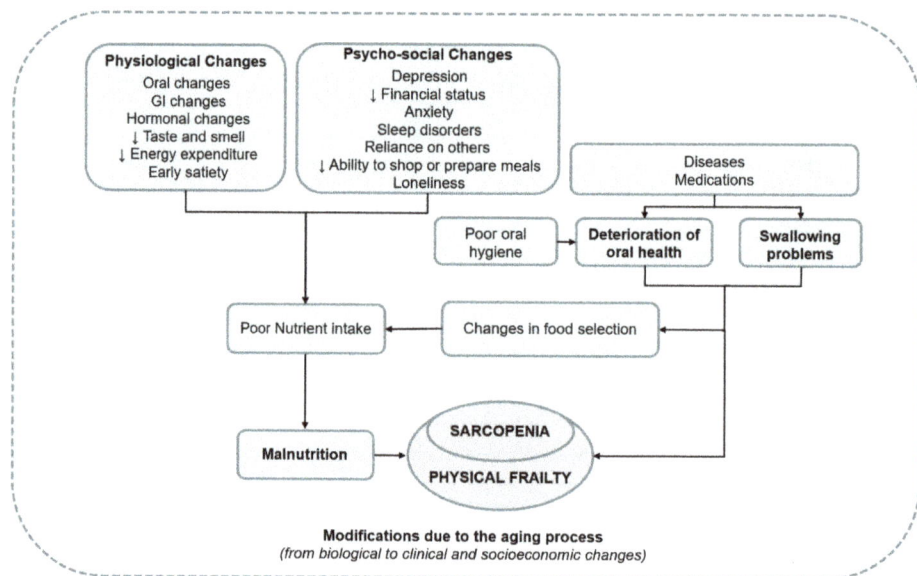

Figure 1. Overview of the interplay between poor oral status, malnutrition, and sarcopenia. GI—gastrointestinal.

2. Oral Changes with Aging

Poor oral health is not an inevitable part of aging since good care throughout the life course can result in the maintenance of functional teeth later in life [24]. Throughout a lifetime, the oral cavity experiences a variety of physiological modifications, such as enamel changes, fractures lines and stains, as well as dentin exposure and darkening of the tooth. At the same time, in the inner part of the tooth, several changes, such as the deposition of secondary dentin reducing the size of the pulp chamber and canals, may also occur [30]. Furthermore, in older people, tooth wear is frequently observed, affecting more than 85% of all the teeth groups in both the mandible and maxilla [31]. Additionally, a loss in terms of elastic fibers in the connective tissue has been documented and, subsequently, the oral mucosa becomes less resilient [32].

However, older people, especially those who are institutionalized or with limited financial resources, may experience problems to access oral care. Furthermore, it has been documented that older people frequently have difficulty expressing complaints and assign low priority to oral health until dental problems become intolerable [33]. Oral problems among older people have been implicated in a high prevalence of tooth loss, dental caries, periodontal disease, xerostomia, and oral precancer/cancer lesions [34]. Periodontitis and dental caries are very common diseases, especially in older people, and are considered the main cause of tooth loss [35].

Around the age of 70, there is also a peak of root/cementum caries, as a result of both tooth retention and major exposure of these surfaces following periodontal support loss. Moreover, older people are at higher risk of periodontitis since it is a cumulative disease, especially with regard to the multirooted teeth [36].

2.1. Edentulism

Edentulism is a pathological condition characterized by multiple missing teeth; it can be partial or total. The etiology of tooth loss includes factors such as predisposition, diet, hormonal status, coexisting diseases, hygiene habits, and use of dental clinics. Additionally, edentulism may result from an unsuccessful periodontal treatment or important carious lesions [37,38]. Dental disease and loss of teeth are not part of normal aging, but if this occurs, it is probably a result of neglected oral hygiene and/or an inadequate treatment [39,40]. Edentulism is exacerbated when masticatory function is not restored with dental prostheses [41]. Tooth loss affects the individual ability to chew determining an alteration of food choices [42]. Indeed, edentulous people are at greater risk of malnutrition than dentate or partially dentate individuals [43], and, consequently, with an increased susceptibility to sarcopenia and frailty [25]. Tooth loss is also a risk factor for disability, since it impedes self-sufficiency and worsens the quality of life [42].

2.2. Dry Mouth

Saliva is pivotal for bolus formation and consequently is also related to the sensory and textural experience. Xerostomia is a clinical condition characterized by an excessive sensation of dryness in the mouth, which is not necessarily linked to salivary gland hypofunction [30,44]. Xerostomia is estimated to affect 25–50% of older individuals [45]. Etiologic factors include polypharmacy (especially with antihypertensives, antidepressants, and antipsychotics) [46], diseases, poor general health, female sex, and older age [47,48]. Furthermore, radiation for head and neck cancers can damage salivary glands, leading to permanent xerostomia [49]. With aging, there is also a reduced salivary flow in salivary glands, which cannot be explained only on the basis of medications [50]. In fact, salivary hypofunction and xerostomia are two distinct constructs that are frequently improperly used interchangeably [33].

However, it has been reported that nearly one third of older adults complaining of xerostomia do not present any reduction of the salivary flow or saliva secretion. This suggests a psychological component may be involved when reporting the symptom [30]. Nonetheless, hyposalivation may seriously compromise chewing function and early digestive process. A reduced quantity of saliva can, in fact, affect the preparation of the alimentary bolus and the swallowing [51].

2.3. Periodontal Disease

Periodontitis is described as a chronic inflammatory disease that affects the supporting tissues of the teeth, leading to a progressive destruction of the periodontium [52]. It can also cause mobility and displacement of the remaining teeth and is often linked to difficulty in chewing. Prevalence of periodontal disease, considering a periodontal index score of 4 (deep pockets), ranges from approximately 5% to 70% among older people [53]. Periodontitis is a cumulative disease; therefore, it becomes increasingly severe as the person ages [30]. Poor oral hygiene is a critical determinant of periodontitis since it leads to the formation of dental plaque containing microorganisms [54]. Systemic risk factors for periodontal disease also include other behaviors, such as smoking, medical conditions (i.e., poorly controlled diabetes, obesity, stress, osteopenia), and inadequate dietary consumption of calcium and vitamin D [55]. Since periodontitis share some characteristics with other systemic inflammatory diseases, a relationship between periodontitis and other inflammatory pathologies (i.e., diabetes, cardiovascular diseases, adverse pregnancy outcomes, and rheumatoid arthritis) has been proposed [56].

In recent years, the role of the diet in periodontitis has been highlighted. To date, it has been documented that a diet poor in fruit and vegetables and therefore in micronutrients may lead to a greater inflammatory response of periodontal tissues that support the tooth. Interestingly, a recent systematic review of the relationship between dietary intake and periodontal health in community-dwelling older adults, reported positive associations between periodontal disease and lower intakes of docosahexaenoic acid, vitamin C, vitamin E, β-carotene, milk, fermented dairy products, dietary fiber, fruits and vegetables, and higher intakes of omega-6/omega-3 ratio and saturated fatty acids [57]. Additionally, micronutrient deficiencies can negatively affect healing following periodontal surgery [58]. At the same time, the loss of dental elements due to periodontitis can negatively affect the nutritional status of the patient, resulting in a discomfort during chewing and leading to a selection of soft and easy-to-chew foods.

2.4. Dental Caries

Dental caries is a multifactorial infectious disease characterized by the demineralization and destruction of the dental substance: enamel, in fact, is susceptible to acid dissolution over time. The pathological changes of the dental structure may have serious consequences, ultimately leading to the breakdown of the teeth themselves [59]. The prevalence of dental caries varies between 20% and 60% in community-dwelling older people and 60% and 80% in care home settings [60–64]. Various predisposing conditions to dental caries have been reported, including carbohydrate (especially simple sugars) consumption, diabetes, and poor socioeconomic conditions [60,65–68].

With increasing age, people may experience physical and cognitive decline, which may result in poor oral hygiene, leading to an increased incidence of caries. Over time, small lesions already filled can need a larger dental restoration, that can lead to a tooth fracture or an endodontic treatment [30]. Endodontic therapy (also known as root canal treatment) is a necessary procedure in case of inflamed or infected dental pulp. It consists in the removal of the pulp, both in the coronal and radicular part of the tooth, and in its replacement with a gutta-percha permanent filling (a substance of vegetable origin such as natural rubber). Xerostomia is closely related to a higher risk for developing caries since loss of saliva may lead to an increased acidity of the mouth. This leads to different situations that may contribute to the development of the dental caries: the proliferation of bacteria, the loss of minerals from the tooth surfaces, and the loss of lubrication [69].

2.5. Impact of Oral Health on Nutritional Status

Nutrition is a key modulator of health in older persons. Inadequate intake of nutrients is a well-known contributing factor in the progression of many diseases. This also has a significant impact in the complex etiology of sarcopenia and frailty [70–72]. Due to a decline in many functions, including poor oral status, dietary intake is often compromised in older people and the risk of malnutrition is increased. Particularly, acute and chronic illnesses and medications as well as poor dentition can exacerbate anorexia [5,70,73]. Oral problems in older individuals are associated with modifications in food selection and, therefore, in nutrient intake [25]. Deterioration of oral health can ultimately lead to the development of chronic conditions such as diabetes [74] and cardiovascular problems [75–77]. Masticatory performance is affected by the number of teeth in functional occlusion [78–80], the maximal biting force [81,82], denture wearing [83] and xerostomia [84]. The functional occlusion during mandibular closure is provided by the even and simultaneous contact of all remaining teeth (at least 20 with 10 contiguous teeth in each arch) [85].

Tooth loss has been implicated in the reduction of chewing ability and in difficulties in bolus formation [86]. To date, it has been reported that as number of remaining teeth decrease, the bolus size increases leading to a dysfunctional swallowing [87]. Edentulous individuals, even when using well-made dentures, may experience more chewing difficulties than dentate people [88]. Therefore, they may be considered as the group more prone to changing their diet [89,90]. Older people who experience dental problems frequently avoid harder foods such as meats, fruits, and vegetables which are typically major sources of proteins, fiber, vitamins, and minerals [41,88,91]. The lack of these latter key nutrients may expose older individuals to an increased risk for malnutrition, frailty, and sarcopenia [24,92]. In addition, it is well established that micronutrient deficiencies, even subtle, may lead to oxidative stress and consequently to inflammation. Therefore, these processes can further exacerbate sarcopenia and frailty and become a clear risk factor for periodontitis. Nutritional deficiencies may also negatively affect the mineralization process, increasing the susceptibility to dental caries [93]. Furthermore, undernutrition can exacerbate the severity of oral infections [94]. Indeed, with advancing age, people show a tendency to select soft foods due to difficulty and fatigue of chewing [10,95]. However, these latter are frequently processed foods that are high in fat and sugar and with a poor content of vitamins and minerals, leading to fat deposition, oxidative stress, inflammation, and, consequently, increased risk of cardiovascular disease and metabolic syndrome [88,95–97]. In fact, it is well established that obesity leads to chronic low-grade inflammation, increasing the susceptibility to dental caries, periodontal disease, and tooth loss [98]. The excess of energy is stored in adipocytes and leads to both hypertrophy and hyperplasia, resulting in an abnormal adipocyte function. This may increase mitochondrial stress and altered endoplasmatic reticulum function. Furthermore, adipocyte-associated inflammatory macrophages can also induce oxidative stress [99]. On the other hand, it is widely recognized that an excessive consumption of simple sugars is a major risk factor for dental caries [100,101].

Large epidemiological studies, such as the UK National Diet and Nutrition Survey (NDNS) [102] and the US National Health and Nutritional Examination Surveys (NHANES) [103,104], reported an association between poor dental status and inadequate dietary intake in older people. In particular, they reported that edentulous subjects, with and without prosthesis, consumed less fruits and vegetables. Moreover, decreased protein and micronutrient intake, together with increased carbohydrate consumption, has been reported in people with less than 21 teeth [104].

3. Sarcopenia and Oral Status

Sarcopenia, defined as the progressive and accelerated loss of muscle mass and function, is a major determinant of several adverse outcomes including frailty, disability, and mortality [13,105]. Although sarcopenia is a condition commonly observed with the aging process, it can also occur earlier in life [106]. Since 2016, sarcopenia has been recognized as an independent condition with an International Classification of Disease, 10th Revision, Clinical Modification (ICD-10-CM) Diagnosis Code [107]. Recently, the European Working Group on Sarcopenia in Older People (EWGSOP) [106] updated their consensus on definition and diagnosis (EWGSOP2). In this revised consensus, low muscle strength is considered a key characteristic of sarcopenia, and poor physical performance is identified as indicative of severe sarcopenia. Moreover, EWGSOP2 have recommended specific cut-off points to identify and characterize the sarcopenic condition, and provide an algorithm that can be used for case-finding.

Sarcopenia has a complex multifactorial pathogenesis, which involves lifestyle habits (i.e., malnutrition, physical inactivity), disease triggers, and age-dependent biological changes (i.e., chronic inflammation, mitochondrial abnormalities, loss of neuromuscular junctions, reduced satellite cell numbers, hormonal alterations) [108,109]. Sarcopenia is a whole-body process, affecting not only lower extremities, but also muscles dedicated to breathing, mastication, and swallowing [14,18–22]. In particular, swallowing is a complex mechanism involving several head and neck muscles simultaneously and in conjunction to coordinate the entire process [110]. Several age-related changes, such as as reduction of tissue elasticity, changes of the head and neck anatomy, reduced oral and pharyngeal sensitivity, and impaired dental status, may contribute to different degrees to a subtle swallowing impairment, the so called "presbyphagia". It is usually an asymptomatic condition in which swallowing function is preserved, but tends to slowly worsen as the aging process advances [16,111]. Presbyphagia may increase the risk of dysphagia and aspiration in older people, especially during acute illnesses and other stressors [112]. Moreover, reductions in muscle mass of the geniohyoid, pterygoid, masseter, tongue, and pharyngeal muscles have been documented in older individuals [20,113–115]. Several authors also reported a decline in the strength of the swallowing muscles with aging or sarcopenia [116]. Maximal tongue strength decreases with aging [116–119], and there is some evidence that aging leads to a decreased jaw-opening force in older men. Several authors also reported an association between tongue strength and handgrip strength [120,121]. A decrease in tongue strength has been associated with a decline of activities of daily living [122], and a reduced tongue thickness has been noted in people with low body weight [20].

Lip function is also important for feeding. In fact, poor lip muscle closure may cause leakage through the corners of the mouth [123]. Additionally, decreased lip strength has been suggested to occur due to sarcopenia and to be related to difficulties in eating and drinking (i.e., dysphagia) [117]. Lip force has been associated with hand grip strength and lip pendency has been associated with aging [117,124].

Indeed, since it has been shown that skeletal muscle mass and strength decline may affect both swallowing and general muscle groups, a new condition, called "sarcopenic dysphagia" has been coined [22,124,125]. Swallowing muscles are characterized by a high percentage of type II fibers, which are more easily affected by malnutrition and sarcopenia than type I muscle fibers [22]. However, some cranial muscles, including the jaw-closers, are very different in fiber-type composition than other skeletal muscle groups (i.e., limbs or abdomen). For instance, the masseter muscle, which originates from the zygomatic arch, contains both type I and type II fibers, but shows a predominance of type I muscle fibers, which are more strongly affected by inactivity rather than aging [126,127]. Given that the meal texture of older people frequently becomes softer, less power of tongue movement and of masseter muscle is required, which may result in decreased activity of these muscles.

Interestingly, poor oral health may predispose one to a chronic low-grade inflammatory state through periodontal disease, which is a well-known risk factor for frailty and sarcopenia [25,128,129]. In fact, the detrimental effects of periodontitis are not confined solely to the oral cavity, but extend systemically, leading to metabolic alterations [130], including insulin resistance [131], diabetes [131,132], arthritis [133], and heart disease [134]. Furthermore, alterations in mitochondrial function leading to oxidative stress through the production of reactive oxygen species (ROS) have also been reported to mediate both oral and systemic pathologies (i.e., sarcopenia) [108,135–137]. Given their regulatory role as signaling molecules in autophagy, it has been speculated that elevated ROS production in periodontal disease could lead to autophagic alterations [138]. Bullon et al. [139] found high levels of mitochondrial-derived ROS, accompanied by mitochondrial dysfunction in peripheral blood mononuclear cells from patients with periodontitis. Moreover, oral gingiva seems to be highly responsive to the lipopolysaccharides (LPS), which are bacterial endotoxins prevalent in periodontal disease. In fact, gingival fibroblasts, which play an important role in remodeling periodontal soft tissues, may directly interact with LPS. In particular, LPS from *Porphyromonas gingivalis* enhances the production of inflammatory cytokines [140]. *Porphyromonas gingivalis* has been found to be responsible for high mitochondrial ROS and coenzyme Q10 levels, and for mitochondrial dysfunction, given its influence on the amount of respiratory chain complex I and III [138,139]. Indeed, LPS-mediated mitochondrial dysfunction could explain the oxidative stress onset in patients with periodontitis. Furthermore, Hamalainen et al. [29] reported an association between periodontitis and quicker declines in handgrip strength.

On the other hand, as discussed in the previous section, the variety of dental problems experienced by older people can lead to a decline in general health through poor nutrient intake, pain, and low quality of life [25]. Poor oral status has been reported to affect 71% of patients in rehabilitation settings [141] and 91% of people in acute-care hospitals [142], and has been associated with malnutrition, dysphagia, and reduced activities of daily living [17]. Hence, poor oral status may lead to sarcopenia through poor nutrient intake. Moreover, inflammation further contributes to malnutrition through various mechanisms, such as anorexia, decreased nutrient intake, altered metabolism (i.e., elevation of resting energy expenditure), and increased muscle catabolism [143]. Chronic inflammation is a common underlying factor, not only in the etiology of sarcopenia, but also for frailty. In fact, sarcopenia and frailty are closely related and show a remarkable overlap especially in the physical function domain [144–146]. The presence of oral problems, alone or in combination with sarcopenia, may thus represent the biological substratum of the disabling cascade experienced by many frail individuals.

4. Interventions

The management of older people should be multimodal and multidisciplinary, especially for those with or at risk of malnutrition [147], in order to improve different conditions (i.e., oral problems and sarcopenia). From a practical point of view, comprehensive geriatric assessment (CGA) is the multidimensional, interdisciplinary diagnostic and therapeutic process aimed at determining the medical, psychological, and functional problems of older people. The CGA's objective is the development of a coordinated and integrated plan for treatment and follow-up in order to maximize overall health with aging [148]. To date, increasing evidence suggests that prosthodontic treatment in combination with personalized dietary counselling may improve the nutritional status of patients [51]. Here, we provide an overview on the management of oral problems, malnutrition, and sarcopenia.

4.1. Oral Management

The stomatognathic system is very vulnerable over time, but with special care, it can be preserved throughout the lifetime [30]. Nevertheless, one of the major challenges in providing both restorative and preventive care for older adults is to check dental status on a regular basis [34]. Prevention is pivotal to detecting oral disease as soon as possible and requires regular patient contact. However, since it has been reported that older people frequently fail to achieve a good oral hygiene, both patients and caregivers should be made more aware about the importance to check dental status as well as oral hygiene.

The oral health-care professionals should develop a personalized program, in order to prevent all the problems related to the aging process. In some cases, it is difficult to provide dental care in the hospital setting in a short time, since in many countries there are long waiting lists (especially in publicly funded hospitals) [149]. Therefore, private dentists also need better awareness concerning the complexity of older people. There is, first and foremost, a need to understand the level of dependency, the medical condition, and the physical or cognitive impairment of the patient. Secondly, it is important to establish an oral healthcare plan that includes both professional and self-care elements [150].

The oral management of older people usually involves different aspects:

(1) For the teeth affected by carious lesions, it must be recommended that prompt treatment be provided in order to prevent tooth loss. It would be equally appropriate for endodontic treatments for teeth with endodontic problems.
(2) It is very important to monitor the periodontal status of the older patient and to provide a proper treatment plan, such as modification of general health-risk factors and oral health-specific risk factors, but professional hygiene or surgical procedures may also be necessary.
(3) Prosthetic rehabilitation of the edentulous patient may help to prevent malnutrition [151] since it restores the chewing function.
(4) In order to prevent problems related to the xerostomia and reduce exacerbation of carious lesions, it may be helpful to treat with saliva substitutes.

4.2. Nutritional Interventions

As discussed above, nutrition is an important determinant of health in older people. Thereby, it is pivotal to provide adequate amounts of energy, proteins, fluid, and micronutrients in order to prevent or treat excess or deficiencies, and therefore improve several health-related outcomes in terms of morbidity and mortality. A personalized approach is pivotal in order to respect individual preferences, needs, and to increase compliance to the diet. Nutritional status should be assessed before each intervention, and the amount of energy and proteins should be individually adjusted with regard to nutritional status, physical activity level, disease status, and tolerance [152]. The European Society for Clinical Nutrition and Metabolism (ESPEN) [152], in its guidelines on clinical nutrition and hydration in geriatrics, recommends a guiding value for energy intake of 30 kcal/kg of body weight/day. However, as stated above, it should be adapted individually. Both ESPEN [153] and the PROT-AGE study group [147] recommend providing a protein intake of at least 1.0 g/kg body weight/day in older people to maintain muscle mass, increasing the intake up to 1.2–1.5 g/kg body weight/day in presence of acute or chronic illness. Additionally, it seems that the per-meal anabolic threshold of protein intake is higher in older individuals (i.e., 25 to 30 g protein/meal, containing about 2.5 to 2.8 g leucine) than young adults [147]. However, since older people may experience difficulty of ingesting large amounts of proteins in a single meal, supplementation should be considered. Since serum vitamin D levels decline gradually with aging [154,155] and have been associated with reduced muscle mass and strength, supplementation should thus be considered in those who are deficient.

Food texture should be adapted depending on the chewing and swallowing condition in order to avoid choking risk [10]. Harder foods may be modified to soft consistencies (i.e., bite-sized, minced, pureed) requiring little chewing, as well as liquids, which may be thickened to render the swallowing process slower and safer [10,156,157]. Controlling the intake of simple sugars is pivotal to prevent both dental caries [101] and metabolic complications [158]. World Health Organization recommends to limit the intake of free sugars to less than 10% of total energy intake to minimize the risk of dental caries [159].

Fruit and vegetables are major sources of minerals and vitamins with antioxidant properties; therefore, their consumption should be promoted both for oral and general health. It has been documented that excessive antioxidant supplementation could compromise both the mechanism of adaption to exercise and have even pro-oxidant effects. Thus, supplementation in people who are not deficient should be regarded carefully [160]. Dietary consumption of fatty fish (i.e., salmon, mackerel, herring, lake trout, sardines, albacore tuna, and their oils), which are a major source of omega-3 fatty acids, has been associated with a greater fat-free mass [161]. Given their antioxidant role, omega-3 fatty acid supplementation has been suggested to improve inflammatory status both in periodontal disease [162] and sarcopenia [163]. However, more studies are needed to further elucidate the exact time and dosage of supplementation as well as long term effects [164]. Nevertheless, consumption of foods rich in omega-3, such as as fatty fish, should be promoted.

4.3. Exercise and Rehabilitative Strategies

Physical inactivity is considered one of the main causes of sarcopenia [165] because it determines a resistance to muscle anabolic stimuli [166]. Moreover, it has been proposed that physically inactive individuals may have a greater risk of periodontal disease [167]. In particular, resistance training seems to be the most effective type of exercise to counteract sarcopenia [168]. Furthermore, since sarcopenia is a systemic process [15,21], it has been recommended to perform a holistic training involving all muscle groups [15]. In fact, it has been documented that both masticatory and swallowing functions can be improved through muscle-strengthening exercises [169,170]. Several studies reported enhancements in subjective chewing ability, swallowing function, salivation, relief of oral dryness, and oral-health quality of life. Indeed, the synergistic effect of nutritional interventions coupled with physical exercise may improve both muscle [164] and oral health [167]. Recently, Kim et al. [171] reported an improvement in oral function following an exercise program which included stretching of the lip, tongue, cheek, masticatory muscle exercise, and swallowing movements. Several studies have been focused on swallowing rehabilitation. To date, a positive effect of expiratory muscle resistance training has been documented in improving suprahyoid muscle activity [172,173]. Furthermore, head lift exercises showed a beneficial impact on swallowing movements [174,175], and tongue strengthening exercises have been reported to enhance tongue strength [176,177]. Yeates et al. [178] demonstrated that isometric tongue strength exercises and tongue pressure accuracy tasks improved isometric tongue strength, tongue pressure generation accuracy, bolus control, and dietary intake by mouth. It has also been reported that tongue exercises prevented general sarcopenia [178,179]. Indeed, swallowing muscles training, despite its focus on swallowing function, may exert its beneficial effects systemically.

5. Conclusions

Aging is characterized by a progressive loss of physiological integrity, leading to a decline in many functions and increased vulnerability to stressors. Many changes in masticatory and swallowing function are subtle but can amplify disease processes seen with aging. Nevertheless, it is often difficult to clearly distinguish the effects of diseases from the underlying age-related modifications. Several stressors, including oral problems, may therefore negatively impact on the increasingly weak homeostatic reserves of older individuals. As a healthy diet may have a systemic beneficial effect, oral care also shows an important role in maintaining and improving not only oral health, but also general health and well-being.

Overall, severe tooth loss, as well as swallowing and masticatory problems, partly contribute to restricted dietary choices and poor nutritional status of older adults, leading to frailty and sarcopenia. On the other hand, oral diseases might be influenced both by frailty and sarcopenia, probably through biological and environmental factors that are linked to the common burden of inflammation and oxidative stress.

A multidisciplinary intervention of dental professionals, geriatricians, nutritionists, and dietitians may help to provide better care and preserve the functional status of older people. Increasing evidence also suggests that oral care, when offered with personalized nutritional advice, may improve the nutritional status of patients. A life course approach to prevention at a younger age, including diet optimization and oral preventive care, as well as physical activity, may help in preserving both oral and muscle function later in life.

Author Contributions: D.A. and P.C.P. equally contributed to conceptualizing and writing the manuscript. P.D.A., G.B.P., A.D. and M.C. edited and revised manuscript. D.A., P.C.P., P.D.A., G.B.P., A.D. and M.C. approved the final version of manuscript.

Funding: This research received no external funding.

Conflicts of Interest: The authors declare no conflict of interest.

References

1. Bales, C.W.; Ritchie, C.S. Sarcopenia, weight loss, and nutritional frailty in the elderly. *Annu. Rev. Nutr.* **2002**, *22*, 309–323. [CrossRef]
2. Palmer, K.; Onder, G.; Cesari, M. The geriatric condition of frailty. *Eur. J. Intern. Med.* **2018**, *56*, 1–2. [CrossRef]
3. López-Otín, C.; Blasco, M.A.; Partridge, L.; Serrano, M.; Kroemer, G. The hallmarks of aging. *Cell* **2013**, *153*, 1194–1217. [CrossRef]
4. Leslie, W.; Hankey, C. Aging, Nutritional Status and Health. *Healthcare* **2015**, *3*, 648–658. [CrossRef]
5. Roberts, H.C.; Lim, S.E.R.; Cox, N.J.; Ibrahim, K. The Challenge of Managing Undernutrition in Older People with Frailty. *Nutrients* **2019**, *11*, 808. [CrossRef]
6. Hickson, M. Malnutrition and ageing. *Postgrad. Med. J.* **2006**, *82*, 2–8. [CrossRef]
7. Schilp, J.; Wijnhoven, H.A.H.; Deeg, D.J.H.; Visser, M. Early determinants for the development of undernutrition in an older general population: Longitudinal Aging Study Amsterdam. *Br. J. Nutr.* **2011**, *106*, 708–717. [CrossRef]
8. Locher, J.L.; Ritchie, C.S.; Roth, D.L.; Sen, B.; Vickers, K.S.; Vailas, L.I. Food choice among homebound older adults: Motivations and perceived barriers. *J. Nutr. Health Aging* **2009**, *13*, 659–664. [CrossRef]
9. Bloom, I.; Lawrence, W.; Barker, M.; Baird, J.; Dennison, E.; Sayer, A.A.; Cooper, C.; Robinson, S. What influences diet quality in older people? A qualitative study among community-dwelling older adults from the Hertfordshire Cohort Study, UK. *Public Health Nutr.* **2017**, *20*, 2685–2693. [CrossRef]
10. Cichero, J.A.Y. Age-Related Changes to Eating and Swallowing Impact Frailty: Aspiration, Choking Risk, Modified Food Texture and Autonomy of Choice. *Geriatrics* **2018**, *3*, 69. [CrossRef]

11. Calvani, R.; Miccheli, A.; Landi, F.; Bossola, M.; Cesari, M.; Leeuwenburgh, C.; Sieber, C.C.; Bernabei, R.; Marzetti, E. Current nutritional recommendations and novel dietary strategies to manage sarcopenia. *J. Frailty Aging* **2013**, *2*, 38–53.
12. Rosenberg, I.H. Sarcopenia: Origins and clinical relevance. *J. Nutr.* **1997**, *127* (Suppl. S5), 990S–991S. [CrossRef]
13. Cruz-Jentoft, A.J.; Landi, F. Sarcopenia. *Clin. Med.* **2014**, *14*, 183–186. [CrossRef]
14. Komatsu, R.; Okazaki, T.; Ebihara, S.; Kobayashi, M.; Tsukita, Y.; Nihei, M.; Sugiura, H.; Niu, K.; Ebihara, T.; Ichinose, M. Aspiration pneumonia induces muscle atrophy in the respiratory, skeletal, and swallowing systems. *J. Cachexia Sarcopenia Muscle* **2018**, *9*, 643–653. [CrossRef]
15. Beckwée, D.; Delaere, A.; Aelbrecht, S.; Baert, V.; Beaudart, C.; Bruyere, O.; de Saint-Hubert, M.; Bautmans, I. Exercise Interventions for the Prevention and Treatment of Sarcopenia. A Systematic Umbrella Review. *J. Nutr. Health Aging* **2019**, *23*, 494–502. [CrossRef]
16. Azzolino, D.; Damanti, S.; Bertagnoli, L.; Lucchi, T.; Cesari, M. Sarcopenia and swallowing disorders in older people. *Aging. Clin. Exp. Res.* **2019**, *22*, 1–7. [CrossRef]
17. Shiraishi, A.; Yoshimura, Y.; Wakabayashi, H.; Tsuji, Y. Prevalence of stroke-related sarcopenia and its association with poor oral status in post-acute stroke patients: Implications for oral sarcopenia. *Clin. Nutr.* **2018**, *37*, 204–207. [CrossRef]
18. Iee Shin, H.; Kim, D.-K.; Seo, K.M.; Kang, S.H.; Lee, S.Y.; Son, S. Relation Between Respiratory Muscle Strength and Skeletal Muscle Mass and Hand Grip Strength in the Healthy Elderly. *Ann. Rehabil. Med.* **2017**, *41*, 686–692. [CrossRef]
19. Fujishima, I.; Fujiu-Kurachi, M.; Arai, H.; Hyodo, M.; Kagaya, H.; Maeda, K.; Mori, T.; Nishioka, S.; Oshima, F.; Ogawa, S.; et al. Sarcopenia and dysphagia: Position paper by four professional organizations. *Geriatr. Gerontol. Int.* **2019**, *19*, 91–97. [CrossRef]
20. Tamura, F.; Kikutani, T.; Tohara, T.; Yoshida, M.; Yaegaki, K. Tongue thickness relates to nutritional status in the elderly. *Dysphagia* **2012**, *27*, 556–561. [CrossRef]
21. Cruz-Jentoft, A.J.; Sayer, A.A. Sarcopenia. *Lancet* **2019**, *393*, 2636–2646. [CrossRef]
22. Wakabayashi, H.; Sakuma, K. Rehabilitation nutrition for sarcopenia with disability: A combination of both rehabilitation and nutrition care management. *J. Cachexia Sarcopenia Muscle* **2014**, *5*, 269–277. [CrossRef] [PubMed]
23. Castrejón-Pérez, R.C.; Jiménez-Corona, A.; Bernabé, E.; Villa-Romero, A.R.; Arrivé, E.; Dartigues, J.-F.; Gutiérrez-Robledo, L.M.; Borges-Yáñez, S.A. Oral Disease and 3-Year Incidence of Frailty in Mexican Older Adults. *J. Gerontol. Ser. A* **2017**, *72*, 951–957. [CrossRef] [PubMed]
24. Woo, J.; Tong, C.; Yu, R. Chewing Difficulty Should be Included as a Geriatric Syndrome. *Nutrients* **2018**, *10*, 2019. Available online: https://www.ncbi.nlm.nih.gov/pmc/articles/PMC6315631/ (accessed on 11 October 2019). [CrossRef] [PubMed]
25. Castrejón-Pérez, R.C.; Borges-Yáñez, S.A.; Gutiérrez-Robledo, L.M.; Avila-Funes, J.A. Oral health conditions and frailty in Mexican community-dwelling elderly: A cross sectional analysis. *BMC Public Health* **2012**, *12*, 773. [CrossRef] [PubMed]
26. Lertpimonchai, A.; Rattanasiri, S.; Arj-Ong Vallibhakara, S.; Attia, J.; Thakkinstian, A. The association between oral hygiene and periodontitis: A systematic review and meta-analysis. *Int. Dent. J.* **2017**, *67*, 332–343. [CrossRef]
27. Dent, E.; Kowal, P.; Hoogendijk, E.O. Frailty measurement in research and clinical practice: A review. *Eur. J. Intern. Med.* **2016**, *31*, 3–10. [CrossRef]
28. Rolland, Y.; Czerwinski, S.; Abellan Van Kan, G.; Morley, J.E.; Cesari, M.; Onder, G.; Woo, J.; Baumgartner, R.; Pillard, F.; Boirie, Y.; et al. Sarcopenia: Its assessment, etiology, pathogenesis, consequences and future perspectives. *J. Nutr. Health Aging* **2008**, *12*, 433–450. [CrossRef]
29. Hämäläinen, P.; Rantanen, T.; Keskinen, M.; Meurman, J.H. Oral health status and change in handgrip strength over a 5-year period in 80-year-old people. *Gerodontology* **2004**, *21*, 155–160. [CrossRef]
30. Lamster, I.B.; Asadourian, L.; Del Carmen, T.; Friedman, P.K. The aging mouth: Differentiating normal aging from disease. *Periodontol 2000* **2016**, *72*, 96–107. [CrossRef]
31. Liu, B.; Zhang, M.; Chen, Y.; Yao, Y. Tooth wear in aging people: An investigation of the prevalence and the influential factors of incisal/occlusal tooth wear in northwest China. *BMC Oral Health* **2014**, *14*, 65. [CrossRef] [PubMed]
32. Klein, D.R. Oral soft tissue changes in geriatric patients. *Bull. N. Y. Acad. Med.* **1980**, *56*, 721–727. [PubMed]
33. MacEntee, M.I.; Donnelly, L.R. Oral health and the frailty syndrome. *Periodontology 2000* **2016**, *72*, 135–141. [CrossRef] [PubMed]

34. Razak, P.A.; Richard, K.M.J.; Thankachan, R.P.; Hafiz, K.A.A.; Kumar, K.N.; Sameer, K.M. Geriatric Oral Health: A Review Article. *J. Int. Oral Health* **2014**, *6*, 110–116. [PubMed]
35. Chapple, I.L.C.; Bouchard, P.; Cagetti, M.G.; Campus, G.; Carra, M.-C.; Cocco, F.; Nibali, L.; Hujoel, P.; Laine, M.L.; Lingstrom, P.; et al. Interaction of lifestyle, behaviour or systemic diseases with dental caries and periodontal diseases: Consensus report of group 2 of the joint EFP/ORCA workshop on the boundaries between caries and periodontal diseases. *J. Clin. Periodontol.* **2017**, *44* (Suppl S18), S39–S51. [CrossRef]
36. Hirotomi, T.; Yoshihara, A.; Yano, M.; Ando, Y.; Miyazaki, H. Longitudinal study on periodontal conditions in healthy elderly people in Japan. *Community Dent. Oral Epidemiol.* **2002**, *30*, 409–417. [CrossRef] [PubMed]
37. Burt, B.A.; Ismail, A.I.; Morrison, E.C.; Beltran, E.D. Risk factors for tooth loss over a 28-year period. *J. Dent. Res.* **1990**, *69*, 1126–1130. [CrossRef]
38. Bahrami, G.; Vaeth, M.; Kirkevang, L.-L.; Wenzel, A.; Isidor, F. Risk factors for tooth loss in an adult population: A radiographic study. *J. Clin. Periodontol.* **2008**, *35*, 1059–1065. [CrossRef]
39. Singh, K.A.; Brennan, D.S. Chewing disability in older adults attributable to tooth loss and other oral conditions. *Gerodontology* **2012**, *29*, 106–110. [CrossRef]
40. Zhang, Q.; Witter, D.J.; Bronkhorst, E.M.; Creugers, N.H. Chewing ability in an urban and rural population over 40 years in Shandong Province, China. *Clin. Oral Investig.* **2013**, *17*, 1425–1435. [CrossRef]
41. Gil-Montoya, J.A.; Ferreira de Mello, A.L.; Barrios, R.; Gonzalez-Moles, M.A.; Bravo, M. Oral health in the elderly patient and its impact on general well-being: A nonsystematic review. *Clin. Interv. Aging* **2015**, *10*, 461–467. [CrossRef] [PubMed]
42. Musacchio, E.; Perissinotto, E.; Binotto, P.; Sartori, L.; Silva-Netto, F.; Zambon, S.; Manzato, E.; Corti, M.C.; Baggio, G.; Crepaldi, G. Tooth loss in the elderly and its association with nutritional status, socio-economic and lifestyle factors. *Acta Odontol. Scand.* **2007**, *65*, 78–86. [CrossRef] [PubMed]
43. Felton, D.A. Complete Edentulism and Comorbid Diseases: An Update. *J. Prosthodont.* **2016**, *25*, 5–20. [CrossRef] [PubMed]
44. Xu, F.; Laguna, L.; Sarkar, A. Aging-related changes in quantity and quality of saliva: Where do we stand in our understanding? *J. Texture Stud.* **2019**, *50*, 27–35. [CrossRef]
45. Nagler, R.M. Salivary glands and the aging process: Mechanistic aspects, health-status and medicinal-efficacy monitoring. *Biogerontology* **2004**, *5*, 223–233. [CrossRef]
46. Scully, C. Drug effects on salivary glands: Dry mouth. *Oral Dis.* **2003**, *9*, 165–176. [CrossRef]
47. Singh, M.L.; Papas, A. Oral implications of polypharmacy in the elderly. *Dent. Clin.* **2014**, *58*, 783–796. [CrossRef]
48. Mortazavi, H.; Baharvand, M.; Movahhedian, A.; Mohammadi, M.; Khodadoustan, A. Xerostomia Due to Systemic Disease: A Review of 20 Conditions and Mechanisms. *Ann. Med. Health Sci. Res.* **2014**, *4*, 503–510.
49. Dumic, I.; Nordin, T.; Jecmenica, M.; Stojkovic Lalosevic, M.; Milosavljevic, T.; Milovanovic, T. Gastrointestinal Tract Disorders in Older Age. *Can. J. Gastroenterol. Hepatol.* **2019**. Available online: https://www.hindawi.com/journals/cjgh/2019/6757524/ (accessed on 11 October 2019). [CrossRef]
50. Affoo, R.H.; Foley, N.; Garrick, R.; Siqueira, W.L.; Martin, R.E. Meta-Analysis of Salivary Flow Rates in Young and Older Adults. *J. Am. Geriatr. Soc.* **2015**, *63*, 2142–2151. [CrossRef]
51. Kossioni, A.E. The Association of Poor Oral Health Parameters with Malnutrition in Older Adults: A Review Considering the Potential Implications for Cognitive Impairment. *Nutrients* **2018**, *10*, 1709. [CrossRef] [PubMed]
52. Saini, R.; Marawar, P.P.; Shete, S.; Saini, S. Periodontitis, a true infection. *J. Glob. Infect. Dis.* **2009**, *1*, 149–150. [CrossRef] [PubMed]
53. WHO. WHO Oral Health Country Area Profile Programe. Available online: https://www.who.int/oral_health/databases/malmo/en/ (accessed on 11 October 2019).
54. Ashimoto, A.; Chen, C.; Bakker, I.; Slots, J. Polymerase chain reaction detection of 8 putative periodontal pathogens in subgingival plaque of gingivitis and advanced periodontitis lesions. *Oral Microbiol. Immunol.* **1996**, *11*, 266–273. [CrossRef] [PubMed]
55. Genco, R.J.; Borgnakke, W.S. Risk factors for periodontal disease. *Periodontol 2000* **2013**, *62*, 59–94. [CrossRef] [PubMed]
56. Hasturk, H.; Kantarci, A. Activation and Resolution of Periodontal Inflammation and Its Systemic Impact. *Periodontol 2000* **2015**, *69*, 255–273. [CrossRef] [PubMed]
57. O'Connor, J.-L.P.; Milledge, K.L.; O'Leary, F.; Cumming, R.; Eberhard, J.; Hirani, V. Poor dietary intake of nutrients and food groups are associated with increased risk of periodontal disease among community-dwelling older adults: A systematic literature review. *Nutr. Rev.* **2019**. [CrossRef]

58. Najeeb, S.; Zafar, M.S.; Khurshid, Z.; Zohaib, S.; Almas, K. The Role of Nutrition in Periodontal Health: An Update. *Nutrients* **2016**, *8*, 530. Available online: https://www.ncbi.nlm.nih.gov/pmc/articles/PMC5037517/ (accessed on 11 October 2019). [CrossRef]
59. Kunin, A.A.; Evdokimova, A.Y.; Moiseeva, N.S. Age-related differences of tooth enamel morphochemistry in health and dental caries. *EPMA J.* **2015**, *6*, 3. [CrossRef]
60. Avlund, K.; Holm-Pedersen, P.; Morse, D.E.; Viitanen, M.; Winblad, B. Tooth loss and caries prevalence in very old Swedish people: The relationship to cognitive function and functional ability. *Gerodontology* **2004**, *21*, 17–26. [CrossRef]
61. Banting, D.W.; Ellen, R.P.; Fillery, E.D. Prevalence of root surface caries among institutionalized older persons. *Community Dent. Oral Epidemiol.* **1980**, *8*, 84–88. [CrossRef]
62. Ellefsen, B.; Holm-Pedersen, P.; Morse, D.E.; Schroll, M.; Andersen, B.B.; Waldemar, G. Caries prevalence in older persons with and without dementia. *J. Am. Geriatr. Soc.* **2008**, *56*, 59–67. [CrossRef] [PubMed]
63. Fure, S.; Zickert, I. Prevalence of root surface caries in 55, 65, and 75-year-old Swedish individuals. *Community Dent. Oral Epidemiol.* **1990**, *18*, 100–105. [CrossRef] [PubMed]
64. Johanson, C.N.; Osterberg, T.; Steen, B.; Birkhed, D. Prevalence and incidence of dental caries and related risk factors in 70- to 76-year-olds. *Acta Odontol. Scand.* **2009**, *67*, 304–312. [CrossRef] [PubMed]
65. Wiktorsson, A.M.; Martinsson, T.; Zimmerman, M. Salivary levels of lactobacilli, buffer capacity and salivary flow rate related to caries activity among adults in communities with optimal and low water fluoride concentrations. *Swed. Dent. J.* **1992**, *16*, 231–237.
66. Lundberg, J.O. Nitrate transport in salivary glands with implications for NO homeostasis. *Proc. Natl. Acad. Sci. USA* **2012**, *109*, 13144–13145. [CrossRef]
67. Guivante-Nabet, C.; Berenholc, C.; Berdal, A. Caries activity and associated risk factors in elderly hospitalised population – 15-months follow-up in French institutions. *Gerodontology* **1999**, *16*, 47–58. [CrossRef]
68. Fure, S. Ten-year cross-sectional and incidence study of coronal and root caries and some related factors in elderly Swedish individuals. *Gerodontology* **2004**, *21*, 130–140. [CrossRef]
69. Su, N.; Marek, C.L.; Ching, V.; Grushka, M. Caries prevention for patients with dry mouth. *J. Can. Dent. Assoc.* **2011**, *77*, 1–8.
70. Morley, J.E. Anorexia of ageing: A key component in the pathogenesis of both sarcopenia and cachexia. *J. Cachexia Sarcopenia Muscle* **2017**, *8*, 523–526. [CrossRef]
71. Clegg, A.; Young, J.; Iliffe, S.; Rikkert, M.O.; Rockwood, K. Frailty in elderly people. *Lancet* **2013**, *381*, 752–762. [CrossRef]
72. Cruz-Jentoft, A.J.; Baeyens, J.P.; Bauer, J.M.; Boirie, Y.; Cederholm, T.; Landi, F.; Martin, F.C.; Michel, J.-P.; Rolland, Y.; Schneider, S.M.; et al. Sarcopenia: European consensus on definition and diagnosis: Report of the European Working Group on Sarcopenia in Older People. *Age Ageing* **2010**, *39*, 412–423. [CrossRef] [PubMed]
73. Agarwal, E.; Miller, M.; Yaxley, A.; Isenring, E. Malnutrition in the elderly: A narrative review. *Maturitas* **2013**, *76*, 296–302. [CrossRef] [PubMed]
74. Mealey, B.L.; Ocampo, G.L. Diabetes mellitus and periodontal disease. *Periodontol 2000* **2007**, *44*, 127–153. [CrossRef] [PubMed]
75. Karnoutsos, K.; Papastergiou, P.; Stefanidis, S.; Vakaloudi, A. Periodontitis as a risk factor for cardiovascular disease: The role of anti-phosphorylcholine and anti-cardiolipin antibodies. *Hippokratia* **2008**, *12*, 144.
76. Syrjälä, A.-M.H.; Ylöstalo, P.; Hartikainen, S.; Sulkava, R.; Knuuttila, M. Number of teeth and selected cardiovascular risk factors among elderly people. *Gerodontology* **2010**, *27*, 189–192. [CrossRef]
77. Touger-Decker, R. Diet, cardiovascular disease and oral health: Promoting health and reducing risk. *J. Am. Dent. Assoc.* **2010**, *141*, 167–170. [CrossRef]
78. Helkimo, E.; Carlsson, G.E.; Helkimo, M. Chewing efficiency and state of dentition. A methodologic study. *Acta Odontol. Scand.* **1978**, *36*, 33–41. [CrossRef]
79. Akeel, R.; Nilner, M.; Nilner, K. Masticatory efficiency in individuals with natural dentition. *Swed. Dent. J.* **1992**, *16*, 191–198.
80. Naka, O.; Anastassiadou, V.; Pissiotis, A. Association between functional tooth units and chewing ability in older adults: A systematic review. *Gerodontology* **2014**, *31*, 166–177. [CrossRef]
81. Tate, G.S.; Throckmorton, G.S.; Ellis, E.; Sinn, D.P. Masticatory performance, muscle activity, and occlusal force in preorthognathic surgery patients. *J. Oral Maxillofac. Surg.* **1994**, *52*, 476–482; discussion 482. [CrossRef]

82. Fontijn-Tekamp, F.A.; Slagter, A.P.; Van Der Bilt, A.; Van 'T Hof, M.A.; Witter, D.J.; Kalk, W.; Jansen, J.A. Biting and chewing in overdentures, full dentures, and natural dentitions. *J. Dent. Res.* **2000**, *79*, 1519–1524. [CrossRef] [PubMed]
83. Kapur, K.K.; Soman, S.D. Masticatory performance and efficiency in denture wearers. *J. Prosthet. Dent.* **2006**, *95*, 407–411. [CrossRef] [PubMed]
84. Pedersen, A.M.; Bardow, A.; Jensen, S.B.; Nauntofte, B. Saliva and gastrointestinal functions of taste, mastication, swallowing and digestion. *Oral Dis.* **2002**, *8*, 117–129. [CrossRef] [PubMed]
85. Clark, J.R.; Evans, R.D. Functional occlusion: I. A review. *J. Orthod.* **2001**, *28*, 76–81. [CrossRef]
86. Furuta, M.; Yamashita, Y. Oral Health and Swallowing Problems. *Curr. Phys. Med. Rehabil. Rep.* **2013**, *1*, 216–222. [CrossRef]
87. Mishellany, A.; Woda, A.; Labas, R.; Peyron, M.-A. The challenge of mastication: Preparing a bolus suitable for deglutition. *Dysphagia* **2006**, *21*, 87–94. [CrossRef]
88. Hutton, B.; Feine, J.; Morais, J. Is there an association between edentulism and nutritional state? *J. Can. Dent. Assoc.* **2002**, *68*, 182–187.
89. Fontijn-Tekamp, F.A.; van 't Hof, M.A.; Slagter, A.P.; van Waas, M.A. The state of dentition in relation to nutrition in elderly Europeans in the SENECA Study of 1993. *Eur. J. Clin. Nutr.* **1996**, *50* (Suppl. S2), S117–S122.
90. Greksa, L.P.; Parraga, I.M.; Clark, C.A. The dietary adequacy of edentulous older adults. *J. Prosthet. Dent.* **1995**, *73*, 142–145. [CrossRef]
91. Hung, H.-C.; Colditz, G.; Joshipura, K.J. The association between tooth loss and the self-reported intake of selected CVD-related nutrients and foods among US women. *Community Dent. Oral Epidemiol.* **2005**, *33*, 167–173. [CrossRef]
92. Takahashi, M.; Maeda, K.; Wakabayashi, H. Prevalence of sarcopenia and association with oral health-related quality of life and oral health status in older dental clinic outpatients. *Geriatr. Gerontol. Int.* **2018**, *18*, 915–921. [CrossRef] [PubMed]
93. Alvarez, J.O. Nutrition, tooth development, and dental caries. *Am. J. Clin. Nutr.* **1995**, *61*, 410S–416S. [CrossRef] [PubMed]
94. Enwonwu, C.O.; Phillips, R.S.; Falkler, W.A. Nutrition and oral infectious diseases: State of the science. *Compend. Contin. Educ. Dent.* **2002**, *23*, 431–434. [PubMed]
95. Friedlander, A.H.; Weinreb, J.; Friedlander, I.; Yagiela, J.A. Metabolic syndrome: Pathogenesis, medical care and dental implications. *J. Am. Dent. Assoc.* **2007**, *138*, 179–187. [CrossRef] [PubMed]
96. Tan, B.L.; Norhaizan, M.E.; Liew, W.-P.-P. Nutrients and Oxidative Stress: Friend or Foe? *Oxid. Med. Cell. Longev.* **2018**, *2018*. Available online: https://www.ncbi.nlm.nih.gov/pmc/articles/PMC5831951/ (accessed on 11 October 2019). [CrossRef]
97. Manzel, A.; Muller, D.N.; Hafler, D.A.; Erdman, S.E.; Linker, R.A.; Kleinewietfeld, M. Role of "Western Diet" in Inflammatory Autoimmune Diseases. *Curr. Allergy Asthma Rep.* **2014**, *14*, 404. Available online: http://link.springer.com/10.1007/s11882-013-0404-6 (accessed on 7 June 2019). [CrossRef]
98. Kang, J.; Smith, S.; Pavitt, S.; Wu, J. Association between central obesity and tooth loss in the non-obese people: Results from the continuous National Health and Nutrition Examination Survey (NHANES) 1999–2012. *J. Clin. Periodontol.* **2019**, *46*, 430–437. [CrossRef]
99. Codoñer-Franch, P.; Valls-Bellés, V.; Arilla-Codoñer, A.; Alonso-Iglesias, E. Oxidant mechanisms in childhood obesity: The link between inflammation and oxidative stress. *Transl. Res.* **2011**, *158*, 369–384. [CrossRef]
100. Hujoel, P.P.; Lingström, P. Nutrition, dental caries and periodontal disease: A narrative review. *J. Clin. Periodontol.* **2017**, *44* (Suppl. S18), S79–S84. [CrossRef]
101. Moynihan, P.J. The role of diet and nutrition in the etiology and prevention of oral diseases. *Bull. World Health Org.* **2005**, *83*, 694–699.
102. Sheiham, A.; Steele, J.G.; Marcenes, W.; Lowe, C.; Finch, S.; Bates, C.J.; Prentice, A.; Walls, A.W. The relationship among dental status, nutrient intake, and nutritional status in older people. *J. Dent. Res.* **2001**, *80*, 408–413. [CrossRef] [PubMed]
103. Nowjack-Raymer, R.E.; Sheiham, A. Numbers of natural teeth, diet, and nutritional status in US adults. *J. Dent. Res.* **2007**, *86*, 1171–1175. [CrossRef] [PubMed]
104. Zhu, Y.; Hollis, J.H. Tooth loss and its association with dietary intake and diet quality in American adults. *J. Dent.* **2014**, *42*, 1428–1435. [CrossRef] [PubMed]

105. Cruz-Jentoft, A.J.; Landi, F.; Topinková, E.; Michel, J.-P. Understanding sarcopenia as a geriatric syndrome. *Curr. Opin. Clin. Nutr. Metab. Care* **2010**, *13*, 1–7. [CrossRef]
106. Cruz-Jentoft, A.J.; Bahat, G.; Bauer, J.; Boirie, Y.; Bruyère, O.; Cederholm, T.; Cooper, C.; Landi, F.; Rolland, Y.; Sayer, A.A.; et al. Sarcopenia: Revised European consensus on definition and diagnosis. *Age Ageing* **2019**, *48*, 16–31. [CrossRef]
107. Anker, S.D.; Morley, J.E.; von Haehling, S. Welcome to the ICD-10 code for sarcopenia. *J. Cachexia Sarcopenia Muscle* **2016**, *7*, 512–514. [CrossRef]
108. Landi, F.; Calvani, R.; Cesari, M.; Tosato, M.; Martone, A.M.; Ortolani, E.; Savera, G.; Salini, S.; Sisto, A.; Picca, A.; et al. Sarcopenia: An Overview on Current Definitions, Diagnosis and Treatment. *Curr. Protein Pept. Sci.* **2018**, *19*, 633–638. [CrossRef]
109. Liguori, I.; Russo, G.; Aran, L.; Bulli, G.; Curcio, F.; Della-Morte, D.; Gargiulo, G.; Testa, G.; Cacciatore, F.; Bonaduce, D.; et al. Sarcopenia: Assessment of disease burden and strategies to improve outcomes. *Clin. Interv. Aging* **2018**, *13*, 913–927. [CrossRef]
110. McCulloch, T.M.; Jaffe, D. Head and neck disorders affecting swallowing. *GI Motil. Online* **2006**. Available online: https://www.nature.com/gimo/contents/pt1/full/gimo36.html (accessed on 11 October 2019).
111. Wirth, R.; Dziewas, R.; Beck, A.M.; Clavé, P.; Hamdy, S.; Heppner, H.J.; Langmore, S.; Leischker, A.H.; Martino, R.; Pluschinski, P.; et al. Oropharyngeal dysphagia in older persons—From pathophysiology to adequate intervention: A review and summary of an international expert meeting. *Clin. Interv. Aging* **2016**, *11*, 189–208. [CrossRef]
112. Robbins, J.; Bridges, A.D.; Taylor, A. Oral, pharyngeal and esophageal motor function in aging. *GI Motil. Online* **2006**. Available online: https://www.nature.com/gimo/contents/pt1/full/gimo39.html (accessed on 11 October 2019).
113. Feng, X.; Todd, T.; Lintzenich, C.R.; Ding, J.; Carr, J.J.; Ge, Y.; Browne, J.D.; Kritchevsky, S.B.; Butler, S.G. Aging-related geniohyoid muscle atrophy is related to aspiration status in healthy older adults. *J. Gerontol. Ser. A* **2013**, *68*, 853–860. [CrossRef] [PubMed]
114. Newton, J.P.; Yemm, R.; Abel, R.W.; Menhinick, S. Changes in human jaw muscles with age and dental state. *Gerodontology* **1993**, *10*, 16–22. [CrossRef] [PubMed]
115. Wakabayashi, H.; Takahashi, R.; Watanabe, N.; Oritsu, H.; Shimizu, Y. Prevalence of skeletal muscle mass loss and its association with swallowing function after cardiovascular surgery. *Nutrition* **2017**, *38*, 70–73. [CrossRef] [PubMed]
116. Machida, N.; Tohara, H.; Hara, K.; Kumakura, A.; Wakasugi, Y.; Nakane, A.; Minakuchi, S. Effects of aging and sarcopenia on tongue pressure and jaw-opening force. *Geriatr. Gerontol. Int.* **2017**, *17*, 295–301. [CrossRef]
117. Sakai, K.; Nakayama, E.; Tohara, H.; Kodama, K.; Takehisa, T.; Takehisa, Y.; Ueda, K. Relationship between tongue strength, lip strength, and nutrition-related sarcopenia in older rehabilitation inpatients: A cross-sectional study. *Clin. Interv. Aging* **2017**, *12*, 1207–1214. [CrossRef]
118. Sporns, P.B.; Muhle, P.; Hanning, U.; Suntrup-Krueger, S.; Schwindt, W.; Eversmann, J.; Warnecke, T.; Wirth, R.; Zimmer, S.; Dziewas, R. Atrophy of Swallowing Muscles Is Associated with Severity of Dysphagia and Age in Patients with Acute Stroke. *J. Am. Med. Dir. Assoc.* **2017**, *18*, 635.e1–635.e7. [CrossRef]
119. Maeda, K.; Akagi, J. Decreased tongue pressure is associated with sarcopenia and sarcopenic dysphagia in the elderly. *Dysphagia* **2015**, *30*, 80–87. [CrossRef]
120. Butler, S.G.; Stuart, A.; Leng, X.; Wilhelm, E.; Rees, C.; Williamson, J.; Kritchevsky, S.B. The relationship of aspiration status with tongue and handgrip strength in healthy older adults. *J. Gerontol. Ser. A* **2011**, *66*, 452–458. [CrossRef]
121. Buehring, B.; Hind, J.; Fidler, E.; Krueger, D.; Binkley, N.; Robbins, J. Tongue strength is associated with jumping mechanography performance and handgrip strength but not with classic functional tests in older adults. *J. Am. Geriatr. Soc.* **2013**, *61*, 418–422. [CrossRef]
122. Tsuga, K.; Yoshikawa, M.; Oue, H.; Okazaki, Y.; Tsuchioka, H.; Maruyama, M.; Yoshida, M.; Akagawa, Y. Maximal voluntary tongue pressure is decreased in Japanese frail elderly persons. *Gerodontology* **2012**, *29*, e1078–e1085. [CrossRef] [PubMed]
123. Ertekin, C.; Aydogdu, I. Neurophysiology of swallowing. *Clin. Neurophysiol.* **2003**, *114*, 2226–2244. [CrossRef]
124. Sakai, K.; Sakuma, K. Sarcopenic Dysphagia as a New Concept. *Frailty Sarcopenia Onset Dev. Clin. Chall.* **2017**. Available online: https://www.intechopen.com/books/frailty-and-sarcopenia-onset-development-and-clinical-challenges/sarcopenic-dysphagia-as-a-new-concept (accessed on 11 October 2019).

125. Wakabayashi, H. Presbyphagia and Sarcopenic Dysphagia: Association between Aging, Sarcopenia, and Deglutition Disorders. *J. Frailty Aging* **2014**, *3*, 97–103. [PubMed]
126. Rowlerson, A.; Raoul, G.; Daniel, Y.; Close, J.; Maurage, C.-A.; Ferri, J.; Sciote, J.J. Fiber-type differences in masseter muscle associated with different facial morphologies. *Am. J. Orthod. Dentofac. Orthop.* **2005**, *127*, 37–46. [CrossRef] [PubMed]
127. Yamaguchi, K.; Tohara, H.; Hara, K.; Nakane, A.; Kajisa, E.; Yoshimi, K.; Minakuchi, S. Relationship of aging, skeletal muscle mass, and tooth loss with masseter muscle thickness. *BMC Geriatr.* **2018**, *18*, 67. [CrossRef]
128. Ferrucci, L.; Fabbri, E. Inflammageing: Chronic inflammation in ageing, cardiovascular disease, and frailty. *Nat. Rev. Cardiol.* **2018**, *15*, 505–522. [CrossRef]
129. Yao, X.; Li, H.; Leng, S.X. Inflammation and immune system alterations in frailty. *Clin. Geriatr. Med.* **2011**, *27*, 79–87. [CrossRef]
130. Napa, K.; Baeder, A.C.; Witt, J.E.; Rayburn, S.T.; Miller, M.G.; Dallon, B.W.; Gibbs, J.L.; Wilcox, S.H.; Winden, D.R.; Smith, J.H.; et al. LPS from, P. gingivalis Negatively Alters Gingival Cell Mitochondrial Bioenergetics. *Int. J. Dent.* **2017**, *2017*. Available online: https://www.ncbi.nlm.nih.gov/pmc/articles/PMC5448046/ (accessed on 11 October 2019). [CrossRef]
131. Taylor, G.W.; Burt, B.A.; Becker, M.P.; Genco, R.J.; Shlossman, M.; Knowler, W.C.; Pettitt, D.J. Severe periodontitis and risk for poor glycemic control in patients with non-insulin-dependent diabetes mellitus. *J. Periodontol.* **1996**, *67* (Suppl. S10), 1085–1093. [CrossRef]
132. Chee, B.; Park, B.; Bartold, P.M. Periodontitis and type II diabetes: A two-way relationship. *Int. J. Evid. Based Healthc.* **2013**, *11*, 317–329. [CrossRef] [PubMed]
133. Fuggle, N.R.; Smith, T.O.; Kaul, A.; Sofat, N. Hand to Mouth: A Systematic Review and Meta-Analysis of the Association between Rheumatoid Arthritis and Periodontitis. *Front. Immunol.* **2016**, *7*, 80. [CrossRef] [PubMed]
134. Beck, J.D.; Offenbacher, S.; Williams, R.; Gibbs, P.; Garcia, R. Periodontitis: A risk factor for coronary heart disease? *Ann. Periodontol.* **1998**, *3*, 127–141. [CrossRef] [PubMed]
135. D'Aiuto, F.; Nibali, L.; Parkar, M.; Patel, K.; Suvan, J.; Donos, N. Oxidative stress, systemic inflammation, and severe periodontitis. *J. Dent. Res.* **2010**, *89*, 1241–1246. [CrossRef]
136. Borges, I.; Moreira, E.A.M.; Filho, D.W.; de Oliveira, T.B.; da Silva, M.B.S.; Fröde, T.S. Proinflammatory and oxidative stress markers in patients with periodontal disease. *Mediat. Inflamm.* **2007**, *2007*, 45794. [CrossRef]
137. Horton, A.L.; Boggess, K.A.; Moss, K.L.; Beck, J.; Offenbacher, S. Periodontal disease, oxidative stress, and risk for preeclampsia. *J. Periodontol.* **2010**, *81*, 199–204. [CrossRef]
138. Bullon, P.; Cordero, M.D.; Quiles, J.L.; del Carmen Ramirez-Tortosa, M.; Gonzalez-Alonso, A.; Alfonsi, S.; García-Marín, R.; de Miguel, M.; Battino, M. Autophagy in periodontitis patients and gingival fibroblasts: Unraveling the link between chronic diseases and inflammation. *BMC Med.* **2012**, *10*, 122. [CrossRef]
139. Bullon, P.; Cordero, M.D.; Quiles, J.L.; Morillo, J.M.; del Carmen Ramirez-Tortosa, M.; Battino, M. Mitochondrial dysfunction promoted by Porphyromonas gingivalis lipopolysaccharide as a possible link between cardiovascular disease and periodontitis. *Free Radic. Biol. Med.* **2011**, *50*, 1336–1343. [CrossRef]
140. Wang, P.-L.; Ohura, K. Porphyromonas gingivalis lipopolysaccharide signaling in gingival fibroblasts-CD14 and Toll-like receptors. *Crit. Rev. Oral Biol. Med.* **2002**, *13*, 132–142. [CrossRef]
141. Andersson, P.; Hallberg, I.R.; Lorefält, B.; Unosson, M.; Renvert, S. Oral health problems in elderly rehabilitation patients. *Int. J. Dent. Hyg.* **2004**, *2*, 70–77. [CrossRef]
142. Hanne, K.; Ingelise, T.; Linda, C.; Ulrich, P.P. Oral status and the need for oral health care among patients hospitalised with acute medical conditions. *J. Clin. Nurs.* **2012**, *21*, 2851–2859. [CrossRef] [PubMed]
143. Cederholm, T.; Jensen, G.L.; Correia, M.I.T.D.; Gonzalez, M.C.; Fukushima, R.; Higashiguchi, T.; Baptista, G.; Barazzoni, R.; Blaauw, R.; Coats, A.; et al. GLIM criteria for the diagnosis of malnutrition—A consensus report from the global clinical nutrition community. *Clin. Nutr.* **2019**, *38*, 1–9. [CrossRef] [PubMed]
144. Cesari, M.; Landi, F.; Vellas, B.; Bernabei, R.; Marzetti, E. Sarcopenia and Physical Frailty: Two Sides of the Same Coin. *Front. Aging Neurosci* **2014**, *6*, 192. Available online: https://www.ncbi.nlm.nih.gov/pmc/articles/PMC4112807/ (accessed on 5 November 2019). [CrossRef] [PubMed]
145. Cruz-Jentoft, A.J.; Kiesswetter, E.; Drey, M.; Sieber, C.C. Nutrition, frailty, and sarcopenia. *Aging Clin. Exp. Res.* **2017**, *29*, 43–48. [CrossRef] [PubMed]
146. Landi, F.; Cherubini, A.; Cesari, M.; Calvani, R.; Tosato, M.; Sisto, A.; Martone, A.M.; Bernabei, R.; Marzetti, E. Sarcopenia and frailty: From theoretical approach into clinical practice. *Eur. Geriatr. Med.* **2016**, *7*, 197–200.

Available online: https://moh-it.pure.elsevier.com/en/publications/sarcopenia-and-frailty-from-theoretical-approach-into-clinical-pr (accessed on 11 October 2019). [CrossRef]

147. Bauer, J.; Biolo, G.; Cederholm, T.; Cesari, M.; Cruz-Jentoft, A.J.; Morley, J.E.; Phillips, S.; Sieber, C.; Stehle, P.; Teta, D.; et al. Evidence-Based Recommendations for Optimal Dietary Protein Intake in Older People: A Position Paper from the PROT-AGE Study Group. *J. Am. Med. Dir. Assoc.* **2013**, *14*, 542–559. [CrossRef]

148. Ellis, G.; Whitehead, M.A.; O'Neill, D.; Langhorne, P.; Robinson, D. Comprehensive geriatric assessment for older adults admitted to hospital. *Cochrane. Database. Syst. Rev.* **2011**, *7*, CD006211.

149. Bollero, P.; Passarelli, P.C.; D'Addona, A.; Pasquantonio, G.; Mancini, M.; Condò, R.; Cerroni, L. Oral management of adult patients undergoing hematopoietic stem cell transplantation. *Eur. Rev. Med. Pharmacol. Sci.* **2018**, *22*, 876–887.

150. Tonetti, M.S.; Bottenberg, P.; Conrads, G.; Eickholz, P.; Heasman, P.; Huysmans, M.-C.; López, R.; Madianos, P.; Müller, F.; Needleman, I.; et al. Dental caries and periodontal diseases in the ageing population: Call to action to protect and enhance oral health and well-being as an essential component of healthy ageing—Consensus report of group 4 of the joint EFP/ORCA workshop on the boundaries between caries and periodontal diseases. *J. Clin. Periodontol.* **2017**, *44* (Suppl. S18), S135–S144.

151. Andreas Zenthöfer, A.; Rammelsberg, P.; Cabrera, T.; Hassel, A. Prosthetic rehabilitation of edentulism prevents malnutrition in nursing home residents. *Int. J. Prosthodont.* **2015**, *28*, 198–200. [CrossRef]

152. Volkert, D.; Beck, A.M.; Cederholm, T.; Cruz-Jentoft, A.; Goisser, S.; Hooper, L.; Kiesswetter, E.; Maggio, M.; Raynaud-Simon, A.; Sieber, C.C.; et al. ESPEN guideline on clinical nutrition and hydration in geriatrics. *Clin. Nutr.* **2019**, *38*, 10–47. [CrossRef] [PubMed]

153. Deutz, N.E.P.; Bauer, J.M.; Barazzoni, R.; Biolo, G.; Boirie, Y.; Bosy-Westphal, A.; Cederholm, T.; Cruz-Jentoft, A.; Krznariç, Z.; Nair, K.S.; et al. Protein intake and exercise for optimal muscle function with aging: Recommendations from the ESPEN Expert Group. *Clin. Nutr.* **2014**, *33*, 929–936. [CrossRef] [PubMed]

154. Johnson, M.A.; Kimlin, M.G. Vitamin D, aging, and the 2005 Dietary Guidelines for Americans. *Nutr. Rev.* **2006**, *64*, 410–421. [CrossRef] [PubMed]

155. Visser, M.; Deeg, D.J.H.; Lips, P. Longitudinal Aging Study Amsterdam. Low vitamin D and high parathyroid hormone levels as determinants of loss of muscle strength and muscle mass (sarcopenia): The Longitudinal Aging Study Amsterdam. *J. Clin. Endocrinol. Metab.* **2003**, *88*, 5766–5772. [CrossRef] [PubMed]

156. Ney, D.M.; Weiss, J.M.; Kind, A.J.H.; Robbins, J. Senescent Swallowing: Impact, Strategies, and Interventions. *Nutr. Clin. Pract.* **2009**, *24*, 395–413. [CrossRef] [PubMed]

157. Sura, L.; Madhavan, A.; Carnaby, G.; Crary, M.A. Dysphagia in the elderly: Management and nutritional considerations. *Clin. Interv. Aging* **2012**, *7*, 287–298.

158. Lutsey, P.L.; Steffen, L.M.; Stevens, J. Dietary intake and the development of the metabolic syndrome: The Atherosclerosis Risk in Communities study. *Circulation* **2008**, *117*, 754–761. [CrossRef]

159. Guideline: Sugars Intake for Adults and Children. Available online: https://apps.who.int/iris/handle/10665/149782 (accessed on 22 October 2019).

160. Gutteridge, J.M.C.; Halliwell, B. Antioxidants: Molecules, medicines, and myths. *Biochem. Biophys. Res. Commun.* **2010**, *393*, 561–564. [CrossRef]

161. Welch, A.A.; MacGregor, A.J.; Minihane, A.-M.; Skinner, J.; Valdes, A.A.; Spector, T.D.; Cassidy, A. Dietary fat and fatty acid profile are associated with indices of skeletal muscle mass in women aged 18-79 years. *J. Nutr.* **2014**, *144*, 327–334. [CrossRef]

162. Woelber, J.P.; Bremer, K.; Vach, K.; König, D.; Hellwig, E.; Ratka-Krüger, P.; Al-Ahmad, A.; Tennert, C. An oral health optimized diet can reduce gingival and periodontal inflammation in humans—A randomized controlled pilot study. *BMC Oral Health* **2016**, *17*, 28. [CrossRef]

163. Dupont, J.; Dedeyne, L.; Dalle, S.; Koppo, K.; Gielen, E. The role of omega-3 in the prevention and treatment of sarcopenia. *Aging Clin. Exp. Res.* **2019**, *31*, 825–836. [CrossRef] [PubMed]

164. Damanti, S.; Azzolino, D.; Roncaglione, C.; Arosio, B.; Rossi, P.; Cesari, M. Efficacy of Nutritional Interventions as Stand-Alone or Synergistic Treatments with Exercise for the Management of Sarcopenia. *Nutrients* **2019**, *11*, 1991. [CrossRef] [PubMed]

165. Dickinson, J.M.; Volpi, E.; Rasmussen, B.B. Exercise and nutrition to target protein synthesis impairments in aging skeletal muscle. *Exerc. Sport Sci. Rev.* **2013**, *41*, 216–223. [CrossRef] [PubMed]

166. Glover, E.I.; Phillips, S.M.; Oates, B.R.; Tang, J.E.; Tarnopolsky, M.A.; Selby, A.; Smith, K.; Rennie, M.J. Immobilization induces anabolic resistance in human myofibrillar protein synthesis with low and high dose amino acid infusion. *J. Physiol.* **2008**, *586*, 6049–6061. [CrossRef]
167. Bawadi, H.A.; Khader, Y.S.; Haroun, T.F.; Al-Omari, M.; Tayyem, R.F. The association between periodontal disease, physical activity and healthy diet among adults in Jordan. *J. Periodont. Res.* **2011**, *46*, 74–81. [CrossRef]
168. Cruz-Jentoft, A.J.; Landi, F.; Schneider, S.M.; Zúñiga, C.; Arai, H.; Boirie, Y.; Chen, L.-K.; Fielding, R.A.; Martin, F.C.; Michel, J.-P.; et al. Prevalence of and interventions for sarcopenia in ageing adults: A systematic review. Report of the International Sarcopenia Initiative (EWGSOP and IWGS). *Age Ageing* **2014**, *43*, 748–759. [CrossRef]
169. Sugiyama, T.; Ohkubo, M.; Honda, Y.; Tasaka, A.; Nagasawa, K.; Ishida, R.; Sakurai, K. Effect of swallowing exercises in independent elderly. *Bull. Tokyo. Dent. Coll.* **2013**, *54*, 109–115. [CrossRef]
170. Argolo, N.; Sampaio, M.; Pinho, P.; Melo, A.; Nóbrega, A.C. Do swallowing exercises improve swallowing dynamic and quality of life in Parkinson's disease? *NeuroRehabilitation* **2013**, *32*, 949–955.
171. Kim, H.-J.; Lee, J.-Y.; Lee, E.-S.; Jung, H.-J.; Ahn, H.-J.; Kim, B.-I. Improvements in oral functions of elderly after simple oral exercise. *Clin. Interv. Aging* **2019**, *14*, 915–924. [CrossRef]
172. Park, J.S.; Oh, D.H.; Chang, M.Y.; Kim, K.M. Effects of expiratory muscle strength training on oropharyngeal dysphagia in subacute stroke patients: A randomised controlled trial. *J. Oral Rehabil.* **2016**, *43*, 364–372. [CrossRef]
173. Park, J.-S.; Oh, D.-H.; Chang, M.-Y. Effect of expiratory muscle strength training on swallowing-related muscle strength in community-dwelling elderly individuals: A randomized controlled trial. *Gerodontology* **2017**, *34*, 121–128. [CrossRef] [PubMed]
174. Park, J.S.; Hwang, N.K.; Oh, D.H.; Chang, M.Y. Effect of head lift exercise on kinematic motion of the hyolaryngeal complex and aspiration in patients with dysphagic stroke. *J. Oral Rehabil.* **2017**, *44*, 385–391. [CrossRef] [PubMed]
175. Antunes, E.B.; Lunet, N. Effects of the head lift exercise on the swallow function: A systematic review. *Gerodontology* **2012**, *29*, 247–257. [CrossRef] [PubMed]
176. Steele, C.M.; Bayley, M.T.; Peladeau-Pigeon, M.; Nagy, A.; Namasivayam, A.M.; Stokely, S.L.; Wolkin, T. A Randomized Trial Comparing Two Tongue-Pressure Resistance Training Protocols for Post-Stroke Dysphagia. *Dysphagia* **2016**, *31*, 452–461. [CrossRef] [PubMed]
177. Kim, H.D.; Choi, J.B.; Yoo, S.J.; Chang, M.Y.; Lee, S.W.; Park, J.S. Tongue-to-palate resistance training improves tongue strength and oropharyngeal swallowing function in subacute stroke survivors with dysphagia. *J. Oral Rehabil.* **2017**, *44*, 59–64. [CrossRef] [PubMed]
178. Yeates, E.M.; Molfenter, S.M.; Steele, C.M. Improvements in tongue strength and pressure-generation precision following a tongue-pressure training protocol in older individuals with dysphagia: Three case reports. *Clin. Interv. Aging* **2008**, *3*, 735–747. [CrossRef]
179. Robbins, J.; Gangnon, R.E.; Theis, S.M.; Kays, S.A.; Hewitt, A.L.; Hind, J.A. The effects of lingual exercise on swallowing in older adults. *J. Am. Geriatr. Soc.* **2005**, *53*, 1483–1489. [CrossRef]

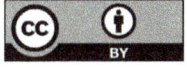

© 2019 by the authors. Licensee MDPI, Basel, Switzerland. This article is an open access article distributed under the terms and conditions of the Creative Commons Attribution (CC BY) license (http://creativecommons.org/licenses/by/4.0/).

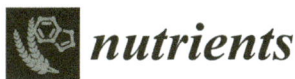

Review

Role of Citrate in Pathophysiology and Medical Management of Bone Diseases

Donatella Granchi [1,*], **Nicola Baldini** [1,2], **Fabio Massimo Ulivieri** [3] **and Renata Caudarella** [4]

1. Laboratory for Orthopedic Pathophysiology and Regenerative Medicine, IRCCS Istituto Ortopedico Rizzoli, via di Barbiano 1/10, 40136 Bologna, Italy; nicola.baldini@ior.it
2. Department of Biomedical and Neuromotor Sciences, Via Pupilli 1, University of Bologna, 40136 Bologna, Italy
3. Nuclear Medicine, Bone Metabolic Unit, IRCCS Ca' Granda Ospedale Maggiore Policlinico, Via F.Sforza 35, 20122 Milano, Italy; ulivieri@gmail.com
4. Maria Cecilia Hospital, GVM Care and Research, Via Corriera 1, 48033 Cotignola (RA), Italy; renata.caudarella@gmail.com
* Correspondence: donatella.granchi@ior.it; Tel.: +39-051-636-6896

Received: 23 September 2019; Accepted: 22 October 2019; Published: 25 October 2019

Abstract: Citrate is an intermediate in the "Tricarboxylic Acid Cycle" and is used by all aerobic organisms to produce usable chemical energy. It is a derivative of citric acid, a weak organic acid which can be introduced with diet since it naturally exists in a variety of fruits and vegetables, and can be consumed as a dietary supplement. The close association between this compound and bone was pointed out for the first time by Dickens in 1941, who showed that approximately 90% of the citrate bulk of the human body resides in mineralised tissues. Since then, the number of published articles has increased exponentially, and considerable progress in understanding how citrate is involved in bone metabolism has been made. This review summarises current knowledge regarding the role of citrate in the pathophysiology and medical management of bone disorders.

Keywords: bone metabolism; bone mineral density; bone remodelling; citrate supplement; osteopenia; osteoporosis; kidney diseases

1. Introduction

Citrate is an intermediate in the tricarboxylic acid cycle (TCA cycle, Krebs cycle), a central metabolic pathway for all aerobic organisms, including animals, plants, and bacteria [1,2]. In humans, citrate is produced in the mitochondria after the condensation of acetyl coenzyme A (acetylCoA) and oxaloacetate, which are catalysed by citrate synthase; it then enters the TCA cycle, thus becoming the primary adenosine 5′-triphosphate (ATP) provider by which living cells harvest the energy they need to accomplish essential and specific functions [1].

The intracellular citrate level reflects the energy status of the cell and acts as a regulator. When the cellular ATP is abundant and the energy demand of the cells is low, the excess citrate can be exported to the cytosol by means of a mitochondrial citrate carrier [3]. It can be used for the lipid biosynthesis of highly proliferating cells [4] or for supporting the tissue-related functions of specialised cells, including the mineralisation of the extracellular matrix by osteoblasts, the bone-forming cells [5]. In this regard, the close association between citrate and bone was pointed out for the first time by Dickens in 1941 [6]. Since then, the number of published articles dealing with this topic has increased exponentially (Figure 1), and considerable progress in understanding how citrate is involved in bone metabolism has been made. This review summarises the current knowledge regarding the relationship between citrate and bone pathophysiology, starting from the link with bone cells and the mineralised matrix, moving through the role of citrate in the onset of bone disorders, and concluding with a critical evaluation of the clinical use of citrate supplements for the medical management of bone diseases.

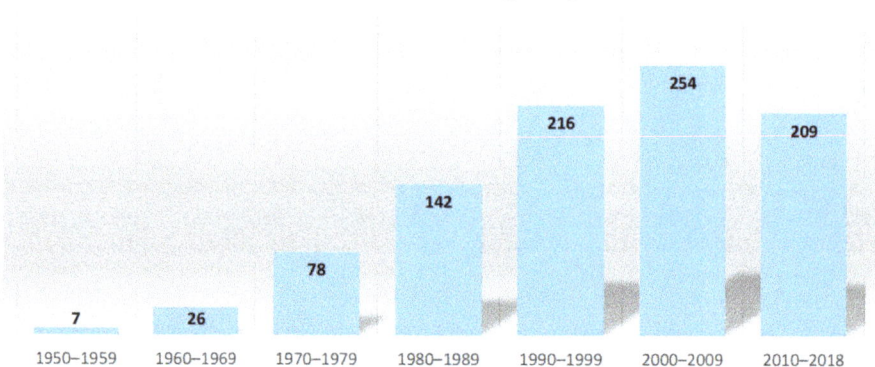

Figure 1. Distribution of the biomedical citations indexed by PubMed over seven decades ($n = 949$, from 1949 to 2018). The search query focused on "citrate" and "bone", with a search restricted to the terms "Title", "Abstract" or "Medical Subject Headings". Only citations related to studies on humans are included with the exception of those dealing with citrate as an anticoagulant.

2. Citrate Homeostasis: General Physiological Concepts

2.1. The Pillars of Citrate Homeostasis

There is a balance between citrate availability and elimination, depending on physiological requirements. Basically, citrate homeostasis depends on four domains, i.e., nutritional intake, renal clearance, cellular metabolism, and bone remodelling (Figure 2).

Citric acid is naturally contained in fruits and vegetables, particularly in citrus fruits, with concentrations ranging from 0.005 mol/L in oranges and grapefruit to 0.30 mol/L in lemons and limes [7,8]. Food citrate may also be produced biotechnologically by many microorganisms through a fermentation process, and of these, Aspergillum Niger has been recognised as the most efficient producer [9]. Industrial-scale citric acid is employed instead of fresh lemon juice in a variety of pre-prepared meals, and it is also used as an additive in foods and beverages since it acts as a preservative, acidity regulator, flavoring substance and emulsifying agent. In fact, due to the variety of applications, citric acid is the most consumed organic acid in the world, leading to high commercial interest as well as motivating scientists to discover new super-producing techniques [10].

The usual nutritional intake of citrate is approximately 4 grams per day [11] and more than 95% of it is absorbed in the small intestine [12] by means of the sodium-dicarboxylate (NaDC) cotransporter similar to that described in the kidney [13]. The total daily consumption of citric acid may exceed 500 mg/kg of body weight, but considering the low citrate amount in foods, both those in which it is naturally contained and those in which it is added in artificial form, the ingestion of excessive doses is very unlikely [14].

The dietary ingestion of citrate is able to enhance the plasma level within thirty minutes; it is then filtered at the glomerular level just as quickly, and eventually reabsorbed according to physiological needs [15]. In healthy individuals, the serum concentration of circulating citrate is relatively constant, ranging from 19 to 50 mg/L with an average of 20 mg/L [16,17]. Citrate in plasma exists as ≈95% tricarboxylate, ≈4% dicarboxylate, and 1% monocarboxylate, and the majority is complexed to divalent ions, such as calcium and magnesium. The high impermeability of the plasma membrane precludes the cellular uptake of citrate from the extracellular fluid. Under special conditions, some cells (i.e., intestinal enterocytes and kidney tubular cells) express a plasma membrane citrate transporter belonging to the "solute carrier" 13 family (Slc13, NaDC), which is essential for uptake from the gastrointestinal tract and tubular fluid.

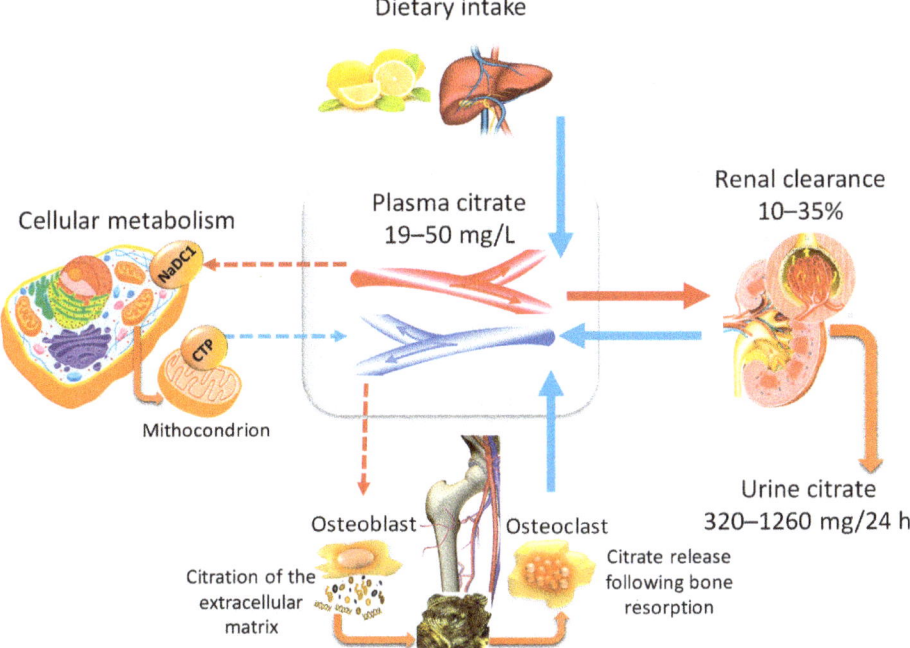

Figure 2. The four domains of citrate homeostasis. The plasma level of citrate mainly depends on four sources, i.e., nutritional intake, renal clearance, cellular metabolism, and bone remodelling. Food citrate is rapidly introduced into the circulation, filtered at the glomerular level, and eventually reabsorbed according to physiological needs. The citrate uptake from the extracellular milieu may occur only when specific transporter proteins are expressed, i.e., sodium-dicarboxylate (NaDC)1 belonging to the "solute carrier" 13 (Slc13) family. The citrate produced by mitochondria only marginally contributes to citrate homeostasis, since it is almost all used by cells as an energy source, or for the synthesis of lipids and other specific functions, i.e., citration of the extracellular matrix by the osteoblasts. In fact, the bulk stored in bone is the main endogenous source of citrate which becomes available following the resorption of the mineralised matrix by the osteoclasts. The mitochondrial citrate-transport protein (CTP) is essential for the release of citrate from the mitochondria to cytosol.

However, the net balance between gastrointestinal absorption and the urinary excretion of citrate suggests that nutritional intake cannot be solely responsible for the maintenance of plasma homeostasis [15,17]. The cellular metabolism also has a scarce impact on citrate availability since almost all the mitochondrial production is consumed by cells as an energy source or for supporting specific cell functions [4,5]. Nowadays, it is well known that the main endogenous bulk of citrate is stored in bone and is mobilised following the resorption of the mineralised matrix by the osteoclasts [17].

2.2. Citraturia as A Marker of Citrate Homeostasis and Bone Health Status

As circulating citrate is freely filtered in the glomerulus, 24-h excretion is considered to be a valid marker for highlighting alterations of citrate homeostasis [11]. The reference values for urinary citrate levels range from 320 to 1260 mg/24 h, with an average in males of 550 mg/24 h and in females of 680 mg/24 h [18,19]. The higher excretion of citrate in females is in relation to the estrogenic rate [20] and explains the lower incidence of nephrolithiasis in premenopausal women, considering that citrate-calcium binding is one of the main mechanisms for inhibiting stone formation [21]. Based on the reference values for lithogenic risk, the threshold for the diagnosis of hypocitraturia is usually fixed as less than 320 mg per day. However, hypocitraturia may be severe (citrate excretion of less than 100 mg per day) or mild-moderate (from 100 to 320 mg), but low excretion (less than 640 mg per day) could also be a significant sign and should be monitored [18]. In general, elevated citrate excretion may be considered a non-pathological condition which reflects the restoration of the acid-base balance and occurs, for instance, after chronic alkali intake [22]. Low citrate excretion is a relatively common finding, and even though the majority of patients have idiopathic hypocitraturia, there are several medical and physiological conditions associated with this abnormality. All the conditions listed in Table 1 may be potentially associated with skeletal disorders or, more broadly, with bone metabolism alterations, even when there are no obvious symptoms.

Table 1. Causes of low citrate excretion.

Cause	Annotation
Acid-base status [16,23]	• Acidosis increases citrate utilization by the mitochondria in the tricarboxylic acid cycle (TCA cycle), thus decreasing intra- and extracellular availability. As a consequence, citrate reabsorption is enhanced and urine excretion is reduced. On the contrary, alkalosis increases citrate elimination.
Hypokalemia [16,23]	• Low potassium levels cause intracellular acidosis (see above).
Diet [24,25]	• Low intake of high-citrate content food (fruit/vegetables). • A diet rich in animal proteins contains sulfate and phosphate moieties which are not metabolised and are excreted as acids which decrease urinary pH and citrate excretion. • High sodium intake, ketosis-promoting diet, and starvation.
Distal renal tubular acidosis (dRTA) [26]	• Complete form (hyperchloremic metabolic acidosis, hypokalemia, elevated urine pH). • Incomplete form (normal serum electrolytes, inability to acidify urine following an ammonium chloride load).
Chronic diarrheal syndrome [16,23]	• The fluid loss and intestinal alkali wasting alter the acid-base status, with low urinary pH and citrate retention.
Medications [16,23,27,28]	• Thiazide diuretics induce hypokalemia with resultant intracellular acidosis. • Acetazolamide (carbonic anhydrase inhibitor) produces changes in urine composition which are similar to those found in dRTA. • Angiotensin-converting enzyme inhibitors cause a reduction in urinary citrate by increasing the adenosine triphosphate (ATP) citrate lyase activity. • Topiramate (carbonic anhydrase inhibitor) exerts a dose-dependent effect on the renal excretion of citrate.
Strenuous physical exercise [23]	• It causes lactic acidosis, producing hypocitraturia.
Hyperuricosuria [23]	• With normouricemia, generally caused by dietary excess of purines (animal proteins). • With hyperuricemia (gouty diathesis), the urinary pH is typically low, with increased citrate reabsorption.

Table 1. *Cont.*

Cause	Annotation
Active urinary tract infection [23]	• Bacteria which degrade citrate lower the urinary citrate concentration.
Chronic kidney disease (CKD) [29]	• The decrease in the glomerular filtration rate causes a stepwise reduction in the amount of filtered citrate. Overt hypocitraturia is usually observed in advanced stages of CKD.
Primary hyperaldosteronism [30]	• Hypocitraturia (and hypercalciuria) occurs via Na-dependent volume expansion and chronic hypokalemia.
Menopause [31–34]	• Estrogen deficiency induces metabolic alteration related to the lowering of estrogen-induced signaling onto the mitochondria which promotes glycolysis and glycolytic-coupled TCA cycle function. Hormone replacement therapy restores the citrate level which is decreased in postmenopausal women.
Genetic defects [16]	• All inheritable diseases, gene defects, and polymorphisms associated with the above mentioned conditions (additional details in Table 2).

Modulation of citrate excretion in the kidney is influenced by multiple factors, but pH regulation, particularly in the proximal tubule, has the strongest impact, and even a small decrease in tubular pH significantly increases tubular reabsorption [16]. Therefore, in response to the elevated acid load occurring in metabolic acidosis, there is a notable increase in citrate recovery with subsequent hypocitraturia; urinary citrate excretion may be used as a laboratory parameter for monitoring the diet- and metabolism-dependent systemic acid-base status, even in subjects without overt metabolic acidosis [29,35,36].

The detrimental effect of acid-base imbalance on bone metabolism has been proven without a doubt [36,37], thus suggesting that citraturia could be a noninvasive and indirect view of bone health status. Actually, the relationship among urinary citrate excretion, bone quality parameters, and circulating levels of bone turnover markers has been demonstrated [34,36], even if its clinical usefulness is still controversial [37].

3. Citrate and Bone Tissue

In 1941 Dickens stated that approximately 90% of the total citrate found in the body of "osteovertebrates" resides in mineralised tissues, but the most valuable insight was that, due to its high binding affinity to calcium stored in the hard tissue, citrate could play a pivotal role in regulating metabolic functions and in maintaining the structural integrity of bone [6]. Moreover, Dickens postulated that the presence of citrate in bone is crucial for preventing calcium precipitation, either when bone tissue is resorbed in response to lowered serum calcium or when the biomineralisation process starts. Over time, data in the literature regarding the relationship between citrate and bone physiology have been increasing exponentially (Figure 1), but the role of citrate in driving the structural and functional properties of healthy bone in humans has only been partially elucidated. Early studies were mainly aimed at searching for the origin and the role of calciotropic hormones (calcitonin, parathyroid hormone (PTH), and vitamin D) in the regulation of its metabolism. However, these issues have remained largely unresolved and/or highly speculative, due to the absence of necessary research methodology and technology. Nowadays, there is adequate knowledge regarding the role of bone cells in producing citrate, how citrate enters the crystalline structure of bone, and how it controls the size and morphology of apatite nanocrystals.

3.1. Citrate and Mineral Structure

Citrate is abundant in bone, representing 1–5 weight percent (wt%) of the organic components with a density of approximately 1 molecule per 2 nm^2, which implies that more than 15% of the apatite surface area available in bone is covered by citrate molecules [38]. Before the introduction of modern analytical techniques, the testing methods to evaluate bone tissue composition were entirely limited to classic wet-chemical analyses. At that time, the evidence of a higher amount of the citrate metabolic activity in bone as compared to other tissues, such as kidney or liver, was a significant breakthrough. These findings allowed hypothesising that bone tissue was endowed with the special capacity of producing and storing a high concentration of citric acid, and suggested the role of citrate in regulating the mineralisation process [39]. On the one hand, citrate may influence the amount of mineral deposition by complexing calcium-phosphate (CaP) and favouring its precipitation; on the other hand, if citrate exceeds the amount incorporated in the bone matrix, it could even reverse the mineralisation phase, thus functioning as a solubilising agent which recalls calcium ions. Hu et al. (2010) have proven that citrate is not a dissolved solubilising agent but is firmly bound to apatite as an integral part of the nanocrystal structure. This could be explained by the fact that the elevated amount of citrate in the organic fraction (5.5 wt%) provides more COO- groups than all the noncollagenous proteins in bone, and therefore, the chances of the binding between citrate and calcium of apatite are proportionally increased [40]. Simultaneously, Xie and Nancollas (2010) proposed a three-phase model to explain how citrate may influence the size, longitudinal growth and thickness of apatite nanocrystals [38]. The biomineralisation process initiates with the formation of the amorphous CaP phase starting from an oversaturated CaP solution [41] (Figure 3A). At the early stage, few citrate molecules can bind with the surface of small-size amorphous CaP clusters, but even so, they are sufficient to slow down particle aggregation (Figure 3B). In the next phase, the noncollagenous proteins released from bone cells promote the amorphous CaP cluster clumping, and apatite nucleation starts within these larger amorphous aggregates. Moreover, the presence of collagen fibrils promotes the self-assembly of the small amorphous CaP clusters and guides their direction on the collagen surface [42] (Figure 3C). At the final stage, the surface of mature apatite nanocrystals is fully covered by citrate, so that the increase in thickness is inhibited whilst the growth may continue in a longitudinal direction, thus explaining the plate-like morphology which apatite crystals exhibit in bone [38]. The final apatite structure has a unique geometry since it does not exceed 30–50 nm in length and maintains 2–6 nm thickness [43].

By using a combination of solid-state Nuclear Magnetic Resonance spectroscopy, powder X-ray diffraction, and the principles of electronic structure calculations, Davies et al. (2014) postulated that citrate anions could be incorporated in a hydrated layer of the CaP structure. This binding configuration favours the growth of the mineral crystals in a plate-like morphology and explains their propensity to form stacks [44,45] (Figure 3D). More recently, Delgado-Lopez et al. (2017) focused on the early mineralisation phase, taking into account the interaction between citrate and collagen [46]. By means of an in-depth characterisation based on X-ray scattering and imaging techniques, they found that collagen and citrate work synergically to favour the platy morphology, since both contributed to maintaining the transient amorphous phase. The amorphous CaP clusters are figured as spherulites or globules which gradually occupy the gap zones of the aligned collagen fibrils [43].

The results of the above-mentioned studies confirmed that citrate is an integral part of the apatite-collagen nanocomposite, and the degree of incorporation into bone mineral, as well as the spatial orientation in the mineral structure, play a key role in maintaining the biomechanic properties of bone, i.e., stability, strength, and resistance to fracture. In light of its structural role, citrate has been used to explain the changes in the bone microarchitecture typical of some diseases [47]. In addition, a series of citrate-based materials for orthopaedic applications have been developed to favour the osteoinductive and osteoconductive properties of scaffolds for bone tissue engineering [48,49], as well as to promote bone healing in other surgical procedures [50–52].

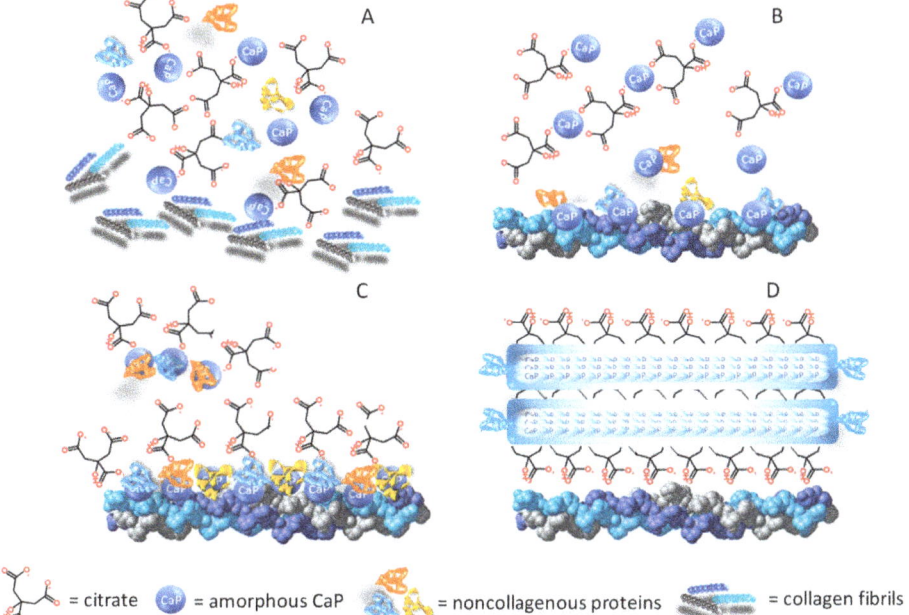

Figure 3. Citrate in the formation of the mineral matrix. The figure combines the theories proposed by different authors regarding the role of citrate in the mineralisation process [38,40,43–45]. (**A**) The amorphous calcium-phosphate (CaP) phase originates from an oversaturated CaP solution, and the mineralisation process starts when the organic phase (citrate, collagen fibrils, and noncollagenous proteins) is available in the bone microenvironment. (**B**) At the early stage, few citrate molecules bind with the amorphous CaP and the particle aggregation is slowed down. (**C**) In the next phase, the noncollagenous proteins released from bone cells favour CaP aggregation and apatite nucleation while the collagen promotes the self-assembly of CaP and guides the aggregate deposition on the collagen surface. (**D**) When the surface is fully covered by citrate, the thickness increase is inhibited (2–6 nm), while longitudinal growth continues up to 30–50 nm, thus explaining the flat morphology of bone mineral platelets. In addition, citrate forms bridges between the mineral platelets which can explain the stacked arrangement which is relevant to the mechanical properties of bone.

3.2. Citrate and Bone Cells

Once the presence of high concentrations of citrate in bone tissue was proven and the role of citrate in the mineralisation process clarified, the main goal of research in this field was to understand what the source of citrate in bone tissue was. Costello et al. (2012) demonstrated that murine osteoblasts were able to secrete citrate [53], thus laying the groundwork for additional studies which elucidated the metabolic process. Basically, the mechanisms were similar to those demonstrated in the prostatic cell, which is the other highly specialised cell capable of releasing high levels of citrate into the extracellular fluid. The elevated level of citrate production is due to the low activity of mitochondrial aconitase. This enzyme activity is suppressed by the zinc (Zn^{2+}) that is accumulated by cells through the solute carrier 39A (SLC39A1), also known as "zinc importer protein 1" (ZIP1) [54–56].

Additional studies have confirmed that human osteoblasts were citrate-producing cells, that ZIP1 expression and intracellular zinc increased during the differentiation of the osteogenic precursors into bone-forming cells, that ZIP1 knockdown prevented the intracellular accumulation of citrate [5], and that ZIP1 expression was promoted by bone morphogenetic protein 2 during the mineralisation process [57]. In addition, the upregulation of the mitochondrial solute carrier 25A (SLC25A1), the citrate transport protein (CTP), was essential for the release of citrate from the mitochondria [56]. In order to define the gene expression patterns underlying the differentiation of mesenchymal stem cells (MSCs) into mature osteoblasts, a large-scale transcriptome analysis starting from the bone-marrow MSCs maintained in osteogenic medium up to deposition of mineral nodules was carried out [58]. While the role of ZIP1 was already described [5,56,59], the microarray analysis showed that solute carrier 13A (SLC39A13), or ZIP13, was upregulated throughout osteogenic differentiation and was also detectable during the mineralisation process [60].

As shown in Figure 4A–E, changes in the citrate metabolism occur during the whole process of differentiation of the MSCs into mature osteoblasts. After the osteogenic commitment of resting MSCs, a highly proliferative phase is expected, and the exportation of citrate into cytosol provides the acetylCoA for the synthesis of the new lipids required for the assembly of the new plasma membranes during cell duplication. Mitochondrial citrate seems to be the preferential source of acetylCoA, since the alternative sources pose some limitations. In fact, extracellular citrate could be used for lipogenesis; however, cellular uptake is subordinated to the expression of the specific transporter, i.e., "sodium-dependent citrate transporter" (NaCT; SLC13A5) [61]. AcetyilCoA could also be obtained from plasma acetate passing through the cell membrane by means of the monocarboxylate transporter (MCT/SLC16A). In order to use this source, the upregulation of acetylCoA synthetase is required, but it is not highly expressed in mammalian cells [56]. Moreover, aconitase inhibition and the lack of mitochondrial citrate affect the energy supply via the Krebs cycle, so that the bioenergetic demand for proliferating/differentiating cells has to be satisfied by alternative sources. For instance, cytosol malate may enter the mitochondrion by CTP in exchange for citrate and may be converted into oxalacetic acid, which in turn may originate new citrate [56].

On the basis of recent studies, citrate released during the bone resorption phase could be considered a matrix-derived signal which contributes to the overall process of bone remodelling within the "basic multicellular unit" [62]. In this regard, Ma et al. have demonstrated that extracellular citrate played a pivotal role regarding the osteogenic differentiation of MSCs [63]. This "metabonegenic" regulation started with citrate uptake through the sodium-citrate transporter SLC13A5 followed by the activation of energy-producing pathways leading to an elevated cell energy status, which in turn fueled the high metabolic demands of MSCs differentiating into osteoblasts. In vitro experiments have shown that the timing and dosage of the citrate supply were critical factors. In fact, the effects were dose-dependent and more evident at the early stages of osteogenic differentiation, with higher proliferation and increased expression of bone-related genes, i.e., alkaline phosphatase and alpha 1 chain of type I collagen [63]. Identical effects have also been observed in a microenvironment hostile to bone cells, for instance using culture conditions which simulated low-grade acidosis [64]. In fact, citrate supplementation opposed the detrimental effects resulting from extracellular acidosis, which inhibited the synthesis of collagen and non-collagen proteins, the activity of alkaline phosphatase, and the formation of mineral nodules [65].

Taken together, studies regarding the role of citrate in the nanocrystal structure and those showing that osteoblasts were the specialised citrate-producing cells in bone have led to a new concept of bone formation related to "citration". Briefly, Costello et al. (2012) stated that … ."when considering the mineralisation role of osteoblasts in bone formation, it now becomes evident that 'citration' must be included in the process. Mineralisation without 'citration' will not result in the formation of normal bone, i.e., bone that exhibits its important properties, such as stability, strength, and resistance to fracture" [53].

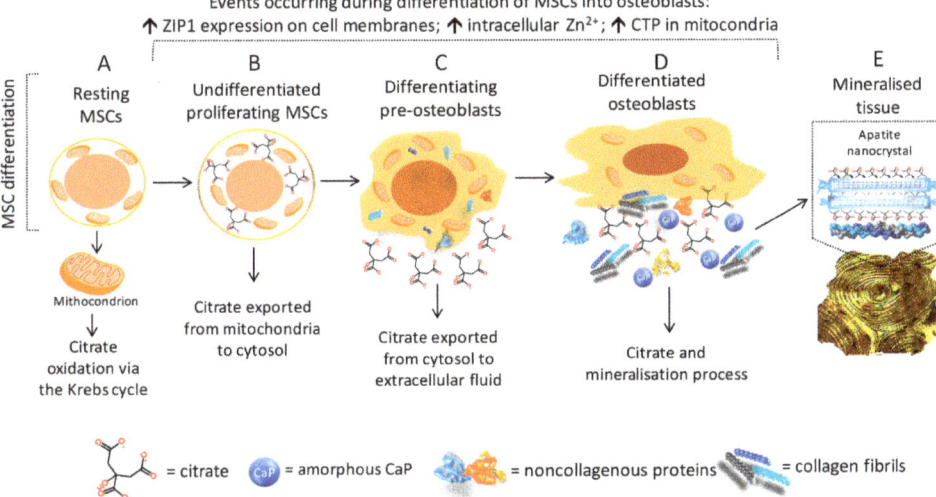

Figure 4. Citrate metabolism, osteoblast differentiation, and mineralisation process. The figure combines the concept of "osteoblast citration" with the main steps of the differentiation of mesenchymal stem cells (MSCs) into bone-forming cells (osteoblasts) [5,53,56]. (**A**) Resting MSCs are quiescent, nonproliferating cells which exhibit the typical mitochondrial metabolism with the oxidation of citrate via the Krebs cycle. (**B**) In the presence of proper stimuli, the undifferentiated MSCs are committed to osteogenic differentiation and, at the early phase, high proliferation is required. To accomplish this goal, the following events are necessary: (1) the upregulation of ZIP1 which promotes the zinc intake, (2) the accumulation of mitochondrial citrate due to the zinc-dependent inhibition of the mitochondrial aconitase, (3) the exportation of citrate into cytosol by means of the "citrate transport protein" (CTP/SLC25A1), (4) the use of cytosol citrate for the lipogenesis process which is essential for cell duplication. (**C,D**) The citrate exportation from cytosol to extracellular fluid starts during cell differentiation, and it is simultaneous for the synthesis and the release of amorphous CaP, collagen, and noncollagenous proteins. (**E**) The "osteoblast citration" is completed when the mineralised matrix is assembled. The role of citrate in growing the apatite nanocrystals and driving the mineralisation process is explained in Figure 3.

4. Citrate Pathophysiology and Bone Diseases

The role of citrate in mineralised tissues poses several questions regarding the consequences of a low bioavailability at the systemic level. For the most part, published data linking citrate alteration with bone metabolism refer to renal diseases, acid-base imbalance or also physiological conditions such as menopause, but there are also inheritable genetic defects which affect the TCA cycle in mitochondria or the citrate transport. In the following paragraphs, the medical conditions in which the association between citrate and bone health status has been implied are discussed.

4.1. Bone Health Status and Alterations of Citrate Homeostasis in Kidney Diseases

With the progressive aging of the population, epidemiological studies have shown a higher rate of elderly-related illnesses, including the impairment of bone quality leading to osteoporosis and decreased renal function with chronic kidney disease (CKD), which in turn may influence bone health status [66–68]. The decrease in renal function may be mild, moderate or severe on the basis of estimated-glomerular filtration rate (GFR) equations and is associated with the simultaneous impairment of mineral homeostasis, including serum and tissue concentrations of phosphorus and calcium, circulating levels of calciotropic hormones (PTH, 25-hydroxyvitamin D, 1,25-dihydroxyvitamin

D), fibroblast growth factor-23, and growth hormone. The modifications of mineral homeostasis may promote a loss of bone mass and an increase in bone fragility [69]. As observed by Malmgren et al. (2015), approximately 95% of women over 75 years of age showed a mild-moderate decrease in renal function (CKD stages 2–3) which may have had a harmful effect on bone health [70]. In a 10-year longitudinal study, the authors evaluated the long-term influence of impaired renal function on bone mineral density (BMD) [71]. They analysed 1044 Caucasian women from the "Osteoporosis Prospective Risk Assessment" (OPRA) cohort and found that renal function was positively correlated with femoral neck BMD in elderly women, although the association attenuated as aging progressed. Women with poor renal function had a higher annual rate of bone loss over 5 years compared to those with normal function, and markers of mineral homeostasis were more frequently altered.

High-throughput "omics" approaches, including metabolomics, have been proposed to identify new biomarkers which could help the management of CKD patients, and TCA cycle-metabolites are emerging as potential candidates [72]. A significantly reduced urinary excretion of citrate (−68%) has been observed in non-diabetic patients with CKD as compared to subjects with normal renal function. The renal expression of genes regulating the TCA cycle was decreased in subjects who had impaired renal function, thus suggesting that mitochondrial dysfunction could be involved in the pathogenesis of CKD [73]. Moreover, GFR positively correlated with citrate excretion, and kidney stone formers with CKD had significantly lower urinary citrate excretion than subjects with kidney stone disease and normal renal function [74].

To the authors' knowledge, the link between CKD, urinary citrate and bone health status has still not been elucidated but, taking into account the information emerging from the previous paragraphs, it is reasonable to assume that the link exists. Some indications have derived from the data regarding kidney stone disease, which is the paradigmatic expression of a relationship between citrate alterations, BMD decrease and fracture risk that has been investigated since the 1970s [75]. In fact, several studies have shown that osteoporotic fractures occurred more frequently in patients with kidney stones than in the general population [76–79].

The connection between kidney stones and bone metabolism is related to several factors. Briefly, kidney stones form when urine becomes supersaturated with respect to its specific components. Since 80% of kidney stones are composed of calcium-oxalate (CaOx) or CaP, the regulation of calcium excretion plays a pivotal role in the etiopathogenesis of nephrolithiasis [80]. As urinary citrate is able to bind calcium and prevent the growth and agglomeration of CaOx and CaP crystals, the close relationship between low citrate excretion and kidney stone formation has been fully established [11]. The incidence of hypocitraturia varies from 20% to 60% in people who have a propensity to form stones, either as a single abnormality or in conjunction with other metabolic disorders [16]. Hypercalciuria may occur either when filtered calcium is abnormally increased or when its reabsorption is abnormally decreased. The former may be associated with enhanced bone resorption which raises calcium bioavailability at the systemic level, while the latter may be the consequence of decreased renal function as occurs in CKD. Theoretically, reduced GFR in CKD should lead to decreased urinary calcium concentration, but the consequences of defective tubular reabsorption are more relevant and are responsible for the supersaturation of calcium salts. In addition, in the distal nephron, calcium reabsorption is a PTH-dependent process, PTH being the hormone capable of stimulating the resorption of the bone matrix in response to low, systemic calcium availability [81]. Therefore, as the decrease in the renal function progresses, PTH levels and bone loss gradually increase, thus explaining why kidney stones are a significant predictor of osteoporotic fracture in patients with CKD [82]. Moreover, when nephrolithiasis occurs, patients are frequently advised to reduce calcium intake, thus favouring a negative calcium balance which is an additional risk factor promoting a decrease in BMD [11].

Recent findings have demonstrated that lithogenic risk factors, including hypocitraturia, are also detectable in patients without kidney stones who exhibit osteoporosis or osteopenia, thus leading to the hypothesis that the evaluation of lithogenic risk could have significant implications for monitoring bone health status [34,83].

4.2. Postmenopausal Osteopenia and "Net Citrate Loss"

Estrogen deficiency and aging are the main factors responsible for the depletion of bone mass [84], but they are also associated with changes in urine composition which are similar to those of subjects having an increased risk of kidney stones [11]. The circulating citrate levels and the citrate content in bone are markedly reduced in animals with age-related or ovariectomy-induced bone loss [85]. A low citrate excretion, less severe than true hypocitraturia fixed at less than 320 mg per day, has been described in postmenopausal women [11,33] and in subjects with a low bone mass [34,83]. Nurses' Health Study II considered an ongoing cohort of 108,639 participants from whom information on menopause and kidney stones was obtained. In general, postmenopausal status was associated with lower BMD and a higher incidence of kidney stones in this cohort. Moreover, small but significant differences in urine composition were found in 658 participants who had pre- and postmenopausal 24-h urine analyses, including a lower citrate excretion [86].

The postmenopausal decline in estrogen concentration influences the activation rate of basic multicellular units composed of bone-resorbing osteoclasts and bone-forming osteoblasts. However, according to Drake et al., resorption increased by 90% while formation increased by only 45% [87] and the final result was a "net bone loss". This imbalanced bone remodelling depends on the effects that the lack of estrogen has on bone cells. On the one hand, the activity of the receptor activator of the nuclear factor-κ B ligand (RANKL) is promoted, a key factor in osteoclast differentiation; on the other hand, the osteogenic precursors are destined to differentiate into adipocytes, and the survival of mature osteoblasts is suppressed [88]. The result is the reduction of mature osteoblasts, and since they are the cells capable of synthesising citrate [5], the consequence is lower citrate production which impairs the quality and the stability of the bone microarchitecture [38,40]. Moreover, osteoclast differentiation and bone resorption are energy-demanding processes, and the citrate which is synthesised cannot be accumulated because it is essentially utilised through the citric acid cycle [89,90]. Similarly, the MSC differentiation towards adipocytes requires more citrate as a source of cytosolic acetylCoA for lipid biosynthesis [85]. In conclusion, according to Granchi et al., estrogen deficiency leads to a "net citrate loss" which could explain the diminished citrate excretion observed in postmenopausal women [91].

4.3. Genetic Variations Influencing Citrate Homeostasis and Skeletal Development

The "Online Mendelian Inheritance in Man®" database (OMIM®) is a comprehensive repository of information on the relationship between genetic variation and phenotypic expression [92]. The annotations connecting citrate homeostasis with skeletal defects are listed in Table 2, and many of these concern Slc proteins, which are a family of solute transporters through the membranes.

Mutations of the Cl2/HCO3·2 exchanger AE1, encoded by SLC4A1 which is expressed in red blood cells and in type A intercalated cells of the renal collecting tubule, may be responsible for distal renal tubular acidosis (dRTA), with or without haemolytic anemia. The corresponding phenotype displays defective urine acidification, nephrocalcinosis, nephrolithiasis, hypercalciuria, and hypocitraturia [93]. The clinical phenotype in patients with inherited dRTA is characterised by stunted growth with bone abnormalities in children, as well as nephrocalcinosis and nephrolithiasis which develop as the consequence of hypercalciuria, hypocitraturia, and relatively alkaline urine.

The same cytogenetic location of SLC4A1 (17q21.31) is involved in Glycogen storage disease Ia which is caused by a deficiency in glucose-6-phosphatase activity that catalyses the synthesis of glucose from glucose-6-phosphate. This enzymopathy results in a failure to maintain normal glucose control with glycogen accumulation in the liver, kidney, and intestine. Low citrate excretion and hypercalciuria have been described by Weinstein et al. (2001), and the combination of these metabolic alterations correlated with the onset of nephrocalcinosis and nephrolithiasis [94]. Furthermore, there is increasing evidence that poor metabolic control, including chronic acidosis (lactic), low muscle mass and delayed puberty, may negatively affect BMD in half of the patients [95].

NaCT is the sodium-coupled tricarboxylate transporter predominantly expressed in the liver, at several-fold lower levels in the testis and the brain, and at weak levels in the kidney and the heart.

The association between the mutations of the SLC13a5 gene on chromosome 17p13 and early infantile epileptic encephalopathy-25 with amelogenesis imperfecta has been clearly recognised [96]. More recently, Irizarry et al. have shown that SLC13a5 deficiency led to decreased BMD and impaired bone formation in homozygote (Slc13a5-/-) and heterozygote (Slc13a5+/-) mice [97]. As shown by Diaz et al. (2017), the epigenetic modulation of SLC13a5 gene may also influence skeletal development, since DNA hypermethylation and low gene expression have been found in the placenta and cord blood of infants born small-for-gestational-age and correlated with low height and weight at birth, low BMD, and low mineral content [98].

Bartter syndrome refers to a group of autosomal recessive disorders characterised by impaired salt reabsorption in the thick ascending limb of the loop of Henle with pronounced salt wasting, e.g., potassium and calcium, and hypokalemic metabolic alkalosis [99]. The antenatal variant or Bartter syndrome type I is caused by a homozygous or compound heterozygous mutation in the sodium-potassium-chloride cotransporter-2 gene [100]. The affected infants develop marked hypercalciuria and, as a secondary consequence, nephrocalcinosis and osteopenia [101]. To the best of the authors' knowledge, low citrate excretion in patients affected by Bartter syndrome has not been described, but citrate potassium administration is able to correct biochemical alterations [102,103].

Familial hypomagnesemia with hypercalciuria and nephrocalcinosis is an autosomal-recessive renal tubular disorder caused by mutations in claudin-16 and claudin-19, which are members of the transmembrane family proteins regulating calcium and magnesium reabsorption in the kidney [104]. Thorleifsson et al. have also identified claudin-14 as a major risk gene of hypercalciuric nephrolithiasis associated with a decrease in BMD [105]. Patients can develop hypomagnesaemia, hypercalciuria, and nephrocalcinosis, and their clinical course is often complicated by the progressive loss of kidney function. Other biochemical anomalies consist of elevated serum PTH levels before the onset of CKD, incomplete distal tubular acidosis, hyperuricemia and hypocitraturia [106]. Additional symptoms may be recurrent urinary tract infections, nephrolithiasis, polyuria, polydipsia and/or failure to thrive [106]. Amelogenesis imperfecta has also been described in some patients [107].

The human gene SLC13A2 encodes the sodium-dicarboxylate cotransporter (NaDC1) which is highly expressed in the brush-border membranes of the renal proximal tubule and intestinal cells, and reabsorbs Krebs cycle intermediates, i.e., succinate and citrate [108]. Although to date no distinctive phenotype has been linked with SLC13A2 variation in the OMIM database, Okamoto et al. (2006) have hypothesised that NaDC1 alterations could play a role in the development of kidney stones by affecting the citrate concentration in the urine [109]. The functional properties and protein expression of eight coding region variants of NaDC1 have recently been characterised; the majority of them appeared to decrease transport activity and were predicted to result in decreased citrate absorption in the intestine and kidney [110]. Even if not investigated, it is reasonable to assume that effects on bone mass may occur since these conditions influence citrate metabolism and predispose to renal stone formation as well.

The mitochondrial CTP, coded by the SLC25A1 gene located on chromosome 22q11.21, is embedded in the inner membrane and determines the efflux of tricarboxylic citrate from the mitochondria to cytosol in exchange for dicarboxylic malate [111]. The high citrate concentration into cytoplasm modulates the lipid synthesis and affects glycolysis by inhibiting phosphofructokinase-1 [112]. Genetic variations of SLC25A1 mainly lead to inheritable diseases featured by alterations of the central nervous system (combined D-2- and L-2-hydroxyglutaric aciduria; OMIM ID: 615182) and skeletal muscle (congenital myasthenic syndrome-23; OMIM ID: 618197) while the presence of bone defects is less relevant. However, SLC25A1 impairment also occurs in the 22q11.2 deletion syndrome which is characterised by congenital absence of the thymus and parathyroid glands as well as cardiac, renal and eye anomalies, developmental delay, and also skeletal defects. As additional evidence of a relationship between citrate transport and bone pathophysiology, it has been shown that SLC25A1 knockout in mice causes a notable decrease in the number of osteoblasts and the amount of osteoid [113].

As mentioned above, zinc plays a crucial role in regulating the extracellular bioavailability of citrate in the formation of new mineralised matrix and, therefore, gene defects involving a zinc transporter may be involved in alterations of the citrate metabolism and bone diseases. Of these, the solute carrier 39A family (SLC39A or ZIP) controls the influx of zinc into the cytoplasm [56]. In a previous study, the authors found that SLC39A13 (ZIP13) is upregulated throughout osteogenic differentiation, and no changes were recorded during the mineralisation process [58]. SLC39A13 gene defects have been associated with low bone mass in knockout mice [56] and spondylodysplastic Ehlers-Danlos syndrome, type 3 (Phenotype MIM number 612350).

Table 2. Genes involved in the regulation of citrate homeostasis with a genotype/phenotype relationship regarding skeletal development and/or bone metabolism (retrieved from the OMIM®database, last access 25 May 2019).

Gene/Locus Name	Gene/Locus	Cytogenetic Location	MIM Number: Phenotype	Inheritance
Solute carrier family 4, anion exchanger, member 1 (erythrocyte membrane protein band 3, Diego blood group)	SLC4A1, AE1, EPB3, SPH4, SAO, CHC	17q21.31	179800: Distal renal tubular acidosis	Autosomal dominant
Solute carrier family 4, anion exchanger, member 1 (erythrocyte membrane protein band 3, Diego blood group)	SLC4A1, AE1, EPB3, SPH4, SAO, CHC	17q21.31	611590: Distal renal tubular acidosis	Autosomal recessive
Glucose-6-phosphatase, catalytic	G6PC, G6PT	17q21.31	232200: Glycogen storage disease Ia	Autosomal recessive
Solute carrier family 13 (sodium-dependent citrate transporter), member 5	SLC13A5, NACT, INDY	17p13.1	615905: Early infantile, epileptic encephalopathy, 25	Autosomal recessive
Solute carrier family 12 (sodium/potassium/chloride transporters), member 1	SLC12A1, NKCC2	15q21.1	60167: Bartter syndrome, type 1	Autosomal recessive
Claudin 16 (paracellin 1)	CLDN16, PCLN1, HOMG3	3q28	248250: Renal hypomagnesemia 3	Autosomal recessive

5. Medical Management of Patients with Metabolic Bone Diseases Associated with Citrate Alterations

5.1. Clinical Work-Up

At present, the guidelines dealing with the clinical management of metabolic bone diseases do not highlight the role of citrate in maintaining bone integrity. Nevertheless, based on research findings, the causes of hypocitraturia should be considered in carrying out a complete evaluation of patients who present BMD alterations; vice versa, the accurate monitoring of BMD is advisable in subjects who have reduced urinary citrate excretion.

Regarding laboratory investigations, citrate homeostasis should be evaluated together with all factors which influence mineral metabolism. Although citrate excretion must be measured over a 24-h period and referred to the 24 h-urine volume, the detection of citrate levels in fasting-morning urine (expressed as creatinine ratios) may be an addional element to complete the metabolic profile. Urine pH can be a valid and simple indicator of acid-base balance. Laboratory testings for evaluation of mineral metabolism have to be carried out on plasma and urine by considering renal function, calcium-phosphorus balance, other electrolytes (in particular, potassium and magnesium), and calciotropic hormones. In addition, bone turnover markers (BTMs), including bone-resorption and bone formation indicators, are considered a useful and inexpensive tool for evaluating turnover rate (high or low) and response to any treatment [114].

Quantitative assessment of BMD is mandatory for evaluating bone health status and for calculating fracture risk [115]. Dual-energy X-ray absorptiometry (DXA), the T score (the number of standard deviations above or below the mean for a healthy 30-year-old adult of the same sex and ethnicity), or the Z-score (the number of standard deviations above or below the mean for the patients of the same age, sex and ethnicity) are employed for measuring areal density ($g \cdot cm^{-2}$) at any skeletal site. The assesment of bone quality may be additionally explored by evaluating the trabecular bone score which reflects bone microarchitecture [116]. "High-resolution peripheral quantitative computed-tomography" allows an accurate assessment of bone strength; however, due to its elevated cost, the diffusion of this technology is still limited.

Even though noninvasive techniques are preferred, bone biopsy remains a valid tool for assessing the tissue quality in metabolic bone diseases, and it is the gold standard for estimating bone impairment in kidney disease and for guiding the clinician in deciding proper treatment [117]. In fact, according to the Kidney Disease Improving Global Outcomes (KDIGO) guidelines, the term renal osteodystrophy may be used exclusively to define the histological alterations in bone morphology associated with CKD, which can be additionally assessed using histomorphometry. Instead, without histological confirmation, the clinical syndrome which develops as a systemic disorder of the mineral and the bone metabolisms is generally called "CKD-Mineral and Bone Disorder" [69,118]. However, bone biopsies in a routine work-up present some drawbacks, which are foremost the availability limited to specialised centres, discomfort for the patients, and the length of time required to process and analyse bone tissue.

Whenever instrumental and laboratory investigations show a significant bone loss, pharmacological treatment has to be planned according to the indications of the current guidelines, eventually adding specific drugs in case of secondary osteoporosis. Moreover, all recommendations related to lifestyle and dietary modifications should be explained to the patient [115]. In the presence of low urine citrate excretion, citrate-based supplements could be recommended to prevent progressive damage to bone and a progressive reduction in BMD.

5.2. Dietary Modification

Since hypocitraturia may depend on food habits (Table 1), dietary modifications should be considered as a first level intervention for the medical management of citrate deficiencies. Diet is aimed at correcting the excessive acid load and, as a consequence, the negative effects that acidosis has on bone metabolism [119]. The acid-ash hypothesis emphasises the role of the skeleton in maintaining the acid-base balance since the hydroxyapatite of the mineral matrix is a reservoir of alkali groups which may be released to neutralise proton excess [120]. Acute and chronic acid loading show distinct effects, with acute acidity first eroding the bone surface to release sodium, potassium and bicarbonate into the circulation, while chronic acidity leads to the release of calcium and phosphate [121]. Moreover, acidosis directly influences the activity of bone cells within the bone remodelling unit by promoting osteoclast-mediated resorption and inhibiting bone formation by osteoblasts [65]. Hypocitraturia is a response to the elevated acid load occurring in metabolic acidosis, since there is a notable increase in citrate reabsorption in the renal proximal tubule when the tubular pH decreases [16]. In this regard, there is consensus in considering citraturia as a biomarker for monitoring diet and the metabolism-dependent systemic acid-base status, even in subjects without overt metabolic acidosis [33–35].

Under physiological conditions, the acid-base balance is strictly controlled by net endogenous acid production related to acid and alkali dietary intake, and incomplete metabolism of organic acids. By using proper methods, such as "net endogenous acid production" (NEAP) [122] and "potential renal acid load" (PRAL) [123], it is possible to determine the production of acids and characterise foods according to their ability to release acids and bases into the bloodstream. The prolonged and excessive consumption of acid precursor foods leads to chronic low-grade metabolic acidosis which reduces the excretion of citrate and predisposes to diseases [124], including alteration of bone health status, especially in older subjects with diminished renal function [125]. Some authors have discarded the acid-ash hypothesis, claiming that the increase in the diet acid load did not promote skeletal bone mineral loss or osteoporosis [126], and the main role in regulating acid-base homeostasis should be attributed to the kidney [127]. However, the above studies did not consider the role played by citrate in preserving the mineralised matrix and it would be interesting to know whether the relationship between acid dietary intake and alterations in the bone metabolism varied according to low or normal urine citrate excretion. As supporting evidence for the link between citrate and bone health, previous studies have demonstrated a positive correlation between citrate excretion and radius densitometric values in pre- and postmenopause, as well as a significant relationship between citraturia and the prevalence of vertebral fracture in postmenopausal women [11].

The general dietary approach to counteract elevated acid load is to limit the intake of foods with a high acidifying potential, i.e., meat (beef, pork, poultry), fish and seafood, eggs, beans and oilseeds, in favour of foods which contribute the most to the release of bases, i.e., fruits and vegetables [128]. However, dietary modifications cannot disregard the medical history of the patients, and the best nutritional approach should be evaluated on a case-by-case basis. For instance, in the elderly, inadequate protein intake could be a greater problem for bone health than protein excess [129], and the intake of high amounts of fruits and vegetables could be contraindicated in patients with CKD due to their high potassium content [130].

The intake of foods with a high citrate content may be a valid approach to compensate for the high demand due to acidosis or other causes of hypocitraturia [24,124]. The daily citrate intake is approximately 4 grams, and almost all citrate introduced by exogenous sources is absorbed into the gastrointestinal tract, arrives in the liver and is metabolised to bicarbonate [11].

Prezioso et al. (2015) examined the relationship between a diet rich in vegetables and urinary citrate excretion [24]. Fruits and vegetables (except for those with high oxalate content) favour citrate excretion; consequently, they decrease urinary saturation for CaOx and CaP, thus having a protective effect on the formation of kidney stones [24]. In general, fruit intake is lower in hypocitraturic than in normocitraturic subjects [131].

In order to provide dietary recommendations aimed at correcting hypocitraturia, Haleblian et al. (2008) carried out an exhaustive analysis of citrate concentrations in citrus juices, noncitrus juices, and commercially available beverages. The highest concentration was found in grapefruit juice (35% more than in lemon juice), and a glass corresponded approximately to a 40 mEq tablet of potassium citrate. In general, commercial beverages had lower amounts of citrate [7].

Several authors have studied the possible influence of the consumption of fruit juices (both citrus and noncitrus) on urinary citrate excretion. Orange juice increased the excretion of urinary oxalate, and therefore, its consumption could result in the biochemical modification of stone risk factors [132]. It should also be noted that grapefruit juice significantly increased urinary oxalate levels, but it was not associated with an increased lithogenic risk probably due to the protective effect of the high citrate content [133]. Regarding noncitrus juices, cranberry juice had a controversial effect on urine citrate (no effect or an increase of 31%), but resulted in a significantly increased concentration of urinary calcium and oxalate. In addition, diluted blackcurrant juice and melon had a positive effect in increasing citraturia [24]. In a recent meta-analysis, Pachaly et al. aimed at systematically investigating the effects of dietary measures on urinary citrate and nephrolithiasis [124]. They searched for randomised controlled and crossover studies which evaluated urine citrate excretion after the intake of citrus-based beverages, including fruit juices and soft drinks, calcium/magnesium rich mineral water, a high-fibre diet, a low-animal-protein diet, and plant extracts. The authors identified thirteen studies involving 358 participants, the majority of whom were stone formers. Summarised estimates showed a significant increase in citraturia levels only in subjects who consumed fruit juice and other beverages while the other dietary modifications did not determine significant changes [7,8].

Clinical trials aimed at evaluating whether an increase in dietary citrate preserved the bone health status are lacking. In a clinical trial, postmenopausal women were randomised into four groups, i.e., a diet (additional daily portion of 300 g of self-selected fruit and vegetables), two doses of potassium citrate (12.5 and 55.5 mEq/day) and a placebo (control group). The participants were followed for two years, and the effects on bone turnover were determined by measuring BTMs and BMD. The authors concluded that neither potassium citrate nor fruit and vegetables influenced bone turnover or prevented BMD loss over 2 years in healthy postmenopausal women (Table 3) [134].

In summary, natural sources of dietary citrate should be considered as a first option for preventing kidney stone recurrence as an alternative to medical treatment [24]. From a theoretical point of view, published data have suggested that dietary modifications could also be effective in preserving bone health. However, at present, there is insufficient evidence supporting the use of natural sources of citrate as the sole treatment for preventing bone loss.

5.3. Citrate-Based Supplements

Nephrolithiasis was the first clinical condition in which oral citrate supplementation showed therapeutic efficacy, particularly in lowering high stone recurrence rate which is more prevalent in people with low urinary citrate levels [11]. The rationale for using citrate salts in kidney stone disease was explained in previous paragraphs and was based on four main issues: (1) citrate salts are rapidly absorbed through the intestine and equally rapidly filtered in the urine; (2) citrate forms calcium citrate complexes, which in turn increase solubility and decrease the amount of free calcium in urine; (3) citrate acts as an inhibitor of CaOx and CaP crystal growth and aggregation, and (4) in the intestine, the complexation between calcium and citrate reduces enteric absorption of calcium, and therefore renal excretion. A recent systematic review has demonstrated that citrate-based therapy reduced recurrent calcium urinary stone formation compared to controls (placebo, usual care) [135]; however, evidence was limited in children [136].

There have also been interventional clinical trials concerning the effect of citrate supplements in preserving bone health status. As stated for dietary modifications, the rationale of the published trials was based on the assumption that citrate-based supplements may be useful as alkalising agents which neutralise the effects of an excessive acid load [16,65,119–121]. Other than diets rich in salt and animal protein [128], several conditions may induce low-grade acidosis, and the majority of them are age-related, such as menopause [33], subclinical inflammatory status [137], and decreased renal function [68]. On the basis of this assumption, Lambert et al. (2015) carried out a meta-analysis aimed at determining whether alkaline potassium salts, including potassium citrate and potassium bicarbonate, had some effect on calcium metabolism and bone health [138]. The seven eligible studies dealing with potassium citrate supplementation did not include subjects with nephrolithiasis and/or other relevant comorbidities in order to avoid confounding factors potentially leading to overestimation or underestimation of the intervention. Citrate salts significantly reduced calcium and acid excretion similarly to potassium bicarbonate, but they seemed to be more effective in preventing collagen resorption. However, insufficient data were available regarding changes in BMD, since it was investigated in only two studies. The authors found major differences in terms of study design, inclusion/exclusion criteria, doses, timing of supplement administration and outcome measures; this heterogeneity represented a notable limitation for translation into a clinical setting.

In the current review, the interventional clinical trials which were primarily aimed at evaluating the effect of citrate supplements on mineral metabolism and bone turnover were reviewed. Sixteen eligible studies were identified which (1) recruited more than 10 subjects, (2) excluded nephrolithiasis and other significant comorbidities and (3) reported the results related to bone health status, including BMD and/or BTMs. Data regarding study design, population, intervention, follow-up, additional supplementation or controlled dietary intake, as well as a summary of results and conclusions, are shown in Table 3.

Table 3. Interventional clinical trials based on the use of citrate supplements with primary or secondary outcomes related to bone health status.

Reference	Study Design; Population	Intervention (Dose/Day) (I) Control (C)	Other Supplements (Dose/Day) and/or Controlled Dietary Intake	Follow Up and Outcomes	BTM Changes (Intragroup)	Changes in BTM and BMD Induced by Intervention (Intergroup)	Conclusion
Dawson-Hughes, 1990 [141]	RCT, controlled vs placebo, double-blind; ≥6 months postmenopausal women (early, <5 years: n = 67; late, >5 years: n = 169); age ≥ 65 years	I1: Ca citrate malate (500 mg Ca), n = 78; I2: Ca carbonate (500 mg Ca), n = 78; C: Placebo (n = 80)	Controlled Ca intake	Baseline, 18, 24, 36 months; BTM (BAP) and BMD	I1: 24 months ↓ BAP; I2: 24 months ↓ BAP; C: 24 months ↓ BAP	BTM: I1 vs. C: 36 months ↓ BAP, related to the Ca intake; I2 vs. C: 36 months ↓ BAP, related to the Ca intake. BMD: I1 vs. C: 12, 24 months ↑ only in late postmenopause and Ca intake ≤400 mg/day; I2 vs C: ↓ in both groups	Adequate Ca intake is essential in preventing postmenopausal bone loss; Ca citrate is more effective than Ca carbonate.
Dawson-Hughes, 1997 [142]	RCT, controlled vs. placebo, double-blind; healthy subjects living in a community (176 M/ 213 F); age ≥ 65 years	I: Ca citrate malate (500 mg Ca) & Vit D3 (700 IU), n = 187; C: Placebo, n = 202	Controlled Ca intake	Baseline, 6, 12, 18, 24, 30, 36 months; BTM (OC, u-NTX) and BMD	I: n.s C: n.s	BTM: I vs. C: 36 months ↓ OC; BMD: I vs. C: 36 months ↑	Ca and vitamin D supplementation leads to a moderate reduction in bone loss and may substantially reduce the risk of nonvertebral fractures among elderly subjects who live in the community.
* Ruml, 1999 [143]	RCT, controlled vs. placebo; postmenopausal women (90% ≤5 years)	I: Ca citrate (800 mg Ca), n = 25; C: Placebo, n = 31		Baseline, 12, 24 months BTM (BAP, OC, u-NTX, u-OH proline) and BMD	I: all BTMs are ↓, at unspecified time points	BMD: I: 24 months, stable	Ca citrate supplementation averted bone loss and stabilised bone density in early postmenopausal women.
Sellmeyer, 2002 [144]	RCT, controlled vs. placebo, double-blind; ≥2 years postmenopausal women; age I: 65 ± 8 years; C: 63 ± 8 years	I: K citrate (90 mmol), n = 26; C: Placebo, n = 26	Ca carbonate (500 mg); controlled salt intake	Baseline, 1 months; BTM (OC, u-NTX)	I: n.s. C: 1 month ↓ OC, ↑ u-NTX	BTM: I vs. C: 1 month ↓ u-NTX	K citrate prevents increased bone resorption due to high salt intake.
Dawson-Hughes, 2002 [145]	RCT, controlled vs. placebo, double-blind; healthy subjects (161 M/ 181F); normal BMD; age ≥ 65 years	I: Ca citrate malate (500 mg Ca), n = 158; C: Placebo, n = 184	Vitamin D3 (700 IU); controlled protein intake	Baseline, 18, 36 months; BTM (OC, u-NTX) and BMD	I: 36 months ↓ u-NTX, related to the protein intake; C: n.s.	BTM: I vs C: 36 months, ↓ u-NTX; BMD: I vs C: 36 month, ↑ related to the protein intake	BMD may be improved by increasing protein intake as long as an adequate intake of Ca and vitamin D is assumed.

Table 3. Cont.

Reference	Study Design; Population	Intervention (Dose/Day) Control (C)	Other Supplements (Dose/Day) and/or Controlled Dietary Intake	Follow Up and Outcomes	BTM Changes (Intragroup)	Changes in BTM and BMD Induced by Intervention (Intergroup)	Conclusion
Marangella, 2004 [146]	Controlled vs. untreated; postmenopausal women; T score: <−1.0; age: 43–72 years	I: K citrate 37–74 mEq (≈1 mEq/kg), $n = 30$; C: No treatment, $n = 24$	Controlled Ca intake	Baseline, 3 months BTM (BAP, OC, u-OH proline, u-DPD)	I: 3 months ↓ OC, u-OH proline, u-DPD; C: 3 months ↑ OC	not shown	K citrate decreases bone resorption thereby contrasting the potential adverse effects caused by chronic acidemia. The implication for the prevention and treatment of postmenopausal osteoporosis has to be confirmed.
Kenny, 2004 [147]	RCT, crossover, open label, 2 phases; 3 months/phase with a washout period of 2 weeks between phases; postmenopausal women; T score: <−1.0 and >−3.5; age: 73 ± 5 years	I1: Ca citrate (1000 mg Ca), $n = 20$; I2: Ca carbonate (1000 mg Ca), $n = 20$	Vitamin D3 (900 IU); controlled Ca intake	Baseline, 1, 3 months (each phase) BTM (BAP, OC, NTX, u-CTX, u-NTX, u-DPD)	I1: 3 months ↓ NTX, u-CTX, u-NTX, u-DPD I2: n.s		Ca citrate inhibits bone resorption more than Ca carbonate.
Sakhaee, 2005 [139]	RCT, crossover, placebo controlled, double-blind, 4 phases; 2 weeks/phase with a washout period of 2 weeks between phases; postmenopausal women; age: 48–76 years	I1: K citrate (40 mEq), $n = 18$; I2: Ca citrate (800 mg), $n = 18$; I3: K citrate (40 mEq) and Ca citrate (800 mg), $n = 18$ C (1st phase): Placebo, $n = 18$	Rigid diet with fixed content of protein, Ca, P, Na, K and fluids	Baseline and at the end of each phase; BTM (BAP, CTX, OC, u-NTX, u-OH proline)	I1: n.s I2: ↓ CTX, u-OH proline I3: ↓ CTX, u-OH proline, u-NTX	I3 vs I1: ↓ u NTX	In postmenopausal women, combined treatment with K citrate and Ca citrate decreases bone resorption by providing an alkali load and increasing absorbed Ca.
Jehle, 2006 [148]	RCT, controlled; ≥5 years postmenopausal women; T score −1/−4; age: ≤70 years	I: K citrate (30 mEq), $n = 82$; C: KCl (30 mmol), $n = 79$	Ca carbonate (500 mg), Vitamin D3 (400 IU); free, nonvegetarian diet	Baseline, 3, 6, 9, 12 months; BTM (BAP, CTX, OC, u-DPD, u-PD) and BMD	I: 3 months, ↓ u-DPD, u-PD; 6 months, ↑ BAP and ↓ OC, u-DPD, u-PD; 9 months, ↓ u-DPD, u-PD; 12 months, ↑ BAP and ↓ OC, u-DPD, u-PD; C: 3 months, ↓ OC, u-DPD, u-PD; 6 months, ↑ BAP, u-DPD, u-PD and ↓ OC; 9 months, ↑ u-DPD, u-PD and ↓ OC; 12 months, ↑ BAP, u-DPD, u-PD and ↓ OC	BTM I vs C: 3 months, ↓ u-DPD BMD I vs C: 12 months ↑	In postmenopausal women, bone mass can be increased significantly by K citrate. The effect on bone resorption seems to be unrelated to K intake.

Table 3. Cont.

Reference	Study Design; Population	Intervention (Dose/Day) (I) Control (C)	Other Supplements (Dose/Day) and/or Controlled Dietary Intake	Follow Up and Outcomes	BTM Changes (Intragroup)	Changes in BTM and BMD Induced by Intervention (Intergroup)	Conclusion
Macdonald, 2008 [134]	RCT, controlled vs. placebo, double-blind for I1 e I2; ≥5 years postmenopausal women; age: 49–54 years	I1: K citrate (55.5 mEq), $n = 70$ I2: K citrate (18.5 mEq), $n = 70$ I3: Diet (300 g fruit = 18.5 mEq alkali), $n = 66$ C: Placebo, $n = 70$	Food diary (free nonvegetarian diet)	Baseline, 3, 6, 12, 18, 24 months; BTM (CTX, P1NP, u-DPD) and BMD	I1: n.s. I2: n.s. I3: n.s. C: n.s	BTM I1, I2, I3 vs. C: n.s BMD I1, I2, I3 vs. C: n.s	In healthy postmenopausal women, neither K citrate at 18.5 or 55.6 mEq/d, nor 300 g self-selected fruit and vegetables influenced bone turnover or prevented BMD loss over 2 years.
Thomas, 2008 [149]	RCT, crossover, double-blind, 2 phases; postmenopausal women for 2 to 6 years; age: 50–60 years	I1: Ca carbonate (1000 mg Ca), $n = 12$ I2: 2) Ca citrate (500 mg Ca), $n = 13$	Controlled Ca intake	Baseline, 7 days; BTM (CTX)	I1: 7 days, ↓ CTX I2: 7 days, ↓ CTX		Ca citrate is at least as effective as Ca carbonate in decreasing PTH and CTX cross-links, at half the dose. All changes are numerically superior after Ca citrate supplementation.
Karp, 2009 [140]	RCT, controlled, 24 h study sessions; women of child-bearing age: 22–30 years	I1: Ca carbonate (1000 mg Ca), $n = 12$ I2: Ca citrate (Ca: 1000 mg; citrate: 3145 mg), $n = 12$ I3: K citrate (K: 57 mEq; citrate: 3145 mg), $n = 12$	4-day diary to estimate food habits before starting the study session; the meals served during each study session were identical	Baseline, 2, 4, 6, 8, 20, 24 h; BTM (BAP, u-NTX) and BMD	I1: 24 h, ↓ u-NTX I2: n.s I3: 24 h, ↓ u-NTX		K citrate supplementation decreases urinary Ca excretion and reduces bone resorption even when the diet is not acidogenic, and reduces the bone resorption marker despite low Ca intake.
Jehle, 2013 [150]	RCT, controlled vs. placebo, double-blind; healthy subjects (79 M/122 F); T score > −2.5; age 65–80 years; women were past the perimenopausal peak turnover	I: K citrate (60 mEq), $n = 101$ C: Placebo, $n = 100$	Ca carbonate (500 mg), Vitamin D3 (400 IU); free nonvegetarian diet	Baseline, 6, 12, 18, 24; BTM (BAP, P1NP, u-NTX) and BMD	I: 6, 12 months, ↓ u-NTX; 18, 24 months, ↑ P1NP C: n.s.	BTM I vs. C: 6 months, ↓ u-NTX BMD I vs. C: 12, 18, 24 months ↑	K citrate administered in a background of vitamin D and Ca supplementation is well tolerated and constitutes an inexpensive intervention to improve BMD and bone microarchitecture in healthy elderly people.
Moseley, 2013 [151]	RCT, controlled vs. placebo, double blind; healthy subjects (17 M/35 F); age ≥ 55 years; women were ≥5 years postmenopause	I1: K citrate (60 mmol), $n = 17$ I2: K citrate (90 mmol), $n = 17$ C: Placebo, $n = 18$	Ca citrate (630 mg), Vitamin D3 (400 IU); controlled Ca, Na, P, protein, fat intake	Baseline, 6 months; BTM, (BAP, CTX)		BTM I1, I2 vs. C: 6 months, ↓ CTX	K citrate decreases markers of bone resorption over 6 months, but a significant improvement in Ca balance is obtained with 90 mmol/day. This dose is well tolerated.

Table 3. Cont.

Reference	Study Design; Population	Intervention (Dose/Day) (I) Control (C)	Other Supplements (Dose/Day) and/or Controlled Dietary Intake	Follow Up and Outcomes	BTM Changes (Intragroup)	Changes in BTM and BMD Induced by Intervention (Intergroup)	Conclusion
Gregory, 2015 [152]	RCT, controlled vs. placebo, double-blind; ≥2 year postmenopausal women s; T score: <−1.0 > −2.5, or <−2.5 unable to take any other medication; age I: 65.1 ± 5.9 years; C: 66.1 ± 7.1 years	I: K citrate (40 mEq), n = 42 C: Placebo, n = 41	Ca citrate (630 mg), Vitamin D3 (400 IU); free nonvegetarian diet	Baseline, 1, 3, 6, 12 months; BTM (BAP, OC, P1NP, u-NTX) and BMD	I: 1 month, ↓ P1NP; 3, 6, 12 months, ↓ P1NP, u-NTX C: I: 6 months, ↓ P1NP u-NTX; 12 months, ↓ P1NP	BTM I vs. C: n.s BMD I: 12 months, stable	In postmenopausal osteopenia, K citrate improves the effect of supplementation with Ca citrate and Vitamin D, as proven by the more rapid decrease in BTM levels.
Granchi, 2018 [91]	RCT, controlled vs. placebo, double-blind; ≥5 years postmenopausal women; T score: <−1.0 and >−2.5; age I: 60.8 ± 1.0 years; C: 58.2 ± 1.1 years	I: K citrate (30 mEq), n = 20 C: Placebo, n = 20	Ca carbonate (500 mg), Vitamin D3 (400 IU); free nonvegetarian diet	Baseline, 3, 6 months; BTM (BAP, CTX, P1NP, TRAcP)	I: 6 months, ↓ BAP, CTX C: 3, 6 months, ↓ BAP, CTX	BTM I vs. C: 6 months ↓ BAP, CTX in subjects with low excretion of K and/or citrate, and/or low urine pH	In postmenopausal osteopenia, K citrate improves the effects of supplementation with Ca carbonate and vitamin D, but only in women with low K and/or citrate excretion and/or low urine pH.

C: control; I: Intervention; RCT: randomised clinical trial; K citrate: potassium citrate; Ca citrate: calcium citrate; KCl: potassium chloride; Na: sodium; P: phosporus; BMD: bone mineral density; BTM: bone turnover markers; n.a.: not applicable; n.s.: not significant; BAP: bone-specific alkaline phosphatase; BMD: bone mineral density; K: tpotassium; Ca: calcium; u-DPD: urinary deoxypyridinoline; u-PYR: urinary pyridinoline; u-OH proline: urinary hydroxyproline; OC: osteocalcin; P1NP: amino-terminal propeptide of type 1 procollagen; u-NTX: urinary N-telopeptide of collagen type 1; M: male; F: female; IU: International Units; PTH: parathyroid hormone; ↓ and ↑ show significant decreases and increases, respectively, according to the criteria indicated by the authors. * Partial data collected from the abstract.

The authors investigated the effect of potassium citrate (one clinical trial, seven randomised clinical trials (RCTs)) [92,134,139–144], calcium citrate (four RCTs and two crossover studies) [145–150], and two studies compared the above-mentioned treatments (one RCT, one crossover study) [139,140]. Regarding the intervention under investigation, doses, timing of administration, and follow-up varied greatly among the trials and, in thirteen studies, the co-administration of additional supplements was planned, i.e., calcium carbonate and/or vitamin D3. The majority of the studies included postmenopausal women ($n = 11$) while, in one study, the participants were of childbearing age. The other trials were designed to recruit healthy individuals, i.e., males and females at least 55 years of age. The dietary intake of calcium and/or protein and/or salts was controlled in ten studies; in five studies, the subject consumed a free nonvegetarian diet; in one study, the management of food habits was not described.

Overall, the studies selected provided more than 1000 experimental cases and more than 900 controls. As Lambert et al. reported previously, very high heterogeneity among the studies was observed, and therefore the meta-analysis lost its inferential value while the descriptive overview was more informative. By examining the conclusions reported by various authors, two recurring key points emerged: (1) an adequate calcium intake was essential in preventing bone loss in elderly subjects and in postmenopausal women, and calcium citrate seemed to be more effective than calcium carbonate [145–150] and (2) potassium citrate prevented the increased bone resorption caused by menopause, chronic acidemia and high salt intake [139–144].

Additional findings regarding potassiun citrate can be summarised as follows: effectiveness may be enhanced by combined treatment with calcium citrate [139]; positive effects have also been observed in young women and in the absence of an excessive acid load [140]. Moreover, supplementation with alkalising potassium citrate improved the beneficial effects of calcium and vitamin D only in osteopenic postmenopausal women who exhibited the target conditions, namely low potassium and/or citrate excretion and/or low urine pH [91]. Finally, one study questioned the beneficial effects of potassium citrate since, at 24 months, no significant modifications in BTMs and BMD were recorded [134]. It should be noted that compliance may decrease by 25% over time, mainly due to gastrointestinal side effects (approximately 10%) and costs [24].

Despite the encouraging results, a consensus statement regarding the use of citrate supplementation for the management of metabolic bone diseases is still lacking since the heterogeneity of the current evidence is a major limitation for identifying the best practice. Interestingly, the identification of subjects who better respond to exogenous citrate supplementation could be the correct way to maximise the beneficial effect of the treatment.

6. Conclusions

Since citrate is a ubiquitous metabolite with a multidimensional role in the human organism, it is not surprising that it is involved in the pathophysiology of tissues, organs and systems. In fact, recent data in the literature have highlighted the relationship between citrate defects and various medical conditions with considerable financial and social impact, e.g., cancer [153], dyslipidemia [154], vascular calcifications [155], and visual disabilities [156].

Overall, this review has highlighted the main functions of citrate, and, more specifically, focused on the role of citrate in the pathophysiology and medical management of metabolic bone diseases, thus identifying some key points which are summarised in Table 4.

Although interest in the role of citrate is spreading, a consensus statement regarding the use of citrate supplementation for the management of metabolic bone diseases is still lacking, since the heterogeneity of the current evidence is a major limitation in identifying the best practice. Even when the study design is well planned, there are some reasons which may explain the difficulty in obtaining unique and compelling results from clinical trials.

First, dietary supplementation cannot be regarded as a pharmacological treatment, and therefore the effects on measurable clinical outcomes are expected to be less prominent. Hence, baseline differences between participants which are beyond the investigator's control become selection biases that attenuate the strength of randomisation and interfere with the interpretation of the results. On the other hand, current scientific knowledge provides a sufficient background, leading the clinician and the researcher to further investigate the beneficial effects of citrate-based treatment in depth, as proven by multiple studies which have dealt with this matter.

At present, it can be argued that the use of citrate supplementation should be considered in the medical management of bone diseases, but it is also reasonable to assume that the effects could be maximised in a personalised approach in which the scientific knowledge and the clinical judgement of practitioners are essential in identifying patients who could reap real benefits.

Table 4. The role of citrate in the pathophysiology and medical management of bone diseases.

Highlights
• Citrate is an essential metabolite and plays a pivotal role in maintaining the acid-base balance. • Citrate is an essential component of bone, and serves to maintain the integrity of the skeletal nano- and microstructures.
• Citrate is produced by osteoblasts but, at the same time, it influences their differentiation and functionality. • Bone tissue is the main source of citrate and is therefore a leading actor in maintaining citrate homeostasis. • Citrate excretion is a significant biomarker of citrate homeostasis.
• Genetic and acquired diseases characterised by an alteration in citrate homeostasis are often accompanied by alterations in the development and/or metabolism of bone tissue. • Exogenous supplementation may be a useful tool in treating medical conditions related to poor citrate bioavailability, including bone diseases.

Author Contributions: All the authors (D.G., N.B., F.M.U., and R.C.) participated in the development of the ideas for this review, contributed to reading the articles, and to the writing and editing the manuscript.

Funding: The research activity of D.G. and N.B. is supported, in part, by grants of Italian Government ("5 per mille 2017" and "Ricerca Corrente 2018–2020").

Acknowledgments: We acknowledge Gerald Goldsmith for his valuable assistance in revising the English language.

Conflicts of Interest: The authors declare no conflict of interest.

Abbreviations

acetylCoA: Acetyl Coenzyme A; ATP: Adenosine 5′-Triphosphate; BMD: Bone Mineral Density; BTM: Bone Turnover Marker; CaOx: Calcium-Oxalate; CaP: Calcium-Phosphate; CKD: Chronic Kidney Disease; CTP: mitochondrial Citrate-Transport Protein; dRTA: distal Renal Tubular Acidosis; DXA: Dual-energy X-ray Absorptiometry; GFR: Glomerular Filtration Rate; KDIGO: Kidney Disease Improving Global Outcomes; MSC: Mesenchymal Stem Cell; NaCT: Sodium-dependent Citrate Transporter; NaDC: Sodium-Dicarboxylate; NEAP: Net Endogenous Acid Production; OMIM: Online Mendelian Inheritance in Man; OPRA: Osteoporosis Prospective Risk Assessment; PRAL: Potential Renal Acid Load; PTH: Parathyroid Hormone; RCT: Randomised Clinical Trial; Slc: Solute Carrier; TCA cycle: Tricarboxylic Acid Cycle or Krebs cycle; ZIP1: Zinc Importer Protein 1.

References

1. Krebs, H.A.; Johnson, W.A. The role of citric acid in intermediate metabolism in animal tissues. *FEBS Lett.* **1980**, *117* (Suppl. 1), K1–K10. [CrossRef]
2. Available online: https://www.genome.jp/kegg-bin/show_pathway?map00020 (accessed on 4 July 2019).
3. Iacobazzi, V.; Infantino, V. Citrate—New functions for an old metabolite. *Biol. Chem.* **2014**, *395*, 387–399. [CrossRef] [PubMed]
4. Mycielska, M.E.; Milenkovic, V.M.; Wetzel, C.H.; Rümmele, P.; Geissler, E.K. Extracellular Citrate in Health and Disease. *Curr. Mol. Med.* **2015**, *15*, 884–891. [CrossRef] [PubMed]
5. Franklin, R.B.; Chellaiah, M.; Zou, J.; Reynolds, M.A.; Costello, L.C. Evidence that Osteoblasts are Specialized Citrate-producing Cells that Provide the Citrate for Incorporation into the Structure of Bone. *Open Bone J.* **2014**, *6*, 1–7. [CrossRef] [PubMed]

6. Dickens, F. The citric acid content of animal tissues, with reference to its occurrence in bone and tumour. *Biochem. J.* **1941**, *35*, 1011–1023. [CrossRef] [PubMed]
7. Haleblian, G.E.; Leitao, V.A.; Pierre, S.A.; Robinson, M.R.; Albala, D.M.; Ribeiro, A.A.; Preminger, G.M. Assessment of citrate concentrations in citrus fruit-based juices and beverages: Implications for management of hypocitraturic nephrolithiasis. *J. Endourol.* **2008**, *22*, 1359–1366. [CrossRef] [PubMed]
8. Penniston, K.L.; Nakada, S.Y.; Holmes, R.P.; Assimos, D.G. Quantitative assessment of citric acid in lemon juice, lime juice, and commercially-available fruit juice products. *J. Endourol.* **2008**, *22*, 567–570. [CrossRef] [PubMed]
9. Schuster, E.; Dunn-Coleman, N.; Frisvad, J.C.; Van Dijck, P.W. On the safety of *Aspergillus niger*—A review. *Appl. Microbiol. Biotechnol.* **2002**, *59*, 426–435. [CrossRef]
10. Hu, W.; Li, W.J.; Yang, H.Q.; Chen, J.H. Current strategies and future prospects for enhancing microbial production of citric acid. *Appl. Microbiol. Biotechnol.* **2019**, *103*, 201–209. [CrossRef]
11. Caudarella, R.; Vescini, F.; Buffa, A.; Stefoni, S. Citrate and mineral metabolism, kidney stones and bone disease. *Front. Biosci.* **2003**, *8*, s1084–s1106.
12. Fegan, J.; Khan, R.; Poindexter, J.; Pak, C.Y. Gastrointestinal citrate absorption in nephrolithiasis. *J. Urol.* **1992**, *147*, 1212–1214. [CrossRef]
13. Pajor, A.M. Sodium-coupled transporters for Krebs cycle intermediates. *Annu. Rev. Physiol.* **1999**, *61*, 663–682. [CrossRef] [PubMed]
14. Poerwono, H.; Higashiyama, K.; Kubo, H.; Poernomo, A.T.; Suharjono, I.; Sudiana, I.K.; Indrayanto, G.; Brittain, H.G. Citric acid. In *Analytical Profiles of Drug Substances and Excipients*, 1st ed.; Brittain, H.G., Ed.; Academic Press: San Diego, CA, USA, 2001; Volume 28, pp. 1–76.
15. Sakhaee, K.; Alpern, R.; Poindexter, J.; Pak, C.Y. Citraturic response to oral citric acid load. *J. Urol.* **1992**, *147*, 975–976. [CrossRef]
16. Zuckerman, J.M.; Assimos, D.G. Hypocitraturia: Pathophysiology and medical management. *Rev. Urol.* **2009**, *11*, 134–144. [CrossRef]
17. Costello, L.C.; Franklin, R.B. Plasma citrate homeostasis, how it is regulated, and its physiological and clinical implications. An important, but neglected, relationship in medicine. *HSOA J. Hum. Endocrinol.* **2016**, *1*, 5. [CrossRef]
18. Pak, C.Y.; Resnick, M. Medical therapy and new approaches to management of urolithiasis. *Urol. Clin. N. Am.* **2000**, *27*, 243–253. [CrossRef]
19. Mayo Clinic Medical Laboratories. Endocrinology Catalog Bone/Minerals. Available online: https://endocrinology.testcatalog.org/show/CITR (accessed on 30 May 2019).
20. Heller, H.J.; Sakhaee, K.; Moe, O.W.; Pak, C.Y. Etiological role of estrogen status in renal stone formation. *J. Urol.* **2002**, *168*, 1923–1927. [CrossRef]
21. Caudarella, R.; Vescini, F. Urinary citrate and renal stone disease: The preventive role of alkali citrate treatment. *Arch. Ital. Urol.* **2009**, *81*, 182–187.
22. Melnick, J.Z.; Preisig, P.A.; Moe, O.W.; Srere, P.; Alpern, R.J. Renal cortical mitochondrial aconitase is regulated in hypo- and hypercitraturia. *Kidney Int.* **1998**, *54*, 160–165. [CrossRef]
23. Lerma, E.V. Hypocitraturia. Updated 5 October 2015. Available online: https://emedicine.medscape.com/article/444968-overview (accessed on 29 July 2019).
24. Prezioso, D.; Strazzullo, P.; Lotti, T.; Bianchi, G.; Borghi, L.; Caione, P.; Carini, M.; Caudarella, R.; Ferraro, M.; Gambaro, G.; et al. Dietary treatment of urinary risk factors for renal stone formation. A review of CLU Working Group. *Arch. Ital. Urol.* **2015**, *87*, 105–120. [CrossRef]
25. Dolan, E.; Sale, C. Protein and bone health across the lifespan. *Proc. Nutr. Soc.* **2019**, *78*, 45–55. [CrossRef] [PubMed]
26. Vallés, P.G.; Batlle, D. Hypokalemic Distal Renal Tubular Acidosis. *Adv. Chronic Kidney Dis.* **2018**, *25*, 303–320. [CrossRef] [PubMed]
27. Melnick, J.Z.; Preisig, P.A.; Haynes, S.; Pak, C.Y.; Sakhaee, K.; Alpern, R.J. Converting enzyme inhibition causes hypocitraturia independent of acidosis or hypokalemia. *Kidney Int.* **1998**, *54*, 1670–1674. [CrossRef]
28. Warner, B.W.; LaGrange, C.A.; Tucker, T.; Bensalem-Owen, M.; Pais, V.M., Jr. Induction of progressive profound hypocitraturia with increasing doses of topiramate. *Urology* **2008**, *72*, 29–32. [CrossRef] [PubMed]

29. Goraya, N.; Simoni, J.; Sager, L.N.; Madias, N.E.; Wesson, D.E. Urine citrate excretion as a marker of acid retention in patients with chronic kidney disease without overt metabolic acidosis. *Kidney Int.* **2019**, *95*, 1190–1196. [CrossRef] [PubMed]
30. Shey, J.; Cameron, M.A.; Sakhaee, K.; Moe, O.W. Recurrent calcium nephrolithiasis associated with primary aldosteronism. *Am. J. Kidney Dis.* **2004**, *44*, e7–e12. [CrossRef]
31. Dey, J.; Creighton, A.; Lindberg, J.S.; Fuselier, H.A.; Kok, D.J.; Cole, F.E.; Hamm, L. Estrogen replacement increased the citrate and calcium excretion rates in postmenopausal women with recurrent urolithiasis. *J. Urol.* **2002**, *167*, 169–171. [CrossRef]
32. Brinton, R.D. The healthy cell bias of estrogen action, mitochondrial bioenergetics and neurological implications. *Trends Neurosci.* **2008**, *31*, 529–537. [CrossRef]
33. Mai, Z.; Li, X.; Jiang, C.; Liu, Y.; Chen, Y.; Wu, W.; Zeng, G. Comparison of metabolic changes for stone risks in 24-hour urine between non- and postmenopausal women. *PLoS ONE* **2019**, *14*, e0208893. [CrossRef]
34. Granchi, D.; Caudarella, R.; Ripamonti, C.; Spinnato, P.; Bazzocchi, A.; Torreggiani, E.; Massa, A.; Baldini, N. Association between markers of bone loss and urinary lithogenic risk factors in osteopenic postmenopausal women. *J. Biol. Regul. Homeost. Agents* **2016**, *30*, S145–S151.
35. Adeva, M.M.; Souto, G. Diet-induced metabolic acidosis. *Clin. Nutr.* **2011**, *30*, 416–421. [CrossRef] [PubMed]
36. Esche, J.; Johner, S.; Shi, L.; Schönau, E.; Remer, T. Urinary Citrate, an Index of Acid-Base Status, Predicts Bone Strength in Youths and Fracture Risk in Adult Females. *J. Clin. Endocrinol. Metab.* **2016**, *101*, 4914–4921. [CrossRef] [PubMed]
37. Shea, M.K.; Dawson-Hughes, B. Association of Urinary Citrate With Acid-Base Status, Bone Resorption, and Calcium Excretion in Older Men and Women. *J. Clin. Endocrinol. Metab.* **2018**, *103*, 452–459. [CrossRef] [PubMed]
38. Xie, B.; Nancollas, G.H. How to control the size and morphology of apatite nanocrystals in bone. *Proc. Natl. Acad. Sci. USA* **2010**, *107*, 22369–22370. [CrossRef]
39. Dixon, T.F.; Perkins, H.R. Citric acid and bone metabolism. *Biochem. J.* **1952**, *52*, 260–265. [CrossRef]
40. Hu, Y.Y.; Rawal, A.; Schmidt-Rohr, K. Strongly bound citrate stabilizes the apatite nanocrystals in bone. *Proc. Natl. Acad. Sci. USA* **2010**, *107*, 22425–22429. [CrossRef]
41. Mahamid, J.; Sharir, A.; Addadi, L.; Weiner, S. Amorphous calcium phosphate is major component of the forming fin bones of zebrafish. Indications for an amorphous precursor phase. *Proc. Natl. Acad. Sci. USA* **2008**, *105*, 12748–12753. [CrossRef]
42. Bradt, J.H.; Mertig, M.; Teresiak, A.; Pompe, W. Biomimetic mineralization of collagen by combined fibril assembly and calcium phosphate formation. *Chem. Mater.* **1999**, *11*, 2694–2701. [CrossRef]
43. Lotsari, A.; Rajasekharan, A.K.; Halvarsson, M.; Andersson, M. Transformation of amorphous calcium phosphate to bone-like apatite. *Nat. Commun.* **2018**, *9*, 4170. [CrossRef]
44. Davies, E.; Müller, K.H.; Wong, W.C.; Pickard, C.J.; Reid, D.G.; Skepper, J.N.; Duer, M.J. Citrate bridges between mineral platelets in bone. *Proc. Natl. Acad. Sci. USA* **2014**, *111*, E1354–E1363. [CrossRef]
45. Costello, L.C.; Chellaiah, M.; Zou, J.; Franklin, R.B.; Reynolds, M.A. The status of citrate in the hydroxyapatite/collagen complex of bone, and Its role in bone formation. *J. Regen. Med. Tissue Eng.* **2014**, *3*, 4. [CrossRef] [PubMed]
46. Delgado-López, J.M.; Bertolotti, F.; Lyngsø, J.; Pedersen, J.S.; Cervellino, A.; Masciocchi, N.; Guagliardi, A. The synergic role of collagen and citrate in stabilizing amorphous calcium phosphate precursors with platy morphology. *Acta Biomater.* **2017**, *49*, 555–562. [CrossRef] [PubMed]
47. Einhorn, T.A.; Boskey, A.L.; Gundberg, C.M.; Vigorita, V.J.; Devlin, V.J.; Beyer, M.M. The mineral and mechanical properties of bone in chronic experimental diabetes. *J. Orthop. Res.* **1988**, *6*, 317–323. [CrossRef] [PubMed]
48. Tran, R.T.; Yang, J.; Ameer, G.A. Citrate-Based Biomaterials and Their Applications in Regenerative Engineering. *Annu. Rev. Mater. Res.* **2015**, *45*, 277–310. [CrossRef]
49. Ma, C.; Gerhard, E.; Lu, D.; Yang, J. Citrate chemistry and biology for biomaterials design. *Biomaterials* **2018**, *178*, 383–400. [CrossRef]
50. Qiu, H.; Yang, J.; Kodali, P.; Koh, J.; Ameer, G.A. A citric acid-based hydroxyapatite composite for orthopedic implants. *Biomaterials* **2006**, *27*, 5845–5854. [CrossRef]
51. Xie, D.; Guo, J.; Mehdizadeh, M.; Tran, R.T.; Chen, R.; Sun, D.; Qian, G.; Jin, D.; Bai, X.; Yang, J. Development of Injectable Citrate-Based Bioadhesive Bone Implants. *J. Mater. Chem. B* **2015**, *3*, 387–398. [CrossRef]

52. Chung, E.J.; Sugimoto, M.J.; Koh, J.L.; Ameer, G.A. A biodegradable tri-component graft for anterior cruciate ligament reconstruction. *J. Tissue Eng. Regen. Med.* **2017**, *11*, 704–712. [CrossRef]
53. Costello, L.C.; Franklin, R.B.; Reynolds, M.A.; Chellaiah, M. The Important Role of Osteoblasts and Citrate Production in Bone Formation: "Osteoblast Citration" as a New Concept for an Old Relationship. *Open Bone J.* **2012**, *4*. [CrossRef]
54. Costello, L.C.; Liu, Y.; Franklin, R.B.; Kennedy, M.C. Zinc inhibition of mitochondrial aconitase and its importance in citrate metabolism of prostate epithelial cells. *J. Biol. Chem.* **1997**, *272*, 28875–28881. [CrossRef]
55. Franklin, R.B.; Ma, J.; Zou, J.; Guan, Z.; Kukoyi, B.I.; Feng, P.; Costello, L.C. Human ZIP1 is a major zinc uptake transporter for the accumulation of zinc in prostate cells. *J. Inorg. Biochem.* **2003**, *96*, 435–442. [CrossRef]
56. Costello, L.C.; Franklin, R.B. A review of the important central role of altered citrate metabolism during the process of stem cell differentiation. *J. Regen. Med. Tissue Eng.* **2013**, *2*, 1. [CrossRef] [PubMed]
57. Costello, L.C.; Chellaiah, M.A.; Zou, J.; Reynolds, M.A.; Franklin, R.B. In vitro BMP2 stimulation of osteoblast citrate production in concert with mineralized bone nodule formation. *J. Regen Med. Tissue Eng.* **2015**, *4*, 2. [CrossRef] [PubMed]
58. Granchi, D.; Ochoa, G.; Leonardi, E.; Devescovi, V.; Baglìo, S.R.; Osaba, L.; Baldini, N.; Ciapetti, G. Gene expression patterns related to osteogenic differentiation of bone marrow-derived mesenchymal stem cells during ex vivo expansion. *Tissue Eng. Part C Methods* **2010**, *16*, 511–524. [CrossRef]
59. Fu, X.; Li, Y.; Huang, T.; Yu, Z.; Ma, K.; Yang, M.; Liu, Q.; Pan, H.; Wang, H.; Wang, J.; et al. Runx2/Osterix and Zinc Uptake Synergize to Orchestrate Osteogenic Differentiation and Citrate Containing Bone Apatite Formation. *Adv. Sci.* **2018**, *5*, 1700755. [CrossRef]
60. Accession Number GSE12267. Available online: https://www.ncbi.nlm.nih.gov/geo (accessed on 4 July 2019).
61. Inoue, K.; Zhuang, L.; Ganapathy, V. Human Na+ -coupled citrate transporter: Primary structure, genomic organization, and transport function. *Biochem. Biophys. Res. Commun.* **2002**, *299*, 465–471. [CrossRef]
62. Sims, N.A.; Martin, T.J. Coupling the activities of bone formation and resorption: A multitude of signals within the basic multicellular unit. *Bonekey Rep.* **2014**, *3*, 481. [CrossRef]
63. Ma, C.; Tian, X.; Kim, J.P.; Xie, D.; Ao, X.; Shan, D.; Lin, Q.; Hudock, M.R.; Bai, X.; Yang, J. Citrate-based materials fuel human stem cells by metabonegenic regulation. *Proc. Natl. Acad. Sci. USA* **2018**, *115*, E11741–E11750. [CrossRef]
64. Granchi, D.; Torreggiani, E.; Massa, A.; Caudarella, R.; Di Pompo, G.; Baldini, N. Potassium citrate prevents increased osteoclastogenesis resulting from acidic conditions: Implication for the treatment of postmenopausal bone loss. *PLoS ONE* **2017**, *12*, e0181230. [CrossRef]
65. Arnett, T.R. Acidosis, hypoxia and bone. *Arch. Biochem. Biophys.* **2010**, *503*, 103–109. [CrossRef]
66. Lindeman, R.D.; Tobin, J.D.; Shock, N.W. Association between blood pressure and the rate of decline in renal function with age. *Kidney Int.* **1984**, *26*, 861–868. [CrossRef] [PubMed]
67. Kanis, J.A.; Johnell, O.; Oden, A.; Sembo, I.; Redlund-Johnell, I.; Dawson, A.; De Laet, C.; Jonsson, B. Long-term risk of osteoporotic fracture in Malmo. *Osteoporos Int.* **2000**, *11*, 669–674. [CrossRef] [PubMed]
68. Jassal, S.K.; von Muhlen, D.; Barrett-Connor, E. Measures of renal function, BMD, bone loss, and osteoporotic fracture in older adults: The Rancho Bernardo study. *J. Bone Min. Res.* **2007**, *22*, 203–210. [CrossRef] [PubMed]
69. Kidney Disease: Improving Global Outcomes (KDIGO) CKD-MBD Update Work Group. KDIGO 2017 Clinical Practice Guideline Update for the Diagnosis, Evaluation, Prevention, and Treatment of Chronic Kidney Disease-Mineral and Bone Disorder (CKD-MBD). *Kidney Int.* **2017**, *7*, 1–59. [CrossRef] [PubMed]
70. Malmgren, L.; McGuigan, F.E.; Berglundh, S.; Westman, K.; Christensson, A.; Akesson, K. Declining estimated glomerular filtration rate and its association with mortality and comorbidity over 10 years in elderly women. *Nephron* **2015**, *130*, 245–255. [CrossRef]
71. Malmgren, L.; McGuigan, F.E.; Christensson, A.; Akesson, K. Reduced kidney function is associated with BMD, bone loss and markers of mineral homeostasis in older women: A 10-year longitudinal study. *Osteoporos. Int.* **2017**, *28*, 3463–3473. [CrossRef]
72. Hocher, B.; Adamski, J. Metabolomics for clinical use and research in chronic kidney disease. *Nat. Rev. Nephrol.* **2017**, *13*, 269–284. [CrossRef]

73. Hallan, S.; Afkarian, M.; Zelnick, L.R.; Kestenbaum, B.; Sharma, S.; Saito, R.; Darshi, M.; Barding, G.; Raftery, D.; Ju, W.; et al. Metabolomics and Gene Expression Analysis Reveal Down-regulation of the Citric Acid (TCA) Cycle in Non-diabetic CKD Patients. *Ebiomedicine* **2017**, *26*, 68–77. [CrossRef]
74. Kang, H.W.; Seo, S.P.; Kim, W.T.; Kim, Y.J.; Yun, S.J.; Lee, S.C.; Kim, W.J. Effect of renal insufficiency on stone recurrence in patients with urolithiasis. *J. Korean Med. Sci.* **2014**, *29*, 1132–1137. [CrossRef]
75. Krieger, N.S.; Bushinsky, D.A. The relation between bone and stone formation. *Calcif. Tissue Int.* **2013**, *93*, 374–381. [CrossRef]
76. Sakhaee, K.; Maalouf, N.M.; Kumar, R.; Pasch, A.; Moe, O.W. Nephrolithiasis-associated bone disease: Pathogenesis and treatment options. *Kidney Int.* **2011**, *79*, 393–403. [CrossRef] [PubMed]
77. Denburg, M.R.; Leonard, M.B.; Haynes, K.; Tuchman, S.; Tasian, G.; Shults, J.; Copelovitch, L. Risk of fracture in urolithiasis: A population-based cohort study using thehealth improvement network. *Clin. J. Am. Soc. Nephrol.* **2014**, *9*, 2133–2140. [CrossRef] [PubMed]
78. Taylor, E.N.; Feskanich, D.; Paik, J.M.; Curhan, G.C. Nephrolithiasis and Risk of Incident Bone Fracture. *J. Urol.* **2016**, *195*, 1482–1486. [CrossRef] [PubMed]
79. Lucato, P.; Trevisan, C.; Stubbs, B.; Zanforlini, B.M.; Solmi, M.; Luchini, C.; Girotti, G.; Pizzato, S.; Manzato, E.; Sergi, G.; et al. Nephrolithiasis, bone mineral density, osteoporosis, and fractures: A systematic review and comparative meta-analysis. *Osteoporos. Int.* **2016**, *27*, 3155–3164. [CrossRef] [PubMed]
80. Khan, S.R.; Pearle, M.S.; Robertson, W.G.; Gambaro, G.; Canales, B.K.; Doizi, S.; Traxer, O.; Tiselius, H.G. Kidney stones. *Nat. Rev. Dis. Primers* **2016**, *2*, 16008. [CrossRef] [PubMed]
81. Muntner, P.; Jones, T.M.; Hyre, A.D.; Melamed, M.L.; Alper, A.; Raggi, P.; Leonard, M.B. Association of serum intact parathyroid hormone with lower estimated glomerular filtration rate. *Clin. J. Am. Soc. Nephrol.* **2009**, *4*, 186–194. [CrossRef] [PubMed]
82. Han, S.G.; Oh, J.; Jeon, H.J.; Park, C.; Cho, J.; Shin, D.H. Kidney Stones and Risk of Osteoporotic Fracture in Chronic Kidney Disease. *Sci. Rep.* **2019**, *9*, 1929. [CrossRef]
83. Arrabal-Polo, M.A.; Girón-Prieto, M.S.; Cano-García Mdel, C.; Poyatos-Andujar, A.; Quesada Charneco, M.; Abad-Menor, F.; Arias-Santiago, S.; Zuluaga-Gomez, A.; Arrabal-Martin, M. Retrospective review of serum and urinary lithogenic risk factors in patients with osteoporosis and osteopenia. *Urology* **2015**, *85*, 782–785. [CrossRef]
84. Khosla, S.; Oursler, M.J.; Monroe, D.G. Estrogen and the skeleton. *Trends Endocrinol. Metab.* **2012**, *23*, 576–581. [CrossRef]
85. Chen, H.; Wang, Y.; Dai, H.; Tian, X.; Cui, Z.K.; Chen, Z.; Hu, L.; Song, Q.; Liu, A.; Zhang, Z.; et al. Bone and plasma citrate is reduced in osteoporosis. *Bone* **2018**, *114*, 189–197. [CrossRef]
86. Prochaska, M.; Taylor, E.N.; Curhan, G. Menopause and Risk of Kidney Stones. *J. Urol.* **2018**, *200*, 823–828. [CrossRef] [PubMed]
87. Drake, M.T.; Clarke, B.L.; Lewiecki, E.M. The Pathophysiology and Treatment of Osteoporosis. *Clin. Ther.* **2015**, *37*, 1837–1850. [CrossRef] [PubMed]
88. Rharass, T.; Lucas, S. Mechanisms in endocrinology: Bone marrow adiposity and bone, a bad romance? *Eur. J. Endocrinol.* **2018**, *179*, R165–R182. [CrossRef] [PubMed]
89. Kim, J.M.; Jeong, D.; Kang, H.K.; Jung, S.Y.; Kang, S.S.; Min, B.M. Osteoclast precursors display dynamic metabolic shifts toward accelerated glucose metabolism at an early stage of RANKL-stimulated osteoclast differentiation. *Cell. Physiol. Biochem.* **2007**, *20*, 935–946. [CrossRef] [PubMed]
90. Lemma, S.; Sboarina, M.; Porporato, P.E.; Zini, N.; Sonveaux, P.; Di Pompo, G.; Baldini, N.; Avnet, S. Energy metabolism in osteoclast formation and activity. *Int. J. Biochem. Cell Biol.* **2016**, *79*, 168–180. [CrossRef] [PubMed]
91. Granchi, D.; Caudarella, R.; Ripamonti, C.; Spinnato, P.; Bazzocchi, A.; Massa, A.; Baldini, N. Potassium Citrate Supplementation Decreases the Biochemical Markers of Bone Loss in a Group of Osteopenic Women: The Results of a Randomized, Double-Blind, Placebo-Controlled Pilot Study. *Nutrients* **2018**, *10*, 1293. [CrossRef]
92. Available online: https://www.omim.org/ (accessed on 4 July 2019).
93. Watanabe, T. Improving outcomes for patients with distal renal tubular acidosis: Recent advances and challenges ahead. *Pediatr. Health Med. Ther.* **2018**, *9*, 181–190. [CrossRef]

94. Weinstein, D.A.; Somers, M.J.; Wolfsdorf, J.I. Decreased urinary citrate excretion in type 1a glycogen storage disease. *J. Pediatr.* **2001**, *138*, 378–382. [CrossRef]
95. Kaiser, N.; Gautschi, M.; Bosanska, L.; Meienberg, F.; Baumgartner, M.R.; Spinas, G.A.; Hochuli, M. Glycemic control and complications in glycogen storage disease type I: Results from the Swiss registry. *Mol. Genet. Metab.* **2019**, *126*, 355–361. [CrossRef]
96. Thevenon, J.; Milh, M.; Feillet, F.; St-Onge, J.; Duffourd, Y.; Jugé, C.; Roubertie, A.; Héron, D.; Mignot, C.; Raffo, E.; et al. Mutations in SLC13A5 cause autosomal-recessive epileptic encephalopathy with seizure onset in the first days of life. *Am. J. Hum. Genet.* **2014**, *95*, 113–120. [CrossRef]
97. Irizarry, A.R.; Yan, G.; Zeng, Q.; Lucchesi, J.; Hamang, M.J.; Ma, Y.L.; Rong, J.X. Defective enamel and bone development in sodium-dependent citrate transporter (NaCT) Slc13a5 deficient mice. *PLoS ONE* **2017**, *12*, e0175465. [CrossRef] [PubMed]
98. Díaz, M.; García, C.; Sebastiani, G.; de Zegher, F.; López-Bermejo, A.; Ibáñez, L. Placental and cord blood methylation of genes involved in energy homeostasis: Association with fetal growth and neonatal body composition. *Diabetes* **2017**, *66*, 779–784. [CrossRef] [PubMed]
99. Cunha, T.D.S.; Heilberg, I.P. Bartter syndrome: Causes, diagnosis, and treatment. *Int. J. Nephrol. Renov. Dis.* **2018**, *11*, 291–301. [CrossRef] [PubMed]
100. Simon, D.B.; Karet, F.E.; Hamdan, J.M.; DiPietro, A.; Sanjad, S.A.; Lifton, R.P. Bartter's syndrome, hypokalaemic alkalosis with hypercalciuria, is caused by mutations in the Na-K-2Cl cotransporter NKCC2. *Nat. Genet.* **1996**, *13*, 183–188. [CrossRef]
101. International Collaborative Study Group for Bartter-like Syndromes. Mutations in the gene encoding the inwardly-rectifying renal potassium channel, ROMK, cause the antenatal variant of Bartter syndrome: Evidence for genetic heterogeneity. *Hum. Molec. Genet.* **1997**, *6*, 17–26.
102. Gross, I.; Siedner-Weintraub, Y.; Simckes, A.; Gillis, D. Antenatal Bartter syndrome presenting as hyperparathyroidism with hypercalcemia and hypercalciuria: A case report and review. *J. Pediatr. Endocrinol. Metab.* **2015**, *28*, 943–946. [CrossRef]
103. Li, D.; Tian, L.; Hou, C.; Kim, C.E.; Hakonarson, H.; Levine, M.A. Association of Mutations in SLC12A1 Encoding the NKCC2 Cotransporter with Neonatal Primary Hyperparathyroidism. *J. Clin. Endocrinol. Metab.* **2016**, *101*, 2196–2200. [CrossRef]
104. Hou, J. Claudins and mineral metabolism. *Curr. Opin. Nephrol. Hypertens.* **2016**, *25*, 308–313. [CrossRef]
105. Thorleifsson, G.; Holm, H.; Edvardsson, V.; Walters, G.B.; Styrkarsdottir, U.; Gudbjartsson, D.F.; Sulem, P.; Halldorsson, B.V.; de Vegt, F.; d'Ancona, F.C.; et al. Sequence variants in the CLDN14 gene associate with kidney stones and bone mineral density. *Nat. Genet.* **2009**, *41*, 926–930. [CrossRef]
106. Claverie-Martin, F. Familial hypomagnesaemia with hypercalciuria and nephrocalcinosis, clinical and molecular characteristics. *Clin. Kidney J.* **2015**, *8*, 656–664. [CrossRef]
107. Bardet, C.; Courson, F.; Wu, Y.; Khaddam, M.; Salmon, B.; Ribes, S.; Thumfart, J.; Yamaguti, P.M.; Rochefort, G.Y.; Figueres, M.L.; et al. Claudin-16 Deficiency Impairs Tight Junction Function in Ameloblasts, Leading to Abnormal Enamel Formation. *J. Bone Min. Res.* **2016**, *31*, 498–513. [CrossRef] [PubMed]
108. Pajor, A.M. Sodium-coupled dicarboxylate and citrate transporters from the SLC13 family. *Pflug. Arch* **2014**, *466*, 119–130. [CrossRef] [PubMed]
109. Okamoto, N.; Aruga, S.; Matsuzaki, S.; Takahashi, S.; Matsushita, K.; Kitamura, T. Associations between renal sodium-citrate cotransporter (hNaDC-1) gene polymorphism and urinary citrate excretion in recurrent renal calcium stone formers and normal controls. *Int. J. Urol.* **2007**, *14*, 344–349. [CrossRef] [PubMed]
110. Pajor, A.M.; Sun, N.N. Single nucleotide polymorphisms in the human Na+-dicarboxylate cotransporter affect transport activity and protein expression. *Am. J. Physiol. Ren. Physiol.* **2010**, *299*, F704–F711. [CrossRef]
111. Catalina-Rodriguez, O.; Kolukula, V.K.; Tomita, Y.; Preet, A.; Palmieri, F.; Wellstein, A.; Byers, S.; Giaccia, A.J.; Glasgow, E.; Albanese, C.; et al. The mitochondrial citrate transporter, CIC, is essential for mitochondrial homeostasis. *Oncotarget* **2012**, *3*, 1220–1235. [CrossRef]
112. Cosso, R.; Falchetti, A. Mitochondriopathies and bone health. *J. Tre. Biol. Res.* **2018**, *1*, 1–7. [CrossRef]
113. Brommage, R.; Liu, J.; Hansen, G.M.; Kirkpatrick, L.L.; Potter, D.G.; Sands, A.T.; Zambrowicz, B.; Powell, D.R.; Vogel, P. High-throughput screening of mouse gene knockouts identifies established and novel skeletal phenotypes. *Bone Res.* **2014**, *2*, 14034. [CrossRef]

114. Lorentzon, M.; Branco, J.; Brandi, M.L.; Bruyère, O.; Chapurlat, R.; Cooper, C.; Cortet, B.; Diez-Perez, A.; Ferrari, S.; Gasparik, A.; et al. Algorithm for the Use of Biochemical Markers of Bone Turnover in the Diagnosis, Assessment and Follow-Up of Treatment for Osteoporosis. *Adv. Ther.* **2019**. [CrossRef]
115. Kanis, J.A.; Cooper, C.; Rizzoli, R.; Reginster, J.Y.; Scientific Advisory Board of the European Society for Clinical and Economic Aspects of Osteoporosis (ESCEO) and the Committees of Scientific Advisors and National Societies of the International Osteoporosis Foundation (IOF). European guidance for the diagnosis and management of osteoporosis in postmenopausal women. *Osteoporos. Int.* **2019**, *30*, 3–44. [CrossRef]
116. Ripamonti, C.; Lisi, L.; Buffa, A.; Gnudi, S.; Caudarella, R. The Trabecular Bone Score Predicts Spine Fragility Fractures in Postmenopausal Caucasian Women Without Osteoporosis Independently of Bone Mineral Density. *Med. Arch.* **2018**, *72*, 46–50. [CrossRef]
117. Damasiewicz, M.J.; Nickolas, T.L. Rethinking Bone Disease in Kidney Disease. *JBMR Plus* **2018**, *2*, 309–322. [CrossRef] [PubMed]
118. Moe, S.; Drüeke, T.; Cunningham, J.; Goodman, W.; Martin, K.; Olgaard, K.; Ott, S.; Sprague, S.; Lameire, N.; Eknoyan, G. Kidney Disease: Improving Global Outcomes (KDIGO). Definition, evaluation, and classification of renal osteodystrophy: A position statement from Kidney Disease: Improving Global Outcomes (KDIGO). *Kidney Int.* **2006**, *69*, 1945–1953. [CrossRef] [PubMed]
119. Jorgetti, V.; Drüeke, T.B.; Ott, S.M. Role of proton receptor OGR1 in bone response to metabolic acidosis? *Kidney Int.* **2016**, *89*, 529–531. [CrossRef] [PubMed]
120. Wachman, A.; Bernstein, D.S. Diet and osteoporosis. *Lancet* **1968**, *1*, 958–959. [CrossRef]
121. Nicoll, R.; McLaren Howard, J. The acid-ash hypothesis revisited: A reassessment of the impact of dietary acidity on bone. *J. Bone Min. Metab.* **2014**, *32*, 469–475. [CrossRef] [PubMed]
122. Frassetto, L.A.; Todd, K.M.; Morris, R.C., Jr.; Sebastian, A. Estimation of net endogenous noncarbonic acidproduction in humans from diet potassium and protein contents. *Am. J. Clin. Nutr.* **1998**, *68*, 576–583. [CrossRef]
123. Remer, T.; Manz, F. Estimation of the renal net acid excretion by adults consuming diets containing variable amounts of protein. *Am. J. Clin. Nutr.* **1994**, *59*, 1356–1361. [CrossRef]
124. Pachaly, M.A.; Baena, C.P.; Buiar, A.C.; de Fraga, F.S.; Carvalho, M. Effects of non-pharmacological interventions on urinary citrate levels: A systematic review and meta-analysis. *Nephrol. Dial. Transpl.* **2016**, *31*, 1203–1211. [CrossRef]
125. Frassetto, L.; Banerjee, T.; Powe, N.; Sebastian, A. Acid Balance, Dietary Acid Load, and Bone Effects-A Controversial Subject. *Nutrients* **2018**, *10*, 517. [CrossRef]
126. Fenton, T.R.; Lyon, A.W.; Eliasziw, M.; Tough, S.C.; Hanley, D.A. Meta-analysis of the effect of the acid-ash hypothesis of osteoporosis on calcium balance. *J. Bone Min. Res.* **2009**, *24*, 1835–1840. [CrossRef]
127. Bonjour, J.P. Nutritional disturbance in acid-base balance and osteoporosis: A hypothesis that disregards the essential homeostatic role of the kidney. *Br. J. Nutr.* **2013**, *110*, 1168–1177. [CrossRef] [PubMed]
128. Carnauba, R.A.; Baptistella, A.B.; Paschoal, V.; Hübscher, G.H. Diet-Induced Low-Grade Metabolic Acidosis and Clinical Outcomes: A Review. *Nutrients* **2017**, *9*, 538. [CrossRef] [PubMed]
129. Hirschfeld, H.P.; Kinsella, R.; Duque, G. Osteosarcopenia: Where bone, muscle, and fat collide. *Osteoporos. Int.* **2017**, *28*, 2781–2790. [CrossRef] [PubMed]
130. Cases, A.; Cigarrán-Guldrís, S.; Mas, S.; Gonzalez-Parra, E. Vegetable-Based Diets for Chronic Kidney Disease? It Is Time to Reconsider. *Nutrients* **2019**, *11*, 1263. [CrossRef] [PubMed]
131. Domrongkitchaiporn, S.; Stitchantrakul, W.; Kochakarn, W. Causes of hypocitraturia in recurrent calcium stone formers: Focusing on urinary potassium excretion. *Am. J. Kidney Dis.* **2006**, *48*, 546–554. [CrossRef]
132. Odvina, C.V. Comparative value of orange juice versus lemonade in reducing stone-forming risk. *Clin. J. Am. Soc. Nephrol.* **2006**, *1*, 1269–1274. [CrossRef]
133. Goldfarb, D.S.; Asplin, J.R. Effect of grapefruit juice on urinary lithogenicity. *J. Urol.* **2001**, *166*, 263–267. [CrossRef]
134. Macdonald, H.M.; Black, A.J.; Aucott, L.; Duthie, G.; Duthie, S.; Sandison, R.; Hardcastle, A.C.; Lanham New, S.A.; Fraser, W.D.; Reid, D.M. Effect of potassium citrate supplementation or increased fruit and vegetable intake on bone metabolism in healthy postmenopausal women: A randomized controlled trial. *Am. J. Clin. Nutr.* **2008**, *88*, 465–474. [CrossRef]

135. Phillips, R.; Hanchanale, V.S.; Myatt, A.; Somani, B.; Nabi, G.; Biyani, C.S. Citrate salts for preventing and treating calcium containing kidney stones in adults. *Cochrane Database Syst. Rev.* **2015**, *10*, CD010057. [CrossRef]
136. Kern, A.; Grimsby, G.; Mayo, H.; Baker, L.A. Medical and dietary interventions for preventing recurrent urinary stones in children. *Cochrane Database Syst. Rev.* **2017**, *11*, CD011252. [CrossRef]
137. Lencel, P.; Magne, D. Inflammaging: The driving force in osteoporosis? *Med. Hypotheses* **2011**, *76*, 317–321. [CrossRef] [PubMed]
138. Lambert, H.; Frassetto, L.; Moore, J.B.; Torgerson, D.; Gannon, R.; Burckhardt, P.; Lanham-New, S. The effect of supplementation with alkaline potassium salts on bone metabolism: A meta-analysis. *Osteoporos. Int.* **2015**, *26*, 1311–1318. [CrossRef] [PubMed]
139. Sakhaee, K.; Maalouf, N.M.; Abrams, S.A.; Pak, C.Y. Effects of potassium alkali and calcium supplementation on bone turnover in postmenopausal women. *J. Clin. Endocrinol. Metab.* **2005**, *90*, 3528–3533. [CrossRef] [PubMed]
140. Karp, H.J.; Ketola, M.E.; Lamberg-Allardt, C.J. Acute effects of calcium carbonate, calcium citrate and potassium citrate on markers of calcium and bone metabolism in young women. *Br. J. Nutr.* **2009**, *102*, 1341–1347. [CrossRef]
141. Dawson-Hughes, B.; Dallal, G.E.; Krall, E.A.; Sadowski, L.; Sahyoun, N.; Tannenbaum, S. A Controlled Trial of the Effect of Calcium Supplementation on Bone Density in Postmenopausal Women. *N. Engl. J. Med.* **1990**, *323*, 878–883. [CrossRef]
142. Dawson-Hughes, B.; Harris, S.S.; Krall, E.A.; Dallal, G.E. Effect of Calcium and Vitamin D Supplementation on Bone Density in Men and Women 65 Years of Age Or Older. *N. Engl. J. Med.* **1997**, *337*, 670–676. [CrossRef]
143. Ruml, L.A.; Sakhaee, K.; Peterson, R.; Adams-Huet, B.; Pak, C.Y. The Effect of Calcium Citrate on Bone Density in the Early and Mid-Postmenopausal Period: A Randomized Placebo-Controlled Study. *Am. J. Ther.* **1999**, *6*, 303–311. [CrossRef]
144. Sellmeyer, D.E.; Schloetter, M.; Sebastian, A. Potassium Citrate Prevents Increased Urine Calcium Excretion and Bone Resorption Induced by a High Sodium Chloride Diet. *J. Clin. Endocrinol. Metab.* **2002**, *87*, 2008–2012. [CrossRef]
145. Dawson-Hughes, B.; Harris, S.S. Calcium Intake Influences the Association of Protein Intake with Rates of Bone Loss in Elderly Men and Women. *Am. J. Clin. Nutr.* **2002**, *75*, 773–779. [CrossRef]
146. Marangella, M.; Di Stefano, M.; Casalis, S.; Berutti, S.; D'Amelio, P.; Isaia, G.C. Effects of potassium citrate supplementation on bone metabolism. *Calcif. Tissue Int.* **2004**, *74*, 330–335. [CrossRef]
147. Kenny, A.M.; Prestwood, K.M.; Biskup, B.; Robbins, B.; Zayas, E.; Kleppinger, A.; Burleson, J.A.; Raisz, L.G. Comparison of the Effects of Calcium Loading with Calcium Citrate Or Calcium Carbonate on Bone Turnover in Postmenopausal Women. *Osteoporos. Int.* **2004**, *15*, 290–294. [CrossRef] [PubMed]
148. Jehle, S.; Zanetti, A.; Muser, J.; Hulter, H.N.; Krapf, R. Partial Neutralization of the Acidogenic Western Diet with Potassium Citrate Increases Bone Mass in Postmenopausal Women with Osteopenia. *J. Am. Soc. Nephrol.* **2006**, *17*, 3213–3222. [CrossRef] [PubMed]
149. Thomas, S.D.; Need, A.G.; Tucker, G.; Slobodian, P.; O'Loughlin, P.D.; Nordin, B.E. Suppression of parathyroid hormone and bone resorption by calcium carbonate and calcium citrate in postmenopausal women. *Calcif. Tissue Int.* **2008**, *83*, 81–84. [CrossRef] [PubMed]
150. Jehle, S.; Hulter, H.N.; Krapf, R. Effect of potassium citrate on bone density, microarchitecture, and fracture risk in healthy older adults without osteoporosis: A randomized controlled trial. *J. Clin. Endocrinol. Metab.* **2013**, *98*, 207–217. [CrossRef] [PubMed]
151. Moseley, K.F.; Weaver, C.M.; Appel, L.; Sebastian, A.; Sellmeyer, D.E. Potassium Citrate Supplementation Results in Sustained Improvement in Calcium Balance in Older Men and Women. *J. Bone Min. Res.* **2013**, *28*, 497–504. [CrossRef] [PubMed]
152. Gregory, N.S.; Kumar, R.; Stein, E.M.; Alexander, E.; Christos, P.; Bockman, R.S.; Rodman, J.S. Potassium Citrate Decreases Bone Resorption in Postmenopausal Women with Osteopenia: A Randomized, Double-Blind Clinical Trial. *Endocr. Pr.* **2015**, *21*, 1380–1386. [CrossRef] [PubMed]
153. Anderson, N.M.; Mucka, P.; Kern, J.G.; Feng, H. The emerging role and targetability of the TCA cycle in cancer metabolism. *Protein Cell* **2018**, *9*, 216–237. [CrossRef]
154. Sathiyakumar, V.; Kapoor, K.; Jones, S.R.; Banach, M.; Martin, S.S.; Toth, P.P. Novel Therapeutic Targets for Managing Dyslipidemia. *Trends Pharm. Sci.* **2018**, *39*, 733–747. [CrossRef] [PubMed]

155. Ou, Y.; Liu, Z.; Li, S.; Zhu, X.; Lin, Y.; Han, J.; Duan, Z.; Jia, L.; Gui, B. Citrate attenuates vascular calcification in chronic renal failure rats. *APMIS* **2017**, *125*, 452–458. [CrossRef]
156. Michalczuk, M.; Urban, B.; Porowski, T.; Wasilewska, A.; Bakunowicz-Łazarczyk, A. Citrate usage in the leading causes of blindness: New possibilities for the old metabolite. *Metabolomics* **2018**, *14*, 82. [CrossRef]

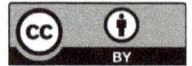

© 2019 by the authors. Licensee MDPI, Basel, Switzerland. This article is an open access article distributed under the terms and conditions of the Creative Commons Attribution (CC BY) license (http://creativecommons.org/licenses/by/4.0/).

MDPI
St. Alban-Anlage 66
4052 Basel
Switzerland
Tel. +41 61 683 77 34
Fax +41 61 302 89 18
www.mdpi.com

Nutrients Editorial Office
E-mail: nutrients@mdpi.com
www.mdpi.com/journal/nutrients

www.ingramcontent.com/pod-product-compliance
Lightning Source LLC
LaVergne TN
LVHW070632100526
838202LV00012B/788